ADVANCES IN

Anesthesia

Editor-in-Chief
Carol L. Lake, MD, MBA, MPH

ELSEVIER
An Imprint of Elsevier, Inc.

PHILADELPHIA   LONDON   TORONTO   MONTREAL   SYDNEY   TOKYO

ADVANCES IN
Anesthesia

VOLUMES 1 THROUGH 22 (OUT OF PRINT)

Vice President, Continuity Publishing: John A. Schrefer
Associate Developmental Editor: Yonah Korngold

Reprints: For copies of 100 or more, of articles in this publication, please contact the Commercial Reprints Department, Elsevier Inc., 360 Park Avenue South, New York, New York 10010-1710. Tel. (212) 633-3813 Fax: (212) 462-1935 email: reprints@elsevier.com.

Printed in the United States of America.
Printing/binding by Sheridan Books, Inc.

Editorial Office:
Elsevier
1600 John F. Kennedy Blvd,
Suite 1800
Philadelphia, PA 19103-2899

International Standard Serial Number: 0737-6146
International Standard Book Number: 0-323-04641-X
978-0-323-04641-1

ADVANCES IN
Anesthesia

Associate Editors

JOEL O. JOHNSON, MD, PhD, Professor and Chair, Department of Anesthesiology and Perioperative Medicine, University of Missouri-Columbia, Columbia, Missouri

THOMAS M. McLOUGHLIN, MD, Chair, Department of Anesthesiology, Lehigh Valley Hospital and Health System, Allentown; and Professor of Clinical Anesthesiology, Penn State College of Medicine, Hershey, Pennsylvania

ADVANCES IN
Anesthesia

CONTRIBUTORS

KEVIN BARRY, MD, President, Anesthesia Associates of Morristown; and PA, Morristown Memorial Hospital, Morristown, New Jersey

JAMES BENONIS, MD, Faculty Fellow, Division of Orthopedics, Plastics, and Regional Anesthesia, Department of Anesthesiology, Duke University Medical Center, Durham, North Carolina

JOANNE CONROY, MD, Executive Vice President, Atlantic Health; and Chief Operating Officer, Morristown Memorial Hospital, Morristown, New Jersey

NANCY L. GLASS, MD, MBA, Professor of Pediatrics and Anethesiology, Baylor College of Medicine; and Department of Pediatric Anesthesiology, Texas Children's Hospital, Houston, Texas

STUART A. GRANT, MBChB, FRCA, Assistant Professor, Division of Orthopedics, Plastics, and Regional Anesthesia, Department of Anesthesiology, Duke University Medical Center, Durham, North Carolina

THOMAS M. HEMMERLING, MD, DEAA, Associate Professor, Department of Anesthesiology, McGill University Health Centre, McGill University, Montreal General Hospital; and Institute of Biomedical Engineering, Université de Montréal, Montreal, Quebec, Canada

JOHN E. FORESTNER, MD, Professor and Director of Education, Department of Anesthesiology and Pain Management, University of Texas Southwestern Medical School, Dallas, Texas

KLAUS KJAER, MD, Associate Professor of Clinical Anesthesiology, Weill Medical College of Cornell University, New York, New York

CAROLE LIN, MD, Assistant Professor of Anethesiology, Department of Pediatric Anesthesia, Texas Children's Hospital, Houston, Texas

LISA McMILLIAN, BBA, Perioperative Enterprise Material Manager, UT MD Anderson Cancer Center, Houston, Texas

ANH-THUY NGUYEN, MD, Associate Professor, Department of Anesthesiology and Pain Medicine, The University of Texas MD Anderson Cancer Center, Houston, Texas

KIM-PHUONG T. NGUYEN, MD, Assistant Professor of Pediatrics and Anesthesiology, Baylor College of Medicine; and Texas Children's Hospital, Houston, Texas

DEBRA NORDMEYER, MD, Fellow in Cardiac Anesthesiology, Department of Anesthesiology and Pain Management, University of Texas Southwestern Medical School, Dallas, Texas

ANAND PATEL, MD, Fellow in Anesthesiology, Division of Pain Medicine, Department of Anesthesiology, Weill Medical College of Cornell University, New York, New York

KEYURI POPAT, MD, Associate Professor, Department of Anesthesiology and Pain Medicine, The University of Texas MD Anderson Cancer Center, Houston, Texas

WANDA M. POPESCU, MD, Assistant Professor, Department of Anesthesiology, Yale University School of Medicine, New Haven, Connecticut

RONALDO PURUGGANAN, MD, Assistant Professor of Anesthesiology, UT MD Anderson Cancer Center, Houston, Texas

THOMAS F. RAHLFS, MD, Professor of Anesthesiology, Department of Anethesiology and Pain Medicine, UT MD Anderson Cancer Center, Houston, Texas

JEFFREY J. SCHWARTZ, MD, Associate Professor, Department of Anesthesiology, Yale University School of Medicine, New Haven, Connecticut

MICHAEL H. WALL, MD, Associate Professor and Chief of Cardiac Anesthesiology, Department of Anesthesiology and Pain Management, University of Texas Southwestern Medical School, Dallas, Texas

ADVANCES IN
Anesthesia

CONTENTS VOLUME 25 • 2007

Advances in Transfusion Medicine
By Debra Nordmeyer, John E. Forestner, and Michael H. Wall

Perioperative Considerations for the Morbidly Obese Patient
By Wanda M. Popescu and Jeffrey J. Schwartz

Impact of Obesity in Pediatric Anesthesia
By Carole Lin

Should Nonanesthesia Providers Be Administering Propofol?
By Klaus Kjaer and Anand Patel

Challenges in Practice Management
By Joanne Conroy and Kevin Barry

Advances in Pediatric Pain Management
By Kim-Phuong T. Nguyen and Nancy L. Glass

The Use of Ultrasound in Regional Anesthesia
By James Benonis and Stuart A. Grant

Airway Management Devices and Approaches
By Anh-Thuy Nguyen and Keyuri Popat

Advances in Anesthesia 25 (2007) 1–16

ADVANCES IN ANESTHESIA

ELSEVIER
MOSBY

Health Care Resource Management: An Introduction and the Role of the Anesthesiologist

Thomas F. Rahlfs, MD[a],*, Ronaldo Purugganan, MD[b],
Lisa McMillian, BBA[b]

[a]Department of Anesthesiology and Pain Medicine, UT MD Anderson Cancer Center,
1515 Holcombe, Box 409, Houston, TX 77030, USA
[b]UT MD Anderson Cancer Center, 1515 Holcombe, Box 25, Houston, TX 77030, USA

This article covers what an anesthesiologist should know and understand if he or she is to engage in matters with anesthetic and/or operating room equipment. It serves as a primer for someone new to the field of resource management. The discussion contains a glossary of terms (Appendix 1) used in resource management and begins with a description of the flow of resources from the manufacturer to the patient. The article discusses inventory management, sourcing and contracts for the procurement of equipment, and a description of value analysis and best practices. It also discusses the use of equipment committees within a department.

It is important for anesthesia groups to have an anesthesiologist who is well-versed in the design and function of anesthesia equipment to be involved in the decisions regarding equipment and supplies. This individual should have a working knowledge of the processes within the institution by which resources are acquired and managed. The day-to-day process of resource procurement and supply chain services should be left to the professional staff whose sole jobs are to ensure that appropriate measures are taken to fulfill institutional requirements and regulatory guidelines. The role of the anesthesiologist is therefore that of a clinical advisor and decision maker for what types of resources are suited best for that institution and its mission.

THE FLOW OF PRODUCT

Fig. 1 shows the flow of product from manufacturer to the health care institution, the patient, and ultimately to disposal. It shows how a facility may obtain its supplies directly from the manufacturer or from a third party. The possible interaction of a group purchasing organization (GPO) is shown with the direction of influence from health care facility to the manufacturer through the GPO.

*Corresponding author. E-mail address: trahlfs@mdanderson.org (T.F. Rahlfs).

0737-6146/07/$ – see front matter
doi:10.1016/j.aan.2007.07.008

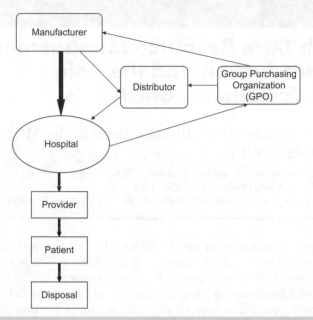

Fig. 1. Material flow from manufacturer to disposal.

DISTINCTION OF CAPITAL EQUIPMENT VERSUS SUPPLIES

Whether devices are considered capital equipment (eg, anesthesia machines) or supplies (eg, anesthesia circuits) will depend on their costs and expected useful lives. Supplies are typically disposable pieces used for each patient, and their cost is passed on to the patient directly. Capital equipment typically has a useful life of more than 1 year, and the long-term depreciation of this equipment is factored into the anesthesia supply charge as a small increment. Whether an item is considered capital equipment also may depend on the operating budget of the institution. For example, a small cerebral function monitor with an initial cost of $3000 and 7-year life expectancy may not meet threshold to be considered capital equipment in the budgeting process of a large institution with a billion dollar revenue stream, but it would be considered capital in a small outpatient surgicenter with six operating rooms. For larger institutions, the threshold for capital may be in the $20,000-50,000 range. Anything of lesser value will be funded out of a maintenance and operations (M&O) budget and not be depreciated over its life by accounting.

INVENTORY MANAGEMENT

Control and management of inventory

The success of any health care institution relies on its care providers having the appropriate medical resources (inventory or stock) on-hand and set for use. Inventory is maintained through two processes: inventory control and inventory management. Inventory control refers to the cataloging of inventory type, quantity, and location. Inventory management deals with the ordering process, from forecasting needs to determining optimal replenishment schedules and quantities. Optimal inventory control must be achieved before effective management; one needs to know the current state of inventory before the acquisition of new or replacement inventory.

Effective inventory management strategies are aimed toward meeting or exceeding end users' expectations of product availability by maintaining an inventory stock that is neither too lean nor too fat, thus saving money, improving customer service, and reducing waste. Inventory problems arise from excess inventory (too much of some products), inadequate or exhausted inventory, inadequate cataloging of inventory, and lack of knowledge of inventory location.

Inventory may be classified as official, unofficial, or consignment. Official inventory refers to products, usually maintained in the stockroom or warehouse, that are documented assets on an institution's balance sheet (the books). Unofficial inventory refers to items that are not carried on the institution's balance sheet, but instead expensed to users when supplied for use. Anesthesia stock typically is handled as unofficial inventory. Consignment inventory usually is stored at the institution but is purchased only upon use. For example, institutions normally consign costly supplies such as implantable pain pumps to minimize their outlay of resources.

Inventory control

Inventory control begins with documenting how much inventory is on hand by manually counting supply items. This count is compared with the amount recorded on the institution's financial records, and any discrepancies are addressed and rectified. Counting may be periodic or cyclic [1]. Periodic counting involves a complete inventory count performed at regular, planned intervals. This counting regimen is inconvenient, because during the count, usage of inventory must be frozen, thus leading to a temporary cessation of services. Cyclic counting, considered best practice for hospitals, involves a count of certain populations of inventory, performed at predetermined intervals so that by the end of the fiscal year the entire inventory has been accounted for. This method allows for inventory to be available for services even during a count [1]. Bar codes/readers may be incorporated in all these counting schemes and may increase efficiency and accuracy. In addition, new technology such as radiofrequency identification (RFID) may provide significant advantages such as inventory and patient tracking without line-of-sight requirements [2].

Once inventory has been accounted for, items should be classified as useful or less useful stock. Useful inventory are those items that are used most during the span of a fiscal period (therefore more logical to keep in stock) [3]. This classification is independent of the cost of service rendered by use of the item. For example, an intravenous kit used 2000 times a year to generate $2000 is more useful to keep in stock than a special central venous catheter (CVC) kit used twice a year to generate $200 in revenue. Less useful stock is maintained if the items are necessary to support the use of useful inventory or if the item would be needed quickly in special cases. Otherwise, minimization of less useful stock by means of location transfer, returns, discounted sales, donation, and discarding is recommended for optimal inventory control [3]. Consolidation of inventory items into one product line from a single vendor can help shift less useful items to become useful inventory. For example, an anesthesia group limits its CVC kits from an assortment of 15 catheters from three vendors to the three or four most commonly used ones in one product line.

Once inventory control procedures are established, their efficiency must be monitored. Efficiency can be calculated by the inventory turn ratio (also called turnover), which is defined as the ratio of total annual inventory purchases divided by the ending inventory value at year's end. A high turn ratio indicates that the inventory is being used efficiently. For anesthesia and operating room stock, an optional inventory turn ratio will be 6 to 12, while for the hospital distribution service it will typically be 15 to 18.

Inventory management

Once inventory control has been achieved, the challenges of inventory management—the ordering process—must be confronted. The goal is to ensure optimal supply on-hand for services without unnecessarily sequestering financial resources. Careful attention must be paid to details regarding order quantity, lead time (the time required from perceived need to the time an order is fulfilled), and safety stock (a buffer against running out, most important for inventory that is critical for on-going operations or providing care) [1].

Organizations usually determine optimal order quantity through a system called ABC analysis [1]. ABC analysis involves classifying inventory items based on annual dollar value of usage (see previous example discussing useful and less useful inventory). Inventory items classified under an A rating are those items with the highest usage; B inventory are those with medium usage, and finally C inventory are items that are seldom used. It is important to stress that ratings are based solely on inventory usage, not on number of items on-hand; therefore, although A inventory may represent a small population of the total inventory, optimizing inventory control and management for this select population is of utmost importance.

For any inventory, regardless of usage, organizations must determine optimal order quantities that will prevent stockpiling but minimize the accessing of safety stock. The most efficient maximum order quantity is defined by the economic order quantity (EOQ) [1] or Q_e [4].

$$EOQ = \sqrt{2FS/CP}$$

F = fixed costs of placing and receiving an order
S = annual usage
C = carrying costs as a percentage of the average inventory value
P = purchase price per unit

The level of a particular inventory item that is kept in supply will depend on the order quantity, lead time, and demand for safety stock. The minimum supply level depends on the safety stock demand and lead time; it also is known as the EOQ threshold, the threshold at which a reorder (EOQ) must be placed to maintain optimal supply levels [5]. The maximum supply level is defined as the minimum supply level plus the order quantity [1]. Thus, greater inventory supply stocks will be correlated with greater order quantities, lead times, and safety stock numbers.

Organizations can assess the effectiveness of ongoing inventory management continually through three types of inventory ratios: not in stock (NIS), fill rate, and percentage of backorders [1]. NIS is the fraction of items requisitioned but not filled (item is out of stock or backordered). Conversely, fill rate is the fraction of items requisitioned and filled. Lastly, percentage of backorder is the fraction of items requisitioned that are awaiting delivery following a backorder; it is more specific than the NIS ratio, which reflects the total fraction of items out of stock and backordered [1].

Inventory valuation

As inventory is used by the organization, its cost must be valued, but this can be complicated by the changing cost of purchased items. For instance, one order may be placed in January at $100 per item and a second order placed in February at $120 per same item. As the items are used, the organization must account for their cost. Three inventory costing methods commonly used in health care scenarios include first in, first out (FIFO), last in, first out (LIFO), and average costing. In FIFO, inventory cost is determined by the cost of the oldest inventory item (each item used in March cost the organization $100). In contrast, LIFO schemes assume that newer inventory is consumed first and that inventory cost is determined by the cost of the newest inventory item ($120). Lastly, average costing involves weighted average—the average cost of all items purchased—to determine unit cost ($110, assuming an equal number of items was purchased at each price).

Inventory receiving and distribution

Receiving operations refers to the physical receipt of inventory, the inspection of items, identification and delivery to end use areas, and preparation of receipt documents. Well-run receiving operations are important to ensure a smooth interaction with the vendor and subsequent distribution to the point of consumption or use.

Health care organizations may use one of two different receiving methods [1]. Centralized systems use a fan-like structure with a single centralized receiving point fanning out and distributing incoming supply to end users. This system is simple, compatible with centralized inventory storage systems, and provides a single point of communication between the organization and vendor. In a decentralized receiving system, delivery of product is at multiple points usually at or near the point of use. In this system, no centralized liaison is established, and implementation may be difficult; however, the decentralized system may be more beneficial to stockless inventory scenarios [1].

Once items are received, they must be distributed to their respective points of use. Seven common distribution methods are described [1]:

1. Random request: A department orders items via requisition and the items are delivered.
2. Emergency requisition: Items are hand-carried to the requesting department on immediate demand.
3. Periodic automatic replenishment (PAR): Items are delivered automatically and periodically to maintain a PAR level that has been predetermined by analyzing lead times, carrying costs, ordering costs, and available storage space (EOQ, as discussed previously). Distribution is not to exceed this predetermined level, which is the maximum volume or quantity established for each item. PAR is used in the anesthesia supply chain for commonly used disposable items such as intravenous kits, endotracheal tubes, and syringes. Typically, inventory technicians keep these items on carts and refill them daily or between cases, depending on the cart's usage and capacity. This system maintains consistent supply and quickly replenishes the anesthesia stock in the operating rooms without being intrusive during a case.
4. Exchange cart: Synonymous with the PAR system; however, prestocked carts are the means of distribution. In this system, the institution keeps identical supply carts at point of use locations and storage locations. At PAR-like intervals, the partially used cart at the point of use is exchanged for the fully stocked cart in storage, and the partially used cart is replenished and ready for the next exchange. A disadvantage of this system includes the cost incurred by redundancy.
5. Case cart: Analogous to the exchange cart concept, except each cart is customized according to physician preference. More effort is needed to use this system with a decentralized receiving system. Case carts typically are used for operation-specific situations (such as blocks, airway management, malignant hyperthermia management, or surgery) or operator-specific situations (such as surgeon-specific cases).
6. Just in time (JIT): Items are delivered frequently on a predetermined schedule and distributed immediately from receiving to the end users without any time in storage. At the authors' institution, each night the supply bins in the anesthesia storeroom are assayed for content. The order is placed to the supplier, who sends the supplies to the hospital. The hospital breaks down the cases and fills the bins to their PAR levels by the start of the next day's business. The success of this system is highly dependent on the performance of a supplier to ship bulk items at predetermined intervals or at request reliably. Supplier performance may benefit from incentives to ensure timely delivery.
7. Stockless: In this scenario, the supplier stores, ships, delivers and charges expenses directly to the requesting department. This system is most compatible with a decentralized receiving operation but can work in special situations within a centralized system. For example, at the authors' institution (centralized), a vendor may bring orthopedic hardware (implants and tools) and serves as a resource for the surgeon.

For JIT and stockless systems to work seamlessly, parameters such as vendor performance (routine and emergency), geographic/meteorological considerations in regards to transport, and materials management sophistication of the vendor and ordering facility must be optimized. So although JIT scenarios appear favorable, successful implementation is usually more difficult. In fact, in a study of operating room expenses where JIT inventory control was used when the operating room schedule was linked with the material management information system, JIT was found to be advantageous only for high-priced and high-volume items; there were no advantages to using JIT for everyday items, and, in fact, JIT was more expensive [5]. This was because of the increased cost of rush orders and the last minute changes in surgery schedules.

Items do not move exclusively one-way (from supplier to the health care facility); sometimes there are returns, recalls, and conversions. Returns occur when an item is sent back because of the end user's dissatisfaction with the item or oversupply of the item. Recalls refer to the request of the distributor/manufacturer to return the item (usually because of a defect). Conversions are product exchanges usually secondary to compatibility issues or changes in the patient care population. Monitoring the incidence of these obstructions to the supply chain can minimize the detrimental financial consequences of wasted inventory and costs involved in performing a return, recall, or conversion. Analysis also may reveal a greater flaw in an organization's system, such as poor inventory control, inadequate practice standardization, or ill-conceived, poorly researched acquisitions.

Inventory storage

A carefully planned layout for a facility's inventory storage area is of utmost importance in optimizing inventory management and control [3]. Traditionally, inventory items are stored together as similar items. When compared with inventory management and control schemes, it is easy to see that this system is antiquated and far from the most efficient. For optimal efficiency, inventory is stored in a hierarchal system in which high-demand patient-critical items are placed as close to the distribution or point-of-use area as possible. Organizations should consider available real estate (location and amount of space) and the physical characteristics of the inventory items themselves (size, shape, weight, etc.) [3]. JIT systems from close (albeit not prime) storage areas may be implemented for the resupply of high-demand inventory. For example, in the operating room environment, intravenous supplies, endotracheal tubes, and blood pressure cuffs should be stored at point-of-use areas, whereas fiberoptic devices may be stored in a more distant site such as the clean core anesthesia supply room.

Inventory standardization

If similar items that perform a redundant function are in inventory, an institution may wish to standardize. Standardization can reduce the overall number of supplies needed, and at the same time increase the negotiating leverage of a customer by increasing the number of standardized items ordered. Standardization also decreases the complexity of one's inventory storage system. When an organization decides to begin standardization, it most likely performs a needs analysis through a value analysis committee [1]. The needs analysis will address issues regarding practice/operating room history, physician preference, specialty requirements, and inventory storage factors. The analysis also will identify personnel who need to be influential in the decision-making process. Physicians should contribute to decisions to standardize high-priced items they prefer. Claims of superior patient care associated with such high-priced items should be supported by formal statistical evidence before the commitment of financial resources.

THE DECISION PROCESS OF PROCURING EQUIPMENT

Anesthesia groups should strive to be critical and objective in choosing new capital equipment and supplies. In large groups and institutions, decisions typically are made by an equipment committee. There may be one committee for both capital equipment and supplies, or in larger institutions, a capital equipment committee and a separate materials use evaluation (MUE) committee may be required. A capital equipment committee is clinically driven in its team approach to review new and emerging technologies. This important role of technology assessment is best practice and involves extended value analysis and cost analysis to include life cycle costing for new equipment. There are five important characteristics of a successful capital equipment committee:

1. A realistic 5-year plan
2. Early materials management involvement
3. All information gathered to make sound decisions
4. Prioritization, grouping, and standardization
5. Appropriate selection practices

For large anesthesia groups within such large institutions, there is usually a committee within the anesthesia group to handle the specific needs for the group. The committee chair, empowered by the department head, oversees the process. The committees should include representatives from all the various groups within the organization that use the equipment (physicians, certified registered nurse anesthetists, anesthesia technicians, and others) or have an interest or influence in the equipment. For example, at the University of Texas M. D. Anderson Cancer Center (MDACC) in the Division of Anesthesiology and Critical Care, the capital equipment committee consists of faculty from anesthesia, critical care and pain management, ICU nursing, post anesthesia care unit (PACU) nursing, anesthesia technicians, the head certified registered nurse anesthetist, biomedical engineering, sourcing and contracts, the perioperative materials manager, infection control, anesthesia billing, a financial analyst, and the anesthesia program coordinator. The equipment committee meets on a quarterly basis to coordinate its decisions with the institution's quarterly planning process for capital expenditures. The committee's mission is to decide on matters of capital equipment for the entire division by addressing the needs of its constituent departments, Critical Care and Anesthesiology and Pain Medicine. This approach results in more consistency and uniformity for the institution.

Most equipment is tested in a trial period before purchase to determine whether it is a good fit for the group and its mission. Trials may initiate in several ways. A sales representative may bring in a new device for the group to trial; one of the clinicians may request the group to assess a product, or it may be time for replacement of older technology. The head of the equipment committee typically meets with all of the vendors to provide consistent critique of each product and to insulate the individual clinicians from interacting with the representatives. After meeting with a particular vendor, the equipment head decides whether the piece of equipment is potentially useful to the group. If it is, the trial begins (Fig. 2). The progress of the trial is overseen by the equipment head or a designee such as the head anesthesia technician or anesthesia program manager. If there are competitors to be considered, those vendors are contacted for a possible side-by-side or comparison trial. At the beginning of the trial period, the vendor(s) complete and sign a vendor release form. At this time, the vendors are briefed on the code of conduct for vendors within the institution and operating rooms. A zero-dollar purchase order is produced for the vendor for the equipment and any supplies to be used in the trial. All disposables should be provided free of charge by the vendor. A specific evaluation form is designed that is to be completed by all those individuals who use the equipment during the trial. The trial begins after an appropriate in-service has been performed, and during the trial the vendor should be present only for in-service support. Only those who use the equipment (ie, not the vendor, because of potential conflict of interest) should complete the evaluations. The trial should have a specific end point (eg, the use of a fixed number of disposables, a fixed time period, number of patient uses). At the end of the trial, the project coordinator (this might be the head technologist, the anesthesia program manager, or a designated member of the committee) collects all of the evaluations and the equipment, and unused supplies are returned to the vendor. The equipment head reviews the evaluations, and, if reviews strongly favor or disfavor a product, he/she makes the decision whether to purchase the product. More difficult decisions fall to the equipment committee, which will review the evaluations, conduct a value analysis, and look at a return on investment (ROI) analysis where appropriate.

VALUE ANALYSIS

The concept of value analysis was conceived in the 1940s by Lawrence Miles to evaluate how to reduce the cost of products. This technique breaks down the product or device into its component parts and relates the components' costs to their contributions to the functions of the device. The result is a shift of attention away from the costs of the components to the costs of the functions provided by the product. Functions can be viewed as basic functions and secondary functions. Basic functions are the main operative functions of the device, and secondary functions are what make that product uniquely attractive.

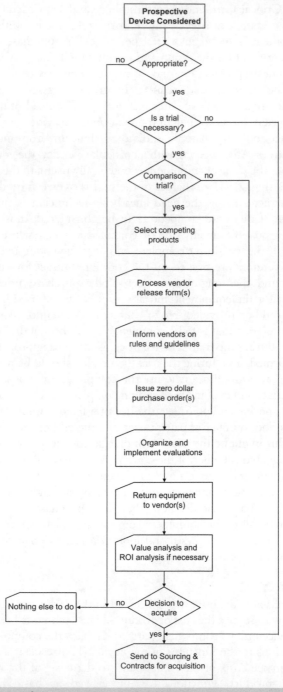

Fig. 2. Decision tree for new equipment trials and purchase.

Both types of functions will have a cost associated with them. Controlling the secondary functions and the sometimes-intangible characteristics of a product that make it attractive (eg, the value of name branding) can reduce costs.

The following is an example of value analysis. Imagine a hospital that is looking to upgrade its pulse oximeters. First, the equipment committee might compare two pulse oximeters (from two manufacturers) head to head (Fig. 3). They likely would identify the basic functions of the monitors to provide clinically reliable SaO2 readings for all sized patients, use disposable probes, and integrate inside each of the institution's existing bedside monitors. Secondary functions include a waveform display, heart rate calculator, good filtering for artifact as a result of patient motion, good filtering from electromagnetic and infrared (EM/IF) interference, and capability to interface with the institution's electronic medical record system. Other tangible factors to include in the value analysis would be the cost of the disposable probes, the rate of failure and the cost of repairs, and the future cost of maintenance contracts, warranties, and upgrades.

Intangible costs to be factored in the value analysis would include the time and effort for staff in-servicing and the potential cost of changing the existing vendor to another. This cost includes not only the time and work to physically change the monitors, but the impact of the different look and feel that a new monitor might have in patient care.

Assume that the only difference between the two monitors is their ability to handle outside interference. At this point, the decision rests on the preference for filtering characteristics of the devices. If monitor B is more expensive than A, but the device will be used predominantly in the ICU environment where

	Monitor A	Monitor B
Basic Functions		
All size patients	√	√
Disposable Probes	√	√
Integration	√	√
Secondary Functions		
Waveform Display	√	√
Heart Rate	√	√
Motion Artifact Filtering		√
EM/IR Filtering	√	
EMR Interface	√	√

Fig. 3. Comparison of basic and secondary functions for two pulse oximeters.

motion artifact can be a problem, the cost of that secondary function would justify the higher cost of monitor B. On the other hand, if the monitors were to be used in the ICU and also in the operating room (an environment rich with EM/IF interference), then the decision becomes evenly balanced. If the possibility of these artifacts is not a factor, then simply taking the cheaper bid might be the best option.

Future expenses for the monitors could be a deciding factor. For instance, the maintenance costs for one may be greater than the other. The cost of the disposable probes may be a factor, depending on the degree of capitation in the environment in which the monitors are to be used. As this example shows, value analysis will take into account various factors unique to the individual institution where the equipment is going to be used; therefore it must be flexible in its design.

RETURN ON INVESTMENT ANALYSIS

For capital equipment, the committee's evaluation often will include a return on investment (ROI) analysis. ROIs typically are done for large ticket capital equipment items (eg, a C-arm and fluoroscopy table for a pain medicine group). The threshold for consideration of an ROI is typically in the $50,000 range, but will vary between institutions. An ROI compares all costs—the initial capital outlay for a piece of equipment, the expense to maintain, and the cost to operate—to the expected revenue generated from the product's use.

The following example illustrates an ROI for a new C-arm in an established outpatient pain clinic. The C-arm would be the first fluoroscopy device in the clinic, which would result in enhanced services and revenue (Fig. 4). The start-up costs include a one-time capital acquisition cost of $150,000, along with installation expense of $15,000. The ongoing expenses include maintenance ($14,000 the first year) and technician salaries ($62,400 the first year). Ongoing expenses are increased in successive years at a rate of 2% per year for maintenance and 4% per year for technician salaries. There are two sources of revenue; the technical revenue for diagnostic imaging ($170 per use) and the professional revenue from the procedures that can be done because the device is available in the clinic ($990 per case on average). The initial estimate for cases is 560 the first year. Growth is factored in successive years at a conservative rate of 2% per year. In this clinic's environment, the overall collection rate is 38%, so gross revenues are adjusted downward by 62%. The forecast is performed 7 years, or the approximate life expectancy of the capital equipment.

In this example, the purchase of a new C-arm for the pain clinic is justified easily (costs over seven years of $763,420 and revenue over seven years of $1,835,138 for a net ROI of $1,071,718). ROI worksheets also can be used to determine the minimum number of cases that would have to be done to cover the expenses of the new service within a specific period of time.

After all analyses have been done, the capital equipment committee rank orders the capital equipment items that have been trialed and that have been

	Year 1	Year 2	Year 3	Year 4	Year 5	Year 6	Year 7	Total
Revenue								
Diagnostic Imaging								
Units	560	571	583	594	606	618	631	4,163
Avg. Charge Per Unit	$170	$170	$170	$170	$170	$170	$170	$170
Gross Patient Revenue	95,200	97,104	99,046	101,027	103,048	105,108	107,211	$707,744
Deduction Percentage	62.00%	62.00%	62.00%	62.00%	62.00%	62.00%	62.00%	62.00%
Total Deductions	59,024	60,204	61,409	62,637	63,889	65,167	66,471	$438,801
Net Patient Revenue (NPR)	36,176	36,900	37,638	38,390	39,158	39,941	40,740	$268,943
Cumulative NPR	36,176	73,076	110,713	149,103	188,261	228,203	268,943	
Professional Fees								
Units	560	571	583	594	606	618	631	4,163
Avg. Charge Per Unit	990	990	990	990	990	990	990	$990.00
Gross Patient Revenue	554,400	565,488	576,798	588,334	600,100	612,102	624,344	$4,121,567
Deduction Percentage	62.00%	62.00%	62.00%	62.00%	62.00%	62.00%	62.00%	62.00%
Total Deductions	343,728	350,603	357,615	364,767	372,062	379,503	387,094	$2,555,371
Net Patient Revenue (NPR)	210,672	214,885	219,183	223,567	228,038	232,599	237,251	$1,566,195
Cumulative NPR	210,672	425,557	644,741	868,307	1,096,346	1,328,944	1,566,195	
Total (NPR)	246,040	251,785	256,821	261,957	267,196	272,540	277,991	$1,835,138
Total Cumulative NPR	246,848	498,633	755,454	1,017,411	1,284,607	1,557,147	1,835,138	
Expenses								
One Time Costs								
Equipment	150,000							$150,000
Installation	15,000							$15,000
Training								$0
Other								$0
Recurring Costs								
Maintenance	14,200	14,484	14,774	15,069	15,371	15,678	15,992	$105,567
Personnel	62,400	64,896	67,492	70,192	72,999	75,919	78,956	$492,854
Other								$0
Total Expenses	241,600	79,380	82,266	85,261	88,370	91,597	94,947	$763,420
Cumulative Expenses	241,600	320,980	403,246	488,506	576,876	668,473	763,420	
ROI								
	5,248	172,405	174,555	176,696	178,827	180,943	183,044	$1,071,718
	5,248	177,653	352,208	520,905	707,731	888,674	1,071,718	

Fig. 4. Return on investment (ROI) analysis for pain clinic c-arm.

deemed appropriate to acquire. This ranked list then is submitted to the institutional budgetary process for funding. For supplies, such ranking is usually not necessary.

For new equipment, any costs for in-services, warranties, and service agreements can be included with the sales pricing at the time of acquisition. However, depending on the institution's accounting practices, however, these things may be paid for from various funding sources and may therefore need to be purchased separately.

GROUP PURCHASING ORGANIZATIONS AND INTEGRATED DELIVERY NETWORKS

Purchased goods and services represent a huge investment for hospitals; in fact, they account for the second largest dollar expenditure [6]. Group purchasing organizations (GPOs) represent a consortium of health care practices customers and function to consolidate purchasing power and contracting services to strengthen the negotiating power of the buyer while increasing sales of a product for a manufacturer. The manufacturer is charged a fee for service to be integrated into a GPO [1]. For the member hospitals, GPOs ensure competitive pricing, price protection, improved quality control programs, reduced contracting cost, and the monitoring of market conditions. In fact, it is estimated that GPOs have saved hospitals $13 to $19 billion (10% to 15%) of total purchasing costs [6]. Although competitive pricing is considered the main advantage of the GPO, these organizations also may offer contracting services, information sharing, clinical and operational benchmarking, and value analysis services that further increase a practice's operational efficiency by freeing personnel who otherwise would be tasked or hired for such purposes [6]. These advantages seem overwhelming, yet member commitment to GPOs is somewhat unreliable, and the cherry picking of advantageous contracts among a GPO's portfolio is common. To meet this trend, GPOs have gone so far as to offer their members a choice between committed and noncommitted options [1].

Integrated delivery networks (IDNs) were conceived in the 1990s as a result of the dual trend of vertical and horizontal integration in the health care industry. IDNs are a horizontal network of hospitals (related by proximity, mergers, multihospital systems, and other factors) that form an alliance with the capability to provide patient services at multiple sites. It is thought that with this super-alliance offering horizontal consolidation of services, consolidation also could occur in purchasing so as to mimic GPO's strength in numbers and eliminate the need for an outside organization. Others argue, however, that GPOs already are entrenched in many hospital-purchasing schemes and have performed admirably, and that IDN consolidation of purchasing is unnecessary. Regardless, some health care experts, particularly physicians, reason that over-dependence on GPOs or IDNs results in the deterioration of the beneficial interaction and exchange of ideas between manufacturer/representative and end user [6].

APPENDIX 1
Glossary of terms

AORN: Association of PeriOperative Nurses

Capital planning: This is a process that looks at the institution's future needs for capital equipment. Most common is a 5-year plan. This involves prioritization, grouping, and standardization. The evaluation process should include a value analysis and a return on investment analysis.

Central Services (CS): This department can contain the sterile processing department (SPD).

Chemical hazard communication standard (CHCS): An OSHA regulation that ensures an employee's right to know about the risks of chemical and hazardous wastes.

Consignment: This is a technique used to decrease the money an institution ties up in expensive inventory items. For example, an operating room will keep one or two implantable pain pumps available, but will not buy them until the time of use so that they are not kept on the books as inventory.

DOT: Department of Transportation

Determination PAR level: The maximum supply level = minimum level + order quantity.

Minimum supply level = safety stock + lead time

EDI: Electronic data interchange

EPA: Environmental Protection Agency

GPO: An organization that combines the total volume of groups of products from multiple health care facilities to bargain/negotiate/leverage the lowest cost from the manufacturer and/or supplier.

Inventory: Items on hand; current assets

Inventory turns: A benchmark for managing inventory. It is calculated by dividing the total annual inventory by the ending inventory value.

JCAHO: Joint Commission on Accreditation of Healthcare Organizations

JIT – A strategy of obtaining supplies near the time of utilization. This results in decreased inventory levels and therefore decreased expense of maintaining inventory.

Lowest unit of measure: Eg, a case of syringes contains six boxes, and each box contains 50 syringes. One syringe is therefore the LUM.

Material safety data sheets (MSDS): This is a database that contains a product's identification, its physical and chemical properties, any fire/explosion/health hazard data, emergency procedures, handling and storage information, manufacturers information, and other information.

MUE: Materials use evaluation; an older term for supplies

NFPA: National Fire Protection Agency

OSHA: Occupational Safety and Health Administration

PAR: Items are maintained in a fixed location and maintained at a maximum established quantity

Sourcing and contracts: This is the department that is responsible for acquiring supplies and equipment through contract negotiation with the vendors. This is another name for procurement services.

SPD: Sterile Processing Department

Supply chain: The process and steps of getting a product from the distributor to the user.

Total deliverable cost: The cost of placing the order. In addition to the purchase price, this includes the administrative costs of receiving, warehousing, inventorying, issuing, and delivering the item. A standard benchmark is to spend an additional $1 in process cost for every $1 spent in product.

Total delivered cost, capital: The cost of the device along with the cost of service and support, any disposables, and the cost of labor to utilize the device throughout the useful life of the device.

Value analysis: A process that determines the best and most economical product, equipment, or service that will meet the needs of the user reliably.

Acknowledgment

The authors thank Mary Purugganan for her help with editing this manuscript.

References

[1] Bryan WC, Cox TK, Fernandez F, et al. In materials management review guide: CMRP examination review guide. 2nd edition. Chicago: Association for Healthcare Resource & Materials Management of the American Hospital Association; 2003. p. 21–34.

[2] Reiner J, Bremer T. Supply chain solutions for healthcare providers. Part 2—supply chain improvement opportunities. White paper: UPS supply chain solutions; 2005. Available at: http://www.ups-scs.com/solutions/white_papers/wp_healthcare2.pdf. Accessed November 1, 2007.

[3] Schreibfeder J. The first steps to achieving effective inventory control. White paper: Microsoft Business Solutions. Available at: http://download.microsoft.com/download/b/f/3/bf334d7f-ad07-458e-a716-fdf46a0cf63c/eimwp1_invcontrol.pdf. Accessed November 1, 2007.

[4] Nowicki M. The financial management of hospitals and healthcare organizations. 2nd edition. Chicago: Health Administration Press; American College of Healthcare Executives; 2001.

[5] Epstein RH, Dexter F. Economic analysis of linking operating room scheduling and hospital material management information systems for just-in-time inventory control. Anesth Analg 2000;91:337–43.

[6] Schneller ES. The value of group purchasing in the healthcare supply chain. White paper: Arizona State University College of Business, School of Health Administration and Policy. Available at: http://www.novationco.com/pressroom/attachments/GroupPurchasing.pdf. Accessed November 1, 2007.

Advances in Anesthesia 25 (2007) 17–39

ADVANCES IN ANESTHESIA

Automated Anesthesia

Thomas M. Hemmerling, MD, DEAA[a,b,*]

[a]Department of Anesthesiology, McGill University Health Center, Montreal General Hospital, McGill University, 1650 Cedar Avenue, Montreal, Quebec H3G 1A4, Canada
[b]Institute of Biomedical Engineering, Université de Montréal, Montreal, Quebec, Canada

F ew specialties are made for the introduction of automation as is anesthesia. Compared with surgery, anesthesiologists do not change the integrity of the human body. Anesthesiologists administer drugs by different access routes into the human body to render it into a state where surgery can be performed. When they work in intensive care, monitoring the different body functions and trying to restore the integrity of these functions or the normal physiological state of the human body are principal tasks. Working in the emergency field—either within the hospital or outside—means to quickly diagnose an immediate and very often life-threatening disorder of the human body and correct it using various interventional pharmacological or nonpharmacological tools.

Therefore, anesthesiology is determined by a fine balance between observing and monitoring body functions for very often a considerable amount of time, be it minutes in the ambulance, hours in the operating room, or days in the ICU, and reacting in the flash of a moment to a life-threatening situation, which, if not recognized and diagnosed correctly and treated accordingly, might kill the patient. For some, this contrast between steady-state anesthesia with stable body functions and rapidly occurring emergencies bears the challenge and fascination of the specialty. For others, it is a constant source of stress.

It is not surprising that anesthesia is one of the specialties with the highest numbers of parameters to constantly monitor, and, if necessary, correct; comparisons often are made with pilots in general aviation, although this might be a bit exaggerated. In recent years, however, the number of monitoring parameters has increased exponentially, and so has the number of precise and sophisticated devices used to display them. One example is the evolution of ventilators. Initially, anesthesiologists started out manually ventilating the patient for hours, then using frugal ventilators with the traditional bag bottle

*Department of Anesthesiology, McGill University Health Center, Montreal General Hospital, McGill University, 1650 Cedar Avenue, Montreal, Quebec H3G 1A4, Canada.
E-mail address: thomas.hemmerling@mcgill.ca

0737-6146/07/$ – see front matter
doi:10.1016/j.aan.2007.07.006

principle of administering tidal volumes and indicating basic parameters like tidal volume, frequency, and inspiratory pressure. The most recent ventilators are extremely sophisticated machines monitoring and displaying up to 100 different parameters.

In addition, the way anesthesia is monitored has changed considerably. The three basic components of general anesthesia are loss of consciousness (or hypnosis), analgesia, and neuromuscular blockade. In the early days of anesthesia, loss of consciousness and analgesia were guessed by looking at clinical signs, such as patients' movement during surgery (in fact, the minimal alveolar concentration [MAC] is defined like that), sweating, or simple heart rate and blood pressure changes, neuromuscular blockade was assessed by either simple clinical signs, such as head lifting, or subjective monitoring using basic neurostimulators and tactile or visual assessment of the motor response. A great effort was done recently to provide anesthesiologists with more precise and objective methods of monitoring. In this area, the arrival of the bispectral index (BIS) monitoring has been a most welcome tool; however artifact prone the technique might be, it has become for many anesthesiologists a standard of care. The greatest advancements were made in the field of neuromuscular monitoring, not only with the development of more easy-to-use and still precise monitoring methods, such as acceleromyography, kinemyography, or, most recently phonomyography, but also with a much better understanding of how muscles react to neuromuscular blocking drugs (NMBD). The assessment of analgesia during general anesthesia is still a very difficult task; however, recent research has explored new ways of monitoring pain while the patient is asleep.

Interestingly, little development has been assigned to the way the increasingly high numbers of parameters are displayed and in which way alarms are used or presented. Monitor development has focused on the way one enters or accesses data—storage systems, touch button screens—but the essentials of display design have not changed dramatically over the years. Once the vital signs are displayed, their display does not change or changes little according to certain situations; one could imagine a monitor which highlights certain parameters when certain limits are passed, and the monitor zooms them into one's field of visual attention. For most parameters, the type of alarms is very much the same: whenever certain limits are exceeded, the parameter will, in general, flash, and an acoustic alarm will follow. One of the most simple and probably best auditory alarm and display systems has been in place for pulse oximetry, where with decreasing saturation, the frequency of the audible signal changes. Many anesthesiologists have developed "an ear" for the saturation signal over the years and can tell just by listening to the sound the range of the displayed saturation with astonishing precision.

Electronic record keeping has been made available for almost all recent monitors; this frees the anesthesiologist's time—so far taken away by hand writing a more or less detailed report of interventions, the drugs administered and the patient's status—to take care of direct patient needs. In addition, these modern systems are very often connected to other hospital networks, therefore allowing immediate access to patient files, radiology, or laboratory reports, and even automatic billing.

Recently, display of anesthetic parameters at distance has been introduced into the clinical practice. Several devices—mostly personal digital assistant device (PDA) based software systems—are commercially available. Initially, regulatory hurdles (problems with the creation of secure data transfer over a distance without disturbing other electric devices in a complex environment of emergency room, ICU, or operating room) inhibited this development, which now has gained almost the speed of other information technology (IT) inventions. More than 40% of physicians in North America, including anesthesiologists, use PDAs for several medical tasks.

BUT WHAT ABOUT THE WAY DRUGS ARE ADMINISTERED?

Initially, most drugs were administered as bolus or repetitive bolus. Loss of consciousness was maintained by applying volatile anesthetics according to clinical signs and the MAC. Then, with the development of syringe pumps, a trend toward total intravenous anesthesia (TIVA) occurred, which in itself opened up the possibility of designing simple and later increasingly sophisticated automation systems to self-administer anesthetic drugs. Because neuromuscular blockade is the most precise and reliable monitoring parameter, it is not suprising that the first completely automated systems of administering anesthetic drugs were conceptualized for NMBDs. Closed-loop drug administration consists of an entity of parameter monitoring, microprocessor controlling system, and syringe pump; it has become available for many research projects, providing astonishing precision to maintain a given state of neuromuscular blockade. However, it was never commercially available for clinicians. This was probably caused by a lack of interest from companies, a lack of more clever designed systems (eg, changing the level of neuromuscular blockade automatically according to the type of surgery and the progress of a given type of surgery) and the fact that a system with friendly and easy-to-use interfaces presenting and controlling the parameters—similar to vital sign monitors—was not available. Some also might argue that, with recent developments in anesthesia—the more widespread use of regional and local anesthetic techniques, the introduction of less invasive forms of anesthesia using laryngeal mask airways, and better and more precise titration of the state of consciousness—less and less neuromuscular blockade is used, even in types of surgeries where traditionally muscle relaxation played a very essential part [1]. In addition, to install an automated closed-loop application of drugs in clinical routine, important regulatory hurdles have to be overcome.

In the last 15 years, the development and routine implementation of BIS monitoring has opened up the development of closed-loop application of drugs providing loss of consciousness. Very interesting systems have been developed to administer propofol and even volatile anesthetics under the automatic guidance of BIS monitoring, and it seems that commercial closed-loop systems might be available in the near future.

Whereas the introduction of pharmacodynamically guided closed-loop systems has been difficult and reserved for research purposes, the pharmacokinetically guided administration of anesthetic drugs is commercially available. Target-controlled systems are available for administering remifentanil or propofol, at least in Europe. This surprises a bit, because the pharmacokinetics vary significantly from one patient to the next; this author has extensive experience with the clinical use of target controlled infusion (TCI)-propofol systems. In my mind, the projected steady-state biophase concentration rather often is accompanied by insufficient depth of anesthesia, patients awakening during surgery, and the target concentration needing constant adjustment—hardly the ideal of an automated system. The integration of pharmacokinetic modelling into closed-loop pharmacodynamic control systems might open up the way to more reliable and precise devices.

Lastly, the way anesthetic training is conducted, be it for medical students, anesthetic technicians and practitioners, or residents, has changed dramatically over the last decade. Although hands-on training was the backbone of anesthetic training—and some patients actually suffered from these training sessions—simulator and virtual reality training has become a reality in many anesthetic departments around the globe. At present, the only thing preventing the widespread use of simulators in training are cost issues, which soon should be resolved. Anesthetic departments and opinion leaders in the field have to propagate the idea of having simulator training available in-house in all anesthetic training departments; simulator training should become a mandatory item on residency programs, as some departments already have done.

SO WHAT IS THE STATUS IN DEVELOPING AUTOMATED ANESTHESIA?

Monitoring display

The way vital signs are displayed has changed very little over the last 20 years. Anesthesiologists constantly are reminded of this fact when they transfer patients from the operating room to the ICU using one of those old transfer monitors showing oxygen saturation, (invasive) blood pressure, and ECG. Some even think that they display the parameters in a better way than most modern monitors. If one compares them with the latest models, there are three main features that have changed, without fundamentally changing its principle:

  Most modern monitors are very large, at least 17 inches or more.
  Most monitors function by touch-screen buttons.
  The amount of parameters displayed has increased significantly, making the
    space for each parameter not much bigger than on those old monitors.

Radical shifts in display design did not make it to commercially available monitors. Most monitor display designs incorporate the principle of a combination of visual and numeric objects, given that using graphical objects, critical errors are detected earlier [2]. Diagnostic errors caused by misinterpreted physiologic data are reduced significantly [3]. Some attempts [4,5] to change the display of monitors more radically [6], such as using more graphically oriented displays, histograms, and polygonal shapes, have shown an increase in anesthesiologists' vigilance. They have not found their way into commercial products despite good results in the National Aeronautics and Space Administration Task Load Index [7], meaning minimal workload, low level of frustration, and high efficiency. The resistance to change the way parameters are displayed in anesthesiology reminds me of the initial response when BMW's I-drive system came into the market; it seemed far too radical and complicated. Now almost all high-end cars use derivatives of this system.

If one looks at displays carefully, there are three different subsets:

> Vital sign parameters, which include not only a five-lead ECG, (invasive) blood pressure, or oxygen saturation, but can include more and more sophisticated parameters, such as cardiac output, pulmonary pressure, central venous pressure, systemic vascular or pulmonary resistance, cerebral oximetry and other parameters. The so-called vital sign monitor, which initially showed only a handful parameters, now carries an increasingly large number of parameters.
>
> The second subset includes all ventilator parameters, such as tidal volumes or frequencies, end-tidal CO_2 pressure, inspiratory pressure, and more sophisticated flow pressure volume curves depending on the technology of the ventilator. Most monitor companies now offer the possibility to display all of these parameters on one screen, which can increase the amount of parameters displayed simultaneously to a range of 40 to 50 or more.
>
> A third subset of parameters gets somehow lost in the vital signs monitor or is displayed in bulky stand-alone devices: the parameters that define the state of general anesthesia: depth of anesthesia, analgesia, and neuromuscular blockade.

As explained before, there are several reliable parameters available in commercial devices to quantify, in real time, the depth of anesthesia (BIS, evoked auditory potentials index, entropy, patient state index and others). Objective quantitative neuromuscular monitoring methods and devices have been available and have been demanded to be mandatory when providing neuromuscular blockade [8]. Electromyography, acceleromyography, kinemyography are available, and phonomyography may soon be available in commercial devices. All of these methods are reliable and precise enough for routine daily use [9].

A novel score, called "Analgoscore", reflecting the state of intraoperative analgesia while the patient is asleep, has recently been proposed [10]. This might open the door for an easy-to-use quantitative method of determining intraoperative pain under general anesthesia.

And yet the question arises: why would the parameters defining the three components of general anesthesia—loss of consciousness, analgesia, and neuromuscular blockade—be scattered over the vital sign monitor? Would it not be better to create a third kind of monitor mainly focusing on the display of these parameters, which would provide a quick but precise glance at the actual state of anesthesia?

Fig. 1 shows a prototype monitor called integrated monitor of anesthesia (IMA), developed by the ITAG group (Intelligent Techniques in Anesthesia group, Department of Anesthesiology, McGill University, Montreal, Canada). It shows a mixture of color-coded graphical–numerical display design integrating the three components of general anesthesia using (for research purposes) BIS as parameter for depth of anesthesia, the "Analgoscore" reflecting intraoperative analgesia and phonomyography for neuromuscular blockade.

A future direction in monitoring design might be to integrate the three subsets of monitoring—vital signs, ventilation parameters, and components of general anesthesia—and make them equally available at distance using PDAs and Bluetooth technology.

Alarms and monitor display

The integration of intelligent alarms is equally important. One study [11] showed that many users turn off alarms because of high prevalence of false alarms, which are regarded as nuisance, and consider that their actions are safer without them. Another problem arises in monitors, which allow users to customize the alarm threshold. Such systems are misleading, because devices with the same external appearance are expected to have a similar operation, thus similar alarm limits. The user might expect the manufacturer's default

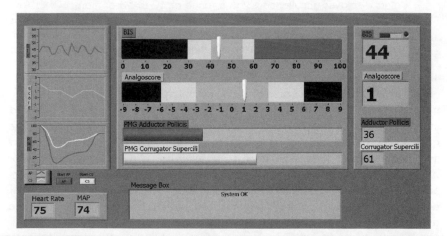

Fig. 1. Integrated monitor of anesthesia (IMA). The IMA is separated in three vertical parts; to the left, there is the trend display of BIS (bispectral index), Analgoscore and phonomyography (PMG, two lines for two different muscles). The middle column shows—color-coded—the actual BIS value, value for Analgoscore at a given time including the exact numerical data. The degree of muscle relaxation also is shown in color-coded columns—two different muscles—without showing the actual numerical value. The right column only shows numerical values for each parameter. Also shown are heart rate and mean arterial blood pressure, as well as a message box.

alarm limits when the device is started, while in fact, alarms have been changed by the previous user [12]. Therefore, intelligent alarm design is important to help cope with the increasing number of parameters. Block and Schaaf [13] performed a study in 50 adult patients under general anesthesia with default alarm settings using an integrated monitor (Cardiocap, Datex, Helsinki). The number of alarms averaged three alarms per case, with a mean frequency of one alarm every 34 minutes. False alarms (those caused by electrocautery, accidental patient movement, or other nonphysiological reasons) represented only 24% of all alarms. Those alarms that were considered as outside the limits occurred at a rate of 53%, and those considered as "patient at risk" occurred at a rate of 23%. Of the alarms, 67% occurred during the beginning and end of anesthesia. The end tidal carbon dioxide accounted for 42% of the alarms, mostly during intubation and extubation. Another study estimated the frequency of false alarms to be between 30% and 76% [12]. A recent study [14] has focused on five areas of alarm concern:

- The number of alarms and its reduction
- False alarm rates and their influence on human reactions
- The design of alarms and the application of research into auditory cognition
- Intelligent alarm systems
- The implementation of alarm designs as a worldwide medical alarms standard

The future of alarm systems might be the development of intelligent alarm systems based on neural networks.

Alarm design has a long way to go, but we finally realize that, in an increasingly complicated workplace, significant changes have to be made to the way data are displayed and alarms are designed. This is not an acceptance of the anesthesiologist's incapability of functioning but rather the equivalent of changes in different other areas of daily and professional life. Do pilots complain that computers are taking over part of their tasks?

Closed-loop administration of drugs in anesthesia

The most important step toward automated anesthesia is the development of a system that can automatically—by regulating the amount of drug given over time according to patients' and surgical needs—administer anesthetic drugs. There have been many studies concerning closed-loop control of anesthesia as opposed to open-loop control (manual control). First, all three components of anesthesia were addressed separately and closed-loop systems developed for each of the three components. Each closed-loop system needs a target control variable, a controller (usually a microprocessor), an established and accepted target value, and the control actuator, a syringe pump or vapor.

The first question is: how definitive is the control variable for the measured effect? Neuromuscular blockade is a classical example of a direct indicator of muscle relaxation, and various different and reliable monitoring methods are available. Processed electroencephalogram (EEG) derivatives or algorithms based on hemodynamic variables are classical examples of indirect indicators of depth of anesthesia or intraoperative pain, respectively. For both direct and indirect indicators, however, various closed-loop systems have been developed.

Depth of anesthesia

The most widely used derivative of EEG as an indicator for depth of anesthesia is BIS, developed by Aspect Medical Company (Norwood, Massachusetts). Usually, levels of 40 to 55 are accepted for a moderate state of hypnosis, whereas BIS lower than 40 indicates a more profound hypnosis. Several closed-loop systems have been developed to administer propofol or inhaled anesthetics using BIS and have been at least as accurate as open-loop systems [15,16]. Several study groups have included target-controlled infusions into the loop [17,18] or adaptive, patient-individualized, model-based control systems [19,20] to increase the controller performance. Using specially configured simulators, BIS-oriented closed-loop systems have been evaluated in more extreme control situations, such as BIS of 30 or 70, and proved good reliability [21].

Neuromuscular blockade

There have been many closed-loop systems over the last 15 years, which were used for research purposes but performed very well, especially in the more profound block range [22–24]. However, the need for profound neuromuscular blockade has decreased significantly over the last decade because of the introduction of different anesthetic techniques (eg, the increased use of laryngeal mask airways, the increased use of regional or local anesthetic techniques, and more reliable titration of anesthetic drugs). Therefore, there are fewer closed-loop systems developed for the newer NMBDs.

Two recent studies presented a closed-loop system for mivacurium [25] and cisatracurium [26] with good reliability. In comparison to administering drugs for depth of anesthesia or analgesia, most anesthesiologists do not administer NMBDs as continuous infusion. There might be less need to develop a closed-loop system to constantly infuse NMBDs, but a far more sophisticated system, which administers NMBDs as bolus, whenever needed for surgical reasons.

Intraoperative analgesia during general anesthesia

There are so far very few closed-loop systems for the administration of analgesics during general anesthesia. First, there is no direct indicator of pain, since the patient is asleep. Most attempts to design closed-loop systems have used surrogate controlling variables, such as blood pressure. One of the first to attack the problem of analgesia-closed-loop systems was Gentilini's group. That group's most recent system uses a pharmacokinetic model together with mean arterial blood pressure, includes safety features such as security algorithms when the controlling variable monitoring is limited by artifacts, and tries to optimize monitoring constantly [27].

The ITAG research group recently presented a novel score of intraoperative pain, the "Analgoscore", based on mean arterial blood pressure and heart rate.

The score varies between -9 and +9, with -3 to +3 reflecting an optimal pain control and negative values analgesia overshoot, positive values analgesia undershoot [10]. Similar to Gentilini's team, the "Analgoscore" was used to control a closed-loop system including similar safety measures, auto-learning processes of the system, and pharmacokinetic models. The first results are very promising, and more studies necd to be performed (Fig. 2).

Putting everything together—an integrated closed-loop system for analgesia, anesthesia, and neuromuscular blockade?

The three components of general anesthesia cannot be regarded separately. Every anesthesiologist uses his or her intellect to balance the effect of drugs toward their impact—direct or indirect—on all three components. If one has the feeling that analgesia might be insufficient, more analgesics can be given or the depth of anesthesia can be increased, depending on the patient, the progress of surgery, and other factors. If one opts for a rather superficial depth of anesthesia, one might increase the analgesic component or take care that the patient is decply relaxed throughout surgery. There are highly complicated intellectual processes based on pharmacological, physiological, or surgical understanding

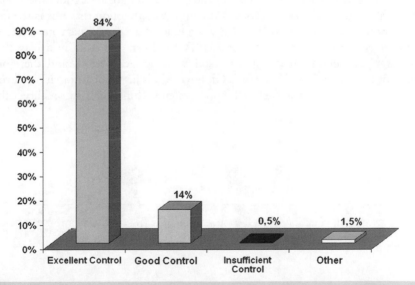

Fig. 2. Analgoscore. Closed-loop control of intraoperative analgesia during general anesthesia using remifentanil controlled by Analgoscore; the score ranges from -9 to +9. The range of -9 to -6 and +6 - +9 are considered as insufficient control; -6 to 3 and +3 - +6 are considered as good control, and -3 - +3 is considered as excellent pain control. The score is based on algorithms incorporating heart rate and mean arterial blood pressure. Results of pain control in percentages are presented for 16 patients undergoing surgery of a mean of 110 minutes, inflicting moderate pain.

and experience, which lead one to react in a certain way, combine different doses and drugs.

It seems logical, that for the future of integrated closed-loop systems, the use of artificial neural networks, which simulate the function of the central nervous system will become important. Future research has to focus on developing integrated closed-loop systems incorporating the experiences made in the development of the three separate components. These integrated systems then will harmonize perfectly with the concept of integrated anesthesia monitoring (Fig. 3).

Target controlled infusion systems

Target controlled infusion (TCI) uses pharmacokinetic algorithms included in a microprocessor to apply automatically intravenous anesthetics or analgesics for induction and maintenance of anesthesia. The first TCI was reported by Schuettler and Schwilden [28,29]; since then, many reports have been published, and TCI systems are commercially available in microprocessor infusion syringe pumps for propofol and remifentanil. In general, TCI works best with drugs that rapidly equilibrate between blood stream and brain; propofol and remifentanil are ideally suited for TCI administration. TCI functions using pharmacokinetic models and manual input, such as patient gender, age, or weight. It then calculates the infusion rates necessary for induction and maintenance of a given target concentration with the assumption that this is the target concentration achieved at steady state in the central nervous system. Supporters of this technique argue that TCI delivers the drug in a way that the target concentration maintains stability for longer period, and therefore depth of anesthesia is more stable. TCI, however, is far from automatic controlling in the same way closed-loop systems function. In reality, the

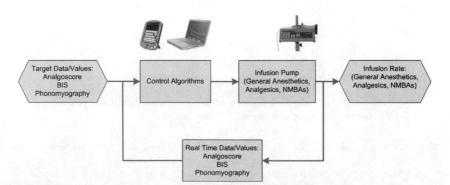

Fig. 3. Integrated closed-loop system for all three components of general anesthesia. Illustration of a closed-loop system integrating all three components of general anesthesia. Abbreviations: BIS, bispectral index; NMBA, neuromuscular blocking agents.

anesthesiologist adjusts frequently the chosen target according to the patient's needs, the progress of surgery, and other factors, such as degree of neuromuscular blockade or analgesic requirements. So far, these systems have not caught on in North America but are popular in Europe. There is no doubt that TCI–especially now with the addition of remifentanil TCI–is a good tool for research purposes. Drug interactions can be examined easily.

Several studies, however, have shown that TCI does not administer propofol in a more precise fashion than manually controlled infusions. In one double-blind, randomized study [30], propofol TCI was tested against manually controlled propofol application (MCI); only clinical parameters, such as heart rate, blood pressure, or other clinical signs were used to adjust TCI concentrations or manual infusion rates. There was no difference in absolute performance errors (BIS derivation from a target of 50) during maintenance of anesthesia with propofol TCI or MCI (23 plus or minus 11% versus 23 plus or minus 9%; $P = .97$). The two groups did not differ significantly in performance error, wobble, or divergence of hemodynamic changes. The authors concluded that TCI and MCI result in similar depth of anesthesia and hemodynamic stability when titrated against traditional clinical signs. Another study in neurosurgical patients [31] also failed to find significant differences in terms of hemodynamic stability or depth of anesthesia between propofol TCI and manually applied propofol TIVA when administered together with remifentanil. The costs for TCI were more than 50% higher than when MCI was used. Another study confirmed the higher costs of TCI versus manually administered propofol, mainly because of an increased amount of propofol infused over time [32]. Costs of TCI systems, however, will decrease with more generic systems being made available.

Though propofol TCI does not present a clear advantage over manually controlled propofol application in terms of hemodynamic or anesthetic stability, and creates still a significantly higher cost, remifentanil TCI has shown some promising results in reducing the remifentanil requirements and improving hemodynamic stability. This has been shown in a recent study in patients undergoing carotid surgery [33]: the study had a limited number of patients $(N = 46)$; the need for remifentanil requirements was almost half in the remifentanil TCI group than when remifentanil was applied manually. It is still too early to predict the usefulness of remifentanil TCI. More controlled studies need to be performed.

TCI systems are interesting tools; their clinical usefulness should be defined more in terms of decreasing the workload of the anesthesiologist than simply reducing drug requirements. More studies should focus on their impact on the time necessary to adjust infusion rates compared with manually administered drugs. Their major pitfall is the inability to automatically adjust the target concentration according to the progress of surgery or other drugs co-administered. A combined remifentanil-propofol TCI might be a useful alternative, based on combined pharmacokinetic models. Future research could use TCI systems as a basis for far more advanced closed-loop systems. At present, it seems that TCI infusion pumps are not very different from conventional infusion pumps.

Automatic anesthesia record keeping

Over 20% of the working hours of anesthesiologists are spent taking care of documentation. Interestingly, right from the start of anesthesia, keeping a patient's chart and record of anesthesia were part of the anesthetic duties. Most of the anesthesiologists in the 1920s kept a written record of what they were doing [34].

Obviously, record keeping helps to keep track of adverse events and documents what was going on during anesthesia; in addition, the mere writing down of anesthetic gestures and pharmacological interventions helps anesthesiologists to keep track of what they are doing and supports patient care. In the current age, automatic record keeping is available from most monitor manufacturers. Electronic record keeping might help in medico–legal cases, better document adverse events, and improve data interpretation simply by offering more time to do so.

Furthermore, automated record keeping might reduce the workload for the anesthesiologist; data will be recorded in greater detail, especially during times when the focus of attention is drawn toward direct patient care such as in vital emergencies or adverse events.

A recent study [35] describes best the current experience of most centers using automatic record keeping. The following account is the result of a 5-year experience of an electronic anesthesia record keeping system (DS 5300 OR, Fukuda Denshi, Tokyo), the first commercially available system combined with an anesthesia monitor in Japan:

> "Although keying in of text with a keyboard on the screen remains to be improved, the user interface of touch screens is easy to use. It seems to be a great advantage that physiologic variables are automatically and accurately captured very minute. The record is more complete, legible, and accurate than a hand-written record. Both long-term storage and search for the data are much easier. The investment in this system is affordable even for small hospitals."

Electronic record keeping in every anesthetic workplace is not a matter of "if" but simply a matter of "when". Computerized and automatic forms of data recording ultimately will affect billing processes [36] and make the anesthesiologist's daily life less bureaucratic or at least more efficient and precise (Fig. 4) [37].

Simulators in anesthesia

Since the introduction of simulator training into anesthetic residency programs, training based on repetitive and frequent exposure to patients and anesthetic situations has been replaced—especially in the early stages of the residency—by achieving goals and manual or intellectual competence facing simulated

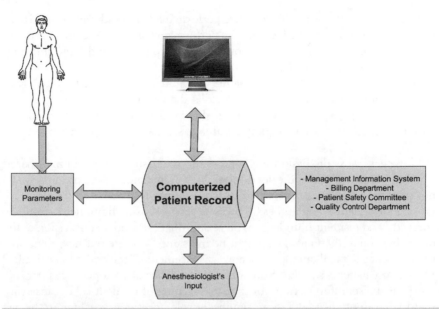

Fig. 4. Electronic anesthetic record keeping. Illustration of electronic anesthetic record keeping showing the possibilities for automatic billing, quality control and other possibilities.

situations [38]. In education as in other areas of anesthesia, technological developments have changed the way one operates. Currently, it is believed that in developed countries 70% to 80% of residents in anesthesia are at various stages of their career exposed to simulator training [39]. The high costs involved in acquiring the simulator, the training of the personnel, and the running costs remain important obstacles. As described for the development of new anesthetic monitors, aviation simulators were the model on which simulator training in anesthesia was based.

The first simulator was introduced in 1969 [40]. Most early simulators focused on pharmacological, anatomical, or physiological teaching and crisis interventions. More full-scale (called high-fidelity) simulators have been introduced into the practice of anesthesia education with the development of CASE (comprehensive anesthesia simulation environment) [41] and TOMS (team-oriented medical simulation) [42].

Most full-scale simulators teach pharmacological and physiological basics and simulate common intraoperative situations and problems. How efficient are these training sessions? Are they superior to conventional human-based training? Very few results are available. There is no doubt that simulator training is beneficial for train anesthesiologists to treat rare events, such as malignant hyperthermia or anaphylactic shock [43]. It is important to know that the feedback of people trained using simulators is generally positive [44,45]. There is equally no doubt that simulators—even very simple ones—can be used as an assessment tool to measure performance of anesthesiologists [46] as long as one is aware of the fact that the performance is related to the parameter that is examined; simulators do not measure experience and have difficulty measuring specific manual skills.

Some controversy still exists whether computer-based simulators are overall more efficient in teaching manual skills than real patient-related training. Recently, however, two studies have shown the supremacy of simulator-based training versus conventional training sessions in emergency medicine [47,48].

However, most discussion might miss the real issue; even if human based training results in the same level of skills as simulator-based training, have not patients possibly been exposed to harm during human-based training programs? If resident A undergoes 30 training sessions using dummies to intubate correctly and resident B undergoes 30 real intubations under supervision in the operating room, the final skills might be the same for both, but how many patients needed several attempts for correct placement of the endotracheal tube? How many patients suffered from a higher incidence of postoperative pharyngolaryngeal discomfort because of the real teaching of resident B? Because simulators have only played a more significant role in resident teaching in the last 10 to 15 years, long-term results comparing residents who underwent training with or without simulators are not available or are difficult to obtain. There is no doubt that simulators are useful tools in training rare complications and improve crisis management.

Full-scale simulators—the most advanced simulators presenting all sorts of scenarios using highly sophisticated mannequins (eg, SimMan or SimBaby [Laerdal Medical, Stavanger, Norway]) or the METI ECS or BabySim (Meti Incorporated, Sarasota, Florida)—are an important tool of teaching and evaluation of skills. However, even their limitations have to be addressed. A simulator is only as good as how real it represents the situation assessed. Constant improvements in software design and especially mannequin realism will further improve their utility. In addition, one has to counterbalance the focus of simulators on rare events and crisis management. One could imagine the following scenario for useful simulator training in an anesthetic teaching department: focus on basic pharmacology, physiology and common anesthetic scenarios in junior residents. The more residents advance in their training, the more specific and focused on rare events the simulator training should become. Staff anesthesiologists can use simulators to refresh their knowledge of basic pharmacology and physiology, equally focusing on rare complications and events, on intercommunicative skills and crisis management, or on organization talents. It is important that simulator training is adapted to the anesthesiologist's level of training and his or her specific needs. Otherwise, the importance of rare events is over-or underestimated.

There is no doubt that full-scale simulators will play an essential part in anesthetic teaching, practice, and performance evaluation, and the goal should be to equip every teaching center with at least one simulator [45].

Timmermann and colleagues [49] has summarized the potential of full-scale simulators as follows:

- Teaching in a secure environment
- Reproducibility of clinical scenarios
- Option for repetitive interruptions to focus on specific topics
- Focus on nontechnical skills, such as communication skills
- Possibility for debriefing by continuous recording
- Adaptability of skill level to skill grades
- Potential to save costs

Personal digital assistant—technological development and use in anesthesia

PDAs are used commonly in medicine in North America, with almost 40% of physicians using them for different purposes. Although some of us still use them mainly as electronic calendars, there are more sophisticated ways to make use of the improved technology. PDAs were introduced in 1986 with the first Palm Pilots being big, bulky and offering very limited power storage capacities. The exponentially fast developments in the IT sectors have produced PDAs that are almost as powerful as standard laptops; most experts predict that PDAs will replace portable computers with hybrid PDA–cell phones possibly replacing PDAs in the future. For anesthesia, PDAs offer software that includes general textbooks, such as Harrison's medical textbook, pharmacologically oriented compendiums, specific small programs, such as programs to aid with blood gas analysis, and even simple, low-fidelity simulation programs. In addition, PDAs present the latest scientific manuscripts and abstracts (eg, Avant Go, Hayward). Modern operating systems let one run almost any program on the PDA; therefore, statistical analysis, data management and other applications are all possible. PDAs can be used directly to perform presentations and lectures.

Whereas the aforementioned tasks are not different from every day use of PDAs, more focused applications are available in terms of billing management (eg, e/MD^2, Houston, Texas) or anesthetic record keeping; many academic centers are providing logbooks to their residents. New technological developments, such as Bluetooth technology, enable wireless connection and fast data transfer between the PDA and local networks; therefore, it creates rapid availability of medical charts and radiological or laboratory results. In the future, some diagnostic measurements will be aided using PDA technologies, such as electronic stethoscopes including automatic ECG interpretation or pulmonary diagnostics. The idea of transferring vital signs or basically all monitored parameters from the operating room to the anesthetic PDA is certainly technically feasible. More powerful PDAs will be the personal link of the anesthesiologist with everything concerning patient care, including medical charts, diagnostic results, connections with electronic anesthetic record keeping, billing, and operating room monitoring. This should lead to an increase in patient safety and higher efficiency of patient management. The near future should make the supervision and, if necessary, manual overriding of closed loop systems in the operating room possible by way of PDA.

SUMMARY
In the near future
Anesthetic monitoring
I believe that the near future will be a system of different monitoring entities; three monitoring subsets are thinkable. There is the subset of vital sign monitoring; this will include the monitoring of basic conventionally measured vital signs, such as heart rate, blood pressure, and pulse oximetry. More modern, less invasive methods will come into place for monitoring invasive blood pressure, such as pulse plethysmography or impedance measurements replacing intra-arterial pressure transducers. In addition, the more widespread introduction of less or non-invasive monitoring methods for cardiac output, pulmonary pressure (eg, ultrasound impedance), and their respective derivative parameters, such as systemic or pulmonary vascular resistance, will add these parameters to the conventional vital signs for almost all standard types of surgery. The less invasive but reliable the method, the more likely it will be to be included in standard monitoring. The inclusion of technologies, such as cerebral oximetry, into standard monitoring devices is just a question of price.

There will be rapid developments of sophisticated but cheaper monitoring devices, similar to developments seen in the car industry, where sophisticated systems, such as cruise control or automatic parking assistance, were reserved for expensive extra lists, but are now standard. Parameters that reflect the patient's metabolic state will be included; continuous blood glucose monitoring comes into mind.

A second subset will be reserved for patients undergoing general anesthesia necessitating ventilation. Ventilatory parameters, such as end-tidal CO_2, tidal frequency or volume, inspiratory pressure, and flow pressure loops will all be part of this second subset of monitoring parameters. In the near future, sophisticated, closed loop systems will control these parameters, automatically adjusting ventilatory settings. One could think of a closed-loop type of change of ventilation from volume control to pressure control according to flow pressure loops and sophisticated compliance or barotrauma calculations [50].

A third subset of parameters is focused on monitoring the actual state of general anesthesia; the three components of general anesthesia, loss of consciousness, analgesia and neuromuscular blockade are displayed here (BIS or equivalent methods, new parameters such as the Analgoscore, and maybe newer more clever forms of neuromuscular monitoring methods. The entity of neuromuscular monitoring is probably the most advanced of these parameters; more than one muscle may be monitored, and various methods are available [9,51].

One could imagine a sort of anesthetic cockpit of advanced monitoring and displaying system incorporating closed-loop systems for all anesthetic drug application and electronic record keeping (Fig. 5).

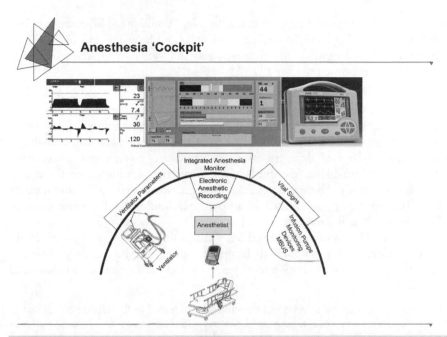

Fig. 5. The anesthesia cockpit. Model of an automated anesthesia workspace; ventilator parameters (*left*), parameters defining the state of general anesthesia (see Fig. 2: Integrated monitor of anesthesia; *middle*) and vital signs monitor (*right*). An additional monitor for electronic anesthetic record keeping and linkage to personal digital assistant device.

Monitoring at distance

Most physicians already heavily rely on PDAs. PDAs will be the constant link to the operating room. This will give us more flexibility and increase patient security. Whether wanted or not, economic forces seen in other areas of the daily life–constant reduction in manpower due to more sophisticated machines–will be a reality in anesthesia. There is a gap between anesthesia practice in North America, especially the United States, and the rest of the world, especially Europe; whereas the constant shortage of anesthesiologists in the United States has led to a system with nurse practitioners and one anesthesiologist often running more than one operating room, this is not the case in Europe. It is not so much a difference of technology–in general, European anesthesia is more technology orientated because of greater budgets–but a difference in availability of manpower–far greater in Europe–and their pay–less in Europe.

Carrying PDAs will increase the safety and contact to the patient. It is very possible that the use of PDAs carries the risk of overloading the anesthesiologist with multitasking; regulatory measures have to limit the amount of multitasking and define what distance is accepted in the interest of safe patient care. Would it be reasonable to be so far away from the operating room that the attending anesthesiologist is not available within minutes to handle life-threatening issues?

PDAs, however, can make life more flexible. Would it not be more comfortable if, when giving a talk to medical students about how exciting anesthesia is, the patient's vital signs, status of anesthesia, and ventilatory parameters were available in real time on your PDA?

Target-controlled infusion systems

TCI systems have been an important tool for researchers to investigate the effect of drugs to the body; modeling systems have increased our knowledge about the amount of drug necessary to achieve a given effect. Potentially, TCI systems can make anesthesia more focused, meaning more titrated to the patient's needs. There is a potential for increased patient safety, but it needs to be proven. Again, one is astonished by the technological difference between Europe and North America.

Whereas TCI systems are used very frequently in Europe and are established, especially for propofol to facilitate routine anesthesia, they have not entered the North American market yet. This has to do with two fundamental problems:

- Any technology or drug not developed and tested in the United States has to undergo vigorous testing and lengthy US Food and Drug Administration approval before it can enter the market.
- TCI systems are part of the concept of total intravenous anesthesia, a concept that has not gained widespread use in North America, (for reasons beyond the scope of this article).

The advancement of TCI systems is certain, TCI of propofol and remifentanil allowing a TCI-TIVA anesthesia. Overshooting and undershooting are very common with all TCI systems, making it necessary to frequently adjust the target site concentration; therefore, TCI systems are far away from the idea of automated anesthesia, in which the system, once initially programmed, runs on its own. It seems that the best approach would be to combine TCI systems—representing drug administration based on pharmacokinetics—with closed-loop systems that add the target parameter (eg, depth of anesthesia or analgesia) to the control process.

Several studies, have stressed the importance of pharmacokinetic–pharmacodynamic modeling to fully understand the pharmacological behavior and control of an anesthetic drug administered to the body [52–55]. However, they have mostly been applied to NMBDs [56,57].

Closed-loop systems

Closed-loop systems present the fascinating advantage of measuring a given parameter, feeding it into a microprocessor controlling system, and finishing the loop, driving the administration of a given drug without manual intervention.

It therefore carries the potential to significantly reduce the anesthesiologist's workload in an ever-increasing complex environment of multitasking and monitoring an increasing number of parameters. Despite a booming IT industry, closed-loop application of anesthetic drugs has been used mainly for research purposes. In contrast to TCI systems, there is no commercially available closed-loop system, not even for neuromuscular blockade. This is astonishing in a world where many daily activities are controlled by closed-loop systems, starting with in-room air conditioning. True, it is more complicated to apply propofol in closed-loop fashion to a patient guided by BIS monitoring than maintaining a given temperature in a room. The main problem with the wide-spread use of closed-loop systems has been the absence of reliable parameters or algorithms for analgesia monitoring in anesthesia. Another problem is that, compared with TCI systems, there is a more dramatic change of anesthetic technique. However, we might feel more comfortable with closed-loop systems than with TCI systems, because we know that the system constantly monitors the target parameter.

In the near future, one has to explore the safety, efficacy, reliability, robustness, and utility of closed-loop anesthesia to develop commercial systems ready to be implemented in daily practice.

The integration of pharmacokinetic programming and closed-loop pharmacodynamic control might lead to more reliable and precise devices.

Simulation and anesthesia

Simulators play an integral part of resident and staff training sessions in many universities and teaching facilities. Almost every aspect of our daily anesthetic life can be simulated; the choice of purchasing a given model of simulator will depend on budget, frequency of use and space. Recently, a classification system to distinguish different simulator types has been proposed [58]. Many residency programs have already implemented intensive training sessions for new residents before they deal with applying anesthesia to patients. It will be very interesting to measure the impact of simulators on the morbidity and mortality in anesthesia; one would expect a significant reduction of morbidity at least. Better trained residents will perform better when they first apply patients; in addition, simulator training provides a golden opportunity to familiarize residents and staff with computer based systems, discussed before: TCI systems, closed-loop systems can be learnt and tested using simulators – although more sophisticated simulators have to be developed.

Further down the road

Robotic anesthesia?

Some anesthesiologists have experience with performing anesthesia for robotic surgery, mainly cardiac surgery. Robotic cardiac surgery is a very complex procedural setup with the goal to semi-automate cardiac surgery. With this technology, the surgeon manipulates the surgical instruments using a computer. An endoscope and various surgical instruments are passed into the thorax using small holes. Instead of manipulating the surgical instruments directly, the surgeon manipulates them by means of a computer console. The computer interprets the surgeon's hand movements and causes the surgical instruments to respond accordingly. This system addresses the major disadvantages to moving the long surgical instruments manually. Computer control of the surgical instruments essentially eliminates the tremor effect and also the nonintuitive feel of maneuvering such instruments. This type of surgery, however, is essentially nothing else than a manual type of procedure where the computer simply assists the surgeon; its major use is to avoid opening the thorax with bigger access ports. Some gestures are aided and stabilized by means of computer control, but the robot cannot perform cardiac surgery on its own. Anesthesia for these procedures is usually—and probably anachronistically—more complex than for open heart surgery necessitating single-lung ventilation and attentive anesthesia, because conversion to open heart surgery can be necessary any time.

And still: what would it take to create the concept of robotic anesthesia?

There are two parts of anesthetic care that each anesthesiologist provides every day. One part includes achieving intravenous or endotracheal access to administer anesthetic drugs, establishing, if necessary, airway control for intermittent positive pressure ventilation and inserting catheters, if necessary, for invasive monitoring. On the other hand, we titrate anesthetic drugs according to the patient's state and surgical needs. For 80% of cases, no more interventions are needed.

Let us suppose that, in the near future, the titration of drugs is performed completely by a mixture of closed-loop pharmacokinetic systems automatically recording the necessary parameters, feeding them into an artificial brain (microprocessor), which then controls and administers the drugs accordingly and with more precision than we ever could.

What about the access route? How far can automation go? It seems to me that the rising use of ultrasound guidance when accessing peripheral or central veins is the first step towards the creation of robots that automatically insert a catheter into these vessels for monitoring—and probably with more precision than we are capable of. Does this sound too Orwellian? I believe not. Analogous to robotic cardiac surgery, initially, manual help might be necessary (eg, ultrasound placement), but ultimately, a robot could take over this task.

The completely automated anesthesia using computers, robots, and artificial brains might appear to some like pure science fiction; embracing technology as a friend who helps provide better care will lead science to meet fiction, very soon indeed.

Acknowledgments

The author wants to thank Nhien Le, Germain Aoun, and Samer Charabati from ITAG and NRG research groups, McGill University, Montreal, for their invaluable help in preparing the manuscript.

References

[1] Gueret G, Rossignol B, Kiss G, et al. Is muscle relaxant necessary for cardiac surgery? Anesth Analg 2004;99(5):1330–3 [table of contents].

[2] Michels P, Gravenstein D, Westenskow DR. An integrated graphic data display improves detection and identification of critical events during anesthesia. J Clin Monit 1997;13(4): 249–59.

[3] Blike GT, Surgenor SD, Whalen K. A graphical object display improves anesthesiologists' performance on a simulated diagnostic task. J Clin Monit Comput 1999;15(1):37–44.

[4] Gurushanthaiah K, Weinger MB, Englund CE. Visual display format affects the ability of anesthesiologists to detect acute physiologic changes. A laboratory study employing a clinical display simulator. Anesthesiology 1995;83(6):1184–93.

[5] Syroid ND, Agutter J, Drews FA, et al. Development and evaluation of a graphical anesthesia drug display. Anesthesiology 2002;96(3):565–75.

[6] Lowe A, Jones RW, Harrison MJ. The graphical presentation of decision support information in an intelligent anaesthesia monitor. Artif Intell Med 2001;22(2):173–91.

[7] Hart SG, Staveland LE. Development of NASA-TLX (Task Load Index): results of empirical and theoretical research. In: Hancock PA, Meshkati N, editors. Human mental workload. Amsterdam: North-Holland; 1988. p. 139–83.

[8] Eriksson LI. Evidence-based practice and neuromuscular monitoring: it's time for routine quantitative assessment. Anesthesiology 2003;98(5):1037–9.

[9] Hemmerling TM, Le N. Brief review: neuromuscular monitoring: an update for the clinician. Can J Anaesth 2007;54(1).58–72.

[10] Salhab E, Deschamps S, Matthieu P, et al. The Analgoscore: a new score for intraoperative pain used for feedback administration of remifentanil [26410]. Canadian Society of Anesthesiology 62nd Annual Meeting. Toronto (Canada), June 2, 2006.

[11] Beneken JE, Van der Aa JJ. Alarms and their limits in monitoring. J Clin Monit 1989;5(3): 205–10.

[12] Block FE Jr, Nuutinen L, Ballast B. Optimization of alarms: a study on alarm limits, alarm sounds, and false alarms, intended to reduce annoyance. J Clin Monit Comput 1999;15(2):75–83.

[13] Block FE Jr, Schaaf C. Auditory alarms during anesthesia monitoring with an integrated monitoring system. Int J Clin Monit Comput 1996;13(2):81–4.

[14] Edworthy J, Hellier E. Alarms and human behaviour: implications for medical alarms. Br J Anaesth 2006;97(1):12–7.

[15] Suzuki Y, Fujino Y, Ianioka Y, et al. Resection of the colon simultaneously with pancreaticoduodenectomy for tumors of the pancreas and periampullary region: short-term and long-term results. World J Surg 2004;28(10):1007–10.

[16] Morley A, Derrick J, Mainland P, et al. Closed-loop control of anaesthesia: an assessment of the bispectral index as the target of control. Anaesthesia 2000;55(10):953–9.

[17] Absalom AR, Kenny GN. Closed-loop control of propofol anaesthesia using bispectral index: performance assessment in patients receiving computer-controlled propofol and manually controlled remifentanil infusions for minor surgery. Br J Anaesth 2003;90(6):737–41.

[18] Absalom AR, Sutcliffe N, Kenny GN. Closed-loop control of anesthesia using bispectral index: performance assessment in patients undergoing major orthopedic surgery under combined general and regional anesthesia. Anesthesiology 2002;96(1):67–73.

[19] Mortier E, Struys M, De Smet T, et al. Closed-loop controlled administration of propofol using bispectral analysis. Anaesthesia 1998;53(8):749–54.

[20] Struys MM, De Smet T, Versichelen LF, et al. Comparison of closed-loop controlled administration of propofol using bispectral index as the controlled variable versus standard practice controlled administration. Anesthesiology 2001;95(1):6–17.

[21] Struys MM, De Smet T, Greenwald S, et al. Performance evaluation of two published closed-loop control systems using bispectral index monitoring: a simulation study. Anesthesiology 2004;100(3):640–7.

[22] Hemmerling TM, Schuettler J, Schwilden H. Desflurane reduces the effective therapeutic infusion rate (ETI) of cisatracurium more than isoflurane, sevoflurane, or propofol. Can J Anaesth 2001;48(6):532–7.

[23] Kansanaho M, Olkkola KT, Wierda JM. Dose–response and concentration–response relation of rocuronium infusion during propofol–nitrous oxide and isoflurane–nitrous oxide anaesthesia. Eur J Anaesthesiol 1997;14(5):488–94.

[24] Kansanaho M, Hynynen M, Olkkola KT. Model-driven closed-loop feedback infusion of atracurium and vecuronium during hypothermic cardiopulmonary bypass. J Cardiothorac Vasc Anesth 1997;11(1):58–61.

[25] Lendl M, Schwarz UH, Romeiser HJ, et al. Nonlinear model-based predictive control of nondepolarizing muscle relaxants using neural networks. J Clin Monit Comput 1999;15(5): 271–8.

[26] Pohl B, Hofmockel R, Simanski O, et al. [Feedback control of muscle relaxation with a varying on-off controller using cisatracurium]. Anaesthesist 2004;53(1):66–72 [in German].

[27] Gentilini A, Schaniel C, Morari M, et al. A new paradigm for the closed loop intraoperative administration of analgesics in humans. IEEE Trans Biomed Eng 2002;49(4): 289–99.

[28] Schuttler J, Schwilden H, Stoekel H. Pharmacokinetics as applied to total intravenous anaesthesia. Practical implications. Anaesthesia 1983;38(Suppl):53–6.

[29] Schuttler J, Stoeckel H, Schwilden H. Pharmacokinetic and pharmacodynamic modeling of propofol (Diprivan) in volunteers and surgical patients. Postgrad Med J 1985;61(Suppl 3): 53–4.

[30] Gale T, Leslie K, Kluger M. Propofol anaesthesia via target controlled infusion or manually controlled infusion: effects on the bispectral index as a measure of anaesthetic depth. Anaesth Intensive Care 2001;29(6):579–84.

[31] Weninger B, Czerner S, Steude U, et al. [Comparison between TCI-TIVA, manual TIVA and balanced anaesthesia for stereotactic biopsy of the brain]. Anasthesiol Intensivmed Notfallmed Schmerzther 2004;39(4):212–9 [in German].

[32] Lehmann A, Boldt J, Thaler E, et al. Bispectral index in patients with target-controlled or manually controlled infusion of propofol. Anesth Analg 2002;95(3):639–44 [table of contents].

[33] De Castro V, Godet G, Mencia G, et al. Target-controlled infusion for remifentanil in vascular patients improves hemodynamics and decreases remifentanil requirement. Anesth Analg 2003;96(1):33–8 [table of contents].

[34] Lumbard JE. The present status of anesthesia as a specialty. Am J Surg Q Suppl Anesth 1922;36:34–7.

[35] Nakamura I, Matsumura C, Niida H, et al. [Introduction of the electronic anesthesia record keeping system]. Masui 2002;51(3):307–13 [in Japanese].

[36] Reich DL, Kahn RA, Wax D, et al. Development of a module for point-of-care charge capture and submission using an anesthesia information management system. Anesthesiology 2006;105(1):179–86 [quiz 231–2].

[37] Abouleish AE, Conlay L. Automated anesthesia charge capture and submission: wave of the future, or bridge to nowhere? Anesthesiology 2006;105(1):5–7.

[38] Carraccio C, Wolfsthal SD, Englander R, et al. Shifting paradigms: from Flexner to competencies. Acad Med 2002;77(5):361–7.

[39] Morgan PJ, Cleave-Hogg D. A worldwide survey of the use of simulation in anesthesia. Can J Anaesth 2002;49(7):659–62.

[40] Chopra V. Anaesthesia simulators. Balliere's Clinical Anesthesiology 1996;10:297–315.

[41] Gaba DM, DeAnda A. A comprehensive anesthesia simulation environment: re-creating the operating room for research and training. Anesthesiology 1988;69(3):387–94.

[42] Helmreich RL, Schafer HG. Turning silk purses into sow's ears: human factors in medicine. In: Henseon LC, Lee AC, editors. Simulators in anesthesiology education. New York: Plenum Pres; 1998. p. 1–7.

[43] Chopra V, Gesink BJ, de Jong J, et al. Does training on an anaesthesia simulator lead to improvement in performance? Br J Anaesth 1994;73(3):293–7.

[44] Gordon JA, Wilkerson WM, Shaffer DW, et al. Practicing medicine without risk: students' and educators' responses to high-fidelity patient simulation. Acad Med 2001;76(5): 469–72.

[45] Timmermann A, Eich C, Russo SG, et al. [Teaching and simulation: methods, demands, evaluation, and visions]. Anaesthesist 2007;56(1):53–62 [in German].

[46] Byrne AJ, Jones JG. Responses to simulated anaesthetic emergencies by anaesthetists with different durations of clinical experience. Br J Anaesth 1997;78(5):553–6.

[47] Lee SK, Pardo M, Gaba D, et al. Trauma assessment training with a patient simulator: a prospective, randomized study. J Trauma 2003;55(4):651–7.

[48] Steadman RH, Coates WC, Huang YM, et al. Simulation-based training is superior to problem-based learning for the acquisition of critical assessment and management skills. Crit Care Med 2006;34(1):151–7.

[49] Timmermann A, Eich C, Nickel E, et al. [Simulation and airway management]. Anaesthesist 2005;54(6):582–7 [in German].

[50] Iotti GA, Braschi A. Closed-loop support of ventilatory workload: the P0.1 controller. Respir Care Clin N Am 2001;7(3):441–64, ix.

[51] Hemmerling TM, Donati F. Neuromuscular blockade at the larynx, the diaphragm, and the corrugator supercilii muscle: a review. Can J Anaesth 2003;50(8):779–94.

[52] Schiere S, Proost JH, Roggeveld J, et al. An interstitial compartment is necessary to link the pharmacokinetics and pharmacodynamics of mivacurium. Eur J Anaesthesiol 2004; 21(11):882–91.

[53] Kabbaj M, Vachon P, Varin F. Impact of peripheral elimination on the concentration–effect relationship of remifentanil in anaesthetized dogs. Br J Anaesth 2005;94(3):357–65.

[54] Wierda JM, Meretoja OA, Taivainen T, et al. Pharmacokinetics and pharmacokinetic–dynamic modeling of rocuronium in infants and children. Br J Anaesth 1997;78(6):690–5.

[55] Mandema JW, Danhof M. Electroencephalogram effect measures and relationships between pharmacokinetics and pharmacodynamics of centrally acting drugs. Clin Pharmacokinet 1992;23(3):191–215.

[56] Stadler KS, Schumacher PM, Hirter S, et al. Control of muscle relaxation during anesthesia: a novel approach for clinical routine. IEEE Trans Biomed Eng 2006;53(3):387–98.

[57] Kern SE, Johnson JO, Westenskow DR. Fuzzy logic for model adaptation of a pharmacokinetic-based closed-loop delivery system for pancuronium. Artif Intell Med 1997;11(1): 9–31.

[58] Cumin D, Merry AF. Simulators for use in anaesthesia. Anaesthesia 2007;62(2):151–62.

Advances in Anesthesia 25 (2007) 41–58

ELSEVIER
MOSBY

Advances in Transfusion Medicine

Debra Nordmeyer, MD, John E. Forestner, MD*, Michael H. Wall, MD

Department of Anesthesiology and Pain Management, University of Texas Southwestern Medical School, 5323 Harry Hines Blvd, Dallas, TX 75390-9068, USA

Transfusion medicine has developed as a specialty by linking rapidly evolving knowledge in areas of physiology and immunology to the vastly expanded clinical requirements for blood products resulting from advances in medicine and surgery. This article covers major developments in transfusion medicine related to anesthesiology and surgery. It will familiarize the anesthesia practitioner with evolving concepts in basic science as they relate to innovations in clinical care in three areas: (1) red cell transfusion, (2) other blood components, and (3) recently introduced massive transfusion protocols.

RED BLOOD CELL TRANSFUSION

Blood component therapy is a limited resource that contributes to overall health care expense. In the United States, four million patients will receive 12 million units of packed red blood cells this year. The estimated hospital cost for a unit of autologous blood ranges from $250 to $750. Actual costs of transfusion therapy, alternatives to transfusion therapy, complications associated with transfusion therapy, and complications associated with anemia are unknown [1].

The Transfusion Requirement in Critical Care trial has shown that a conservative strategy of red blood cell transfusion (transfusion for a hemoglobin of less than 7 g/dL) is as effective, if not superior to, a liberal transfusion strategy (transfusion for a hemoglobin less than 9 g/dL) in normovolemic critically ill patients [2]. Following a conservative transfusion strategy, institutions may decrease costs by limiting perioperative erythrocyte transfusions and their complications [2]. Erythrocytes compose an estimated 25 trillion of the 100 trillion cells that are found in the human body [3]. The major function of the erythrocyte is to transport hemoglobin, which in turn carries oxygen from the lungs to the tissues. Along with oxygen transporting capacity, hemoglobin acts as an acid–base buffer. The buffering capacity of hemoglobin provides about 70% of the buffering capacity of whole blood. Red blood cells also remove carbon dioxide from the body by using carbonic anhydrase, an enzyme that catalyzes

*Corresponding author. E-mail address: john.forestner@utsouthwestern.edu (J.E. Forestner).

0737-6146/07/$ – see front matter
doi:10.1016/j.aan.2007.07.005

the reaction between carbonic acid and water. This reaction allows the red blood cell to transport carbon dioxide from the tissues to the lungs for elimination [4].

Each red blood cell contains 270 million hemoglobin molecules. Each molecule of hemoglobin carries four heme groups, and each heme group can bind with one molecule of oxygen. Four separate oxygen molecules bind to one molecule of hemoglobin, and each gram of hemoglobin carries 1.38 L of oxygen.

The formula for the oxygen delivery capacity of blood is: $DO_2 = CO *$ CaO_2, where DO_2 is oxygen delivery; CO is cardiac output, and CaO_2 is the oxygen-carrying capacity of blood, and 10 changes volume % from O_2/dL to ml O_2/L.

Cardiac output (CO) is recognized as: $CO = HR * SV$, where HR is heart rate, and SV is stroke volume of the left ventricle.

CaO_2 is derived in the following way: $(1.38*hemoglobin* SaO_2)$ + $(0.0031*PaO_2)$, where SaO_2 is the percent of hemoglobin saturated with oxygen in the arterial circuit; 0.0031 is the coefficient for oxygen solubility in blood. This equation illustrates PaO_2 as a minimal part of oxygen delivery at sea level unless the hemoglobin or arterial blood saturation is decreased severely [5]. The purpose of erythrocyte transfusion is to maintain or increase the oxygen carrying capacity of blood. There is almost no indication to transfuse a hemoglobin level greater than 10 g/dL but there is almost always an indication for hemoglobin less than 6 g/dL. Preoperative hematocrit and estimated blood volume can be used to predict transfusion requirements intraoperatively. One unit of packed red blood cells will increase the hematocrit by approximately 3% and the hemoglobin 1 g/dL in the average adult [6]. Estimated total blood volume is about 65 cc/kg of blood for women and 75 cc/kg of blood for men. The estimated total blood volume then is multiplied by the percent hematocrit ($\times/100$), which gives the estimated red blood cell volume.

The estimated red blood cell volume at a hematocrit of 30 (previously used as a hematocrit target for patients with cardiac disease) is the estimated total blood volume multiplied by 30/100. Subtracting the estimated blood volume at a hematocrit of 30 from the blood volume at the normal hematocrit gives the volume of blood the patient can lose to reach a hematocrit of 30 and gives a baseline at which to consider blood transfusion.

For example, a 70 kg man has 70 kg * 75 cc/kg of blood volume = 5250 cc of blood volume. If his hematocrit is 45, then 45% of his blood volume will be erythrocytes. His blood volume of 5250 cc multiplied by .45 will yield 2362.5 cc of erythrocytes. Using 30 as the previously targeted hemoglobin, his blood volume of 5250 *.30 will be 1575. Using these numbers, he will need to lose 2362.5 − 1575 = 787.5 cc before his hematocrit decreases to 30.

Red blood cell transfusions are indicated in symptomatic anemic patients to restore oxygen-carrying capacity and delivery. Blood viscosity is determined primarily by erythrocyte concentration. In anemia, blood viscosity can decrease severely, which, in turn, decreases the resistance to blood flow in peripheral blood vessels. The decrease in peripheral resistance returns larger than normal quantities of blood from the tissues to the heart, which greatly increases cardiac output. Hypoxemia also results from the decreased transport of erythrocytes, which further decreases peripheral vascular resistance, allowing more blood return to the heart, further increasing CO and myocardial oxygen consumption. Not only does anemia decrease oxygen delivery, it also increases cardiac output, myocardial oxygen consumption, and possibly the risk of end organ ischemia [4].

The lowest limit of hemoglobin tolerated in people is not known, as critical limits for tissue oxygenation remain poorly defined [7]. Even with the detrimental effects of anemia, recent trials have indicated that transfusion is not necessarily the best treatment. Current opinion holds that a universal hemoglobin or hematocrit transfusion trigger is inappropriate for all patients or situations. Therefore, the historical transfusion triggers of hemoglobin of 10 and a hematocrit of 30 have fallen out of favor intraoperatively, postoperatively, and in ICU patients [2].

Blood loss should be replaced with crystalloid or colloid solutions to maintain normovolemia until the danger of anemia outweighs the risks of transfusion. Patients who have low hemoglobin levels before surgery are at higher risk of receiving allogeneic transfusion.

COMPATIBILITY TESTING

The ABO-Rh type, crossmatch, and antibody screen are compatibility tests. These tests were designed to demonstrate harmful antigen–antibody interactions in vitro so harmful in vivo interactions could be prevented [8]. Pretransfusion testing is performed to ensure ABO compatibility between the donor and the recipient. The ABO group remains the most important factor tested, because the most likely cause of death secondary to transfusion therapy is ABO incompatibility [9].

There are three common alleles present on the ABO locus on chromosome 9. ABO is based on inheritance of genes that encode for glycosyltransferases that add specific sugars to make an A or B antigen. The genes are codominant, so an individual inheriting both genes is designated as having AB blood type. Homozygous AA and heterozygous AO are both known as type A blood. The inheritance of O does not create a functional enzyme. Patients make antibodies to the antigens that they lack. Type O people lack A and B antigens on their red cells, so they will have anti-A and anti-B antibodies in their plasma. These naturally occurring antibodies occur in patients even with no prior blood exposure. The antibodies produced against ABO antigens are IgM and capable of causing intravascular hemolysis if incompatible blood is transfused.

In ABO testing, a sample of whole blood is centrifuged to separate red cells from serum. This process allows the red cells and serum to be tested separately and allows the type to be double-checked. The ABO group is determined by mixing the patient's red cells using anti-A and anti-B reagents and by reverse-typing the patient's serum against A and B reagent cells. If agglutination occurs with anti-A reagent, then the patient has type A blood. If agglutination occurs with anti-B reagent, then it is type B blood. If both cause agglutination, it is type AB, and if there is no agglutination, then it is type O blood. The patient's serum is screened for the presence of unexpected antibodies by incubating it with selected reagent red cells (screen cells) using an antihuman globulin (AHG) technique (indirect antiglobulin or Coombs test.) (Table 1).

The type and screen test looks only for the ABO-Rh type and screens for any unexpected antibodies. The Rh system has more than 40 red blood cell (RBC) antigens, but D, C, E, c, and e are the most significant of these antigens. Clinically, the D antigen is the most immunogenic RBC antigen and is known as the Rh factor. The antibody screen consists of detecting abnormal red blood cell antibodies to clinically significant antigens. There are more than 600 antigens, but only a fraction of these are noted to be clinically significant [9].

If the antibody screen is negative, and the patient has no past history of unexpected antibodies, it can be predicted that more than 99.99% of ABO-compatible red blood cell units would be compatible with an AHG crossmatch. If the antibody screen is positive (approximately 1% of patients), the unexpected antibody or antibodies must be identified before antigen negative-compatible RBCs can be found. This process usually takes several hours [10].

The type and cross includes the ABO-Rh type and antibody, screen but it also includes mixing donor red blood cells and recipient serum to inspect for any reactions. The crossmatch takes between 45 to 60 minutes and is characterized by three phases, immediate, incubation, and antiglobulin phases. The two most important phases are the incubation and antiglobulin phases, because the antibodies that appear in these phases can cause severe hemolytic reactions. Once donor blood is crossmatched with recipient blood, that blood is made unavailable to anyone other than the crossmatched recipient by the blood bank for up to 48 hours [8].

Emergent blood supplies should be ABO type O, as this is the least antibody-inducing type of blood. Donor blood used for emergency transfusion of group-specific blood must be screened for both hemolytic anti-A or anti-B antibodies. The Rh factor should be negative, but Rh factor positive blood can be used in men, and postmenopausal women with a small risk of reaction. Rh factor

Table 1
ABO compatibility testing

Blood group	Red cells tested with		Serum tested with	
	Anti-A	Anti-B	A cells	B cells
A	+	−	−	+
B	−	+	+	−
AB	+	+	−	−
O	−	−	+	+

Abbreviations: +, agglutination; −, no agglutination.
　　Reprinted from Miller R, Cucchiara R, Miller ED, editors. Miller's anesthesia. 6th edition. New York: Churchill Livingstone; 2002. p. 1801–2; with permission from Elsevier.

positive blood should not be used in premenopausal women because of the risk of transfusing Rh-positive blood into an Rh-negative female and causing erythroblastosis fetalis in subsequent pregnancies [8].

Table 2 summarizes donor blood groups that patients may safely receive.

RISKS ASSOCIATED WITH CONVENTIONAL RED BLOOD CELL TRANSFUSIONS

There are many complications associated with blood transfusion. Transfused blood has been shown to cause immunomodulation, systemic inflammatory response, occlusion of microvasculature, and an increased risk of postoperative low-output heart failure when transfusion occurs during coronary artery bypass surgery [11].

Allogeneic red blood cell transfusions can induce immunomodulation in the recipient of the transfusion. Allogeneic donor leukocytes appear to mediate significant immunomodulating effects. Leukocyte depletion may reduce the immunomodulation. Immunomodulation caused by transfusion can increase the incidence of postoperative infections and increase the risk of tumor recurrence in patients who have resected malignancies [12]. There is a dose–response relationship showing immunomodulation increases with the increasing number of allogeneic erythrocyte transfusions administered [13].

Immunomodulation can be beneficial for transplant patients. Allogeneic blood transfusions have been shown to improve allograft survival in renal transplants [14]. The mechanism of immunomodulation is suspected to be caused by up-regulation of humoral immunity and down-regulation of cell mediated immunity [15].

TRANSFUSION REACTIONS

Three types of allergic reactions to erythrocyte transfusions are mild, moderate, and anaphylaxis. If any of these transfusion reactions are noted, the transfusion should be stopped, and a new sample of blood should be sent for retype and cross.

A mild allergic reaction will cause focal urticaria that occurs in approximately 3% of patients. It is characterized by well-circumscribed, localized, erythematous, raised, urticarial lesions or hives, and is not associated with other symptoms.

Table 2
Donor blood groups that patients can receive

Donor	Recipient
O	O, A, B, AB
A	A, AB
B	B, AB
AB	AB

Reprinted from Miller R, Cucchiara R, Miller ED, editors. Miller's anesthesia. 6th edition. New York: Churchill Livingstone; 2002. p. 1801–3; with permission from Elsevier.

The transfusion should be held to administer antihistamines and resumed if the reaction stops. A moderate allergic reaction is seen clinically as a more widespread skin rash and a respiratory component, including bronchospasm or stridor. The transfusion should be stopped, and the patient may require steroids and vasopressors [9].

Anaphylaxis is the most severe systemic allergic reaction and is a medical emergency. It occurs in 1 in 20,000 to 47,000 blood transfusions. It has multiple organ system involvement. The symptoms generally begin with hives, dyspnea, flushing, wheezing, and they progress to coughing, stridor, and cardiovascular collapse. The transfusion must be stopped immediately, and the patient should be treated with epinephrine, diphenhydramine, histamine 2 receptor antagonist, steroids, and intravenous fluids [9].

The febrile nonhemolytic transfusion reaction is one of the most common causes of temperature change during blood transfusions. The temperature must change by more than 1°C or 2° F. This reaction can be accompanied by chills or anxiety, and it is seen most often in patients who have multiple transfusions and in multiparous women. Once fever is detected, the transfusion should be stopped, and the patient should be treated with antipyretics [16]. Once the temperature begins to decrease and the suspicion of septic transfusion reaction or acute hemolytic transfusion reaction is eliminated, the transfusion may be started again.

Bacterial contamination of transfused RBCs can cause sepsis in the transfusion recipient. The most common organism associated with contamination is *Yersinia enterocolitica* and other gram-negative organisms. Bacterial contamination of RBC units is related directly to the length of storage [17].

Contamination with gram-negative organisms is the result of occult asymptomatic transient donor bacteremia occurring during collection. The growth of the cryophilic bacteria *Yersinia, Serratia,* and *Pseudomonas* is enhanced by the refrigerated storage conditions of RBCs. Endotoxin produced by these organisms also can induce fulminant sepsis in the recipient. Septic transfusion reactions caused by gram-negative rods can be rapidly fatal, with a mortality rate of 60% [9]. It can evolve over several hours and go unrecognized. Clinically, a temperature increase of greater than 2 or 3°C, severe hypotension, hypertension, disseminated intravascular coagulation, and shock are seen. These signs and symptoms may be absent in a cold surgical patient or a patient who has a postoperative fever. If these symptoms occur, the transfusion should be stopped and a sample of blood sent for culture from the patient and from the donor unit. If there is a high suspicion, treatment should be initiated immediately without waiting for cultures. Broad-spectrum antibiotics, treatment for shock, acute renal failure (ARF), and disseminated intravascular coagulation (DIC) should be initiated immediately. Although restricting the use of antibiotics and particularly broad-spectrum antibiotics is important for limiting superinfection and for decreasing the development of antibiotic-resistant pathogens, patients who have severe sepsis warrant empirical therapy until the causative organ is identified [18].

The acute hemolytic transfusion reaction is a frequent cause of a fatal transfusion reaction caused by ABO incompatibility. The incidence is 1 per 250,000 to 1,000,000 transfusions [17]. Half of all deaths from acute hemolytic transfusion reactions are secondary to administrative errors. The severity of this reaction is related to the amount of blood transfused. If acute hemolytic transfusion reaction is suspected, the transfusion must be stopped and the untransfused blood returned to the blood bank along with a sample of the patient's blood for retyping and crossmatching. Supportive care should ensue.

Transfusion-related acute lung injury, more commonly known as TRALI, is an acute severe respiratory distress syndrome with an incidence of 1 per 5000 units transfused [18]. It usually occurs within 4 hours after transfusion and is characterized by the acute onset of dyspnea and hypoxemia, and it progresses to noncardiogenic pulmonary edema requiring mechanical ventilation and ICU treatment. The PaO_2 to FIO_2 ratio will be less than 300, the SpO_2 less than 90% on room air, and the chest radiograph will show bilateral pulmonary infiltrates.

Donor leukoagglutinins and donor antibodies to human leukocyte antigens (HLA), which react with the recipient leukocytes and monocytes, are hypothesized to cause TRALI. This reaction activates complement, which in turn leads to neutrophil aggregation and increased permeability of the pulmonary microcirculation. Multiparous female donors typically carry these leukoagglutinins [19].

Treatment of TRALI includes supportive measures, supplemental oxygen, tracheal intubation, mechanical ventilation, and positive end-expiratory pressure (PEEP) as indicated. The reaction usually resolves within 48 hours, and 90% of patients experience a complete recovery. Most cases resolve within 4 days of transfusion, but there is a high (5 in 100) incidence of fatal reaction. The incidence of pulmonary edema and acute respiratory distress syndrome (ARDS) is higher in patients who are transfused liberally [20].

DELAYED TRANSFUSION REACTIONS

Delayed transfusion reactions consist of viral contamination, delayed hemolytic transfusion reactions, and graft versus host disease (GVHD). Viral risks include HIV, hepatitis viruses A, B, and C (HAV, HBV, HCV), and human T-cell lymphotrophic virus types I and II. Some new viruses include hepatitis G virus, Torque teno (TT) virus, and human herpes virus 8 (associated with Kaposi's sarcoma) [21]. For HIV transmission, there is an incidence of 1 in 676,000; for HCV, the incidence is 1 in 103,000, and for HBV the incidence is 1 in 63,000. Along with multiple viruses, there is the risk of transmission of bacteria, parasites, and malaria. To date, malaria, Chagas disease, severe acute respiratory syndrome, and variant Creuzfeldt Jakob disease cannot be detected by screening tests [22].

GVHD is a rare complication resulting from foreign lymphocytes, and 90% of patients die. GVHD is T-lymphocyte mediated and usually occurs within

2 weeks of the transfusion. GBHD targets the host endothelium and bone marrow, which results in an aplastic anemia and pancytopenia. It usually is seen in immunosuppressed patients. The only known prevention of this reaction is radiograph or gamma radiation of the donor RBCs to inactivate all donor T cells [16].

METABOLIC COMPLICATIONS OF TRANSFUSIONS

Hyperkalemia, hypocalcemia, and acid-base alterations are the most commonly noted metabolic complications induced by blood transfusion. Hyperkalemia usually is seen in massive transfusions with increased red cell lysis or in renal failure. When red cells are stored, they leak potassium into their storage fluid, but leakage is corrected with transfusion and replenishment of cell energy stores.

Hypocalcemia can occur, because citrate binds calcium and is used as an anticoagulant in stored blood products. Rapidly transfusing RBCs may decrease the level of ionized calcium in the recipient. The liver should metabolize the citrate, but in clinical scenarios with impaired liver function, liver transplantation, or hypothermia, citrate metabolism may be decreased. Ionized calcium levels should be followed, because total serum calcium measures the citrate-bound calcium and may not reflect free serum calcium accurately.

Alterations in acid–base status occur, because stored blood is becomes more acidic secondary to the accumulation of RBC metabolites. The acid load is minimal when transfused. Alkalosis following a massive transfusion is common secondary to metabolism of citrate to bicarbonate by the liver [6].

ALTERNATIVES TO ALLOGENEIC BLOOD TRANSFUSION

Reasons to seek alternatives to allogeneic blood transfusions are numerous, including infectious risks, short supply, rare blood phenotypes, massive transfusion settings, and patient refusal of allogeneic blood transfusion. Blood conservation strategies include autologous blood transfusion, acute normovolemic hemodilution, and intraoperative blood recycling. Future options may include artificial oxygen carriers.

BLOOD CONSERVATION STRATEGIES

There are several ways to perform autologous blood donation. The techniques include acute normovolemic hemodilution, preoperative blood donation, and intraoperative blood salvage. When considering perioperative autologous blood donation, it is mandatory to carefully select patients to reduce the rate of discarded autologous units. Autologous blood donation is one of the simplest, most economical ways to decrease the amount of allogenic blood transfusion used [23].

Acute normovolemic hemodilution uses intraoperative venous drainage of one or more units of blood, with intraoperative storage of this blood. The blood removed is replaced milliliter for milliliter with colloid or 3 cc of crystalloid to 1 cc of blood removed. Blood replacement with dextran or hetastarch may result in coagulation defects. Crystalloid and colloid volume replacement also decreases the risk of anaphylaxis associated with dextran. The volume replacement allows the blood lost intraoperatively to have a lower hematocrit, with the idea that more dilute blood may be lost and then replaced with the more concentrated blood removed at the beginning of the case [24].

The amount of blood that can be removed during hemodilution is calculated using the formula V = EBV x Hi-Hf/Hav, where V is the volume of blood expected to be removed; EBV is estimated blood volume (TBW(kg) * 60 cc/kg (female) or 70 cc/kg (male). Hi is the patient's initial hematocrit level before onset of hemodilution; Hf is the desired hematocrit at the end of hemodilution, and Hav is the average hematocrit level during hemodilution (Hi + Hf/2) [21].

Acute normovolemic hemodilution is useful and cost-effective in procedures where expected estimated blood loss is greater than 1000 mL. It is less expensive than perioperative autologous blood donation, and it eliminates the risk of administrative errors that may occur anytime blood is banked.

PREOPERATIVE AUTOLOGOUS BLOOD DONATION

The ability of the patient to donate sufficient blood depends on his or her total blood volume and ability to regenerate red blood cells. Autologous blood donation is something that can be performed in patients who are stable before donation and are having elective surgery known to require transfusion. Criteria for self-donation as outlined by the American Association of Blood Banks includes a donor hemoglobin of greater than or equal to 11 g/dL, or a hematocrit of 33%. There is no age or weight requirement. The amount a patient can donate for him/herself is 10.5 mL/kg body weight. The limitation includes no donation at least 72 hours before the procedure to allow the patient to recover his or her intravascular volume status before surgery and to allow the blood bank to process the donated blood [25].

Poor candidates for autologous blood donation include patients with significant heart disease or those with preoperative anemia. Autologous blood donation is not recommended in patients who are to undergo procedures where the incidence of blood transfusion is low. Contraindications to autologous blood donation include: evidence of infection, risk of bacteremia, surgery to correct aortic stenosis, unstable angina, acute seizure disorder, myocardial ischemia or cerebrovascular accident within 6 months of donation, patients with cardiac or pulmonary disease who have not been cleared for surgery by their primary physician, high-grade left main coronary artery disease, cyanotic heart disease, or uncontrolled hypertension [26].

Another form of autologous blood donation is intraoperative blood salvage (cell saver), which includes the retrieval of blood from the surgical patient and return of that blood to the patient. A suction device used by the surgeon aspirates shed blood that is anticoagulated with citrate or heparin and returned to a disposable sterile centrifugal bowl. The collected blood then is washed with normal saline, concentrated to a hemoglobin of 50%, and returned to a second bag, which then is returned to the patient [27].

Cell salvage may cause a metabolic acidosis secondary to the loss of bicarbonate associated with a parallel increase in the chloride concentration (hyperchloremic acidosis), because the red blood cells recovered are washed with normal saline. Calcium and magnesium concentrations also may decrease with progressive cell salvage transfusions. The processed erythrocyte suspension never should be administered under pressure, as the bag contains air. If the bag is placed under pressure, the risk for venous air embolism is increased greatly, causing a potentially fatal complication. Because the washed blood is solely erythrocytes and may contain residual heparin, patients may develop a coagulopathy after a liter of transfused salvaged cells. RBC salvage should not be used in operations with nonsterile fields or during an oncologic surgery based on the risks of infusing bacteria or tumor cells into the patient [26].

Erythrocyte production is regulated by the secretion of erythropoietin by the kidney in response to renal hypoxia. If there are adequate supplies of folate, iron, and vitamin B12, erythropoietin will stimulate an increase in red cell production by marrow and an increase in oxygen-carrying capacity. Exogenous erythropoietin affects erythropoiesis in the same way. For elective postsurgical patients, erythropoietin will stimulate the rate of erythropoiesis to return RBC mass to a steady state. Exogenous erythropoietin will increase RBC mass in many anemic states and has been shown to do the same for preoperative surgical patients undergoing autologous blood transfusions. It has been demonstrated to decrease transfusion requirements in the postoperative period when patients are given erythropoietin preoperatively, provided there is iron available. It also can be given to anemic postoperative patients to increase the rate of recovery to normal hemoglobin levels. Perioperative erythropoietin is expensive but generally well tolerated, and with low doses costs may be comparable to preoperative autologous blood donation. This option increases the patient's red cell mass before surgery with exogenous erythropoietin. The efficacy of erythropoietin in reducing the volume of allogeneic blood transfused per patient and reducing the number of patients requiring transfusions is documented well in certain populations (renal insufficiency, anemia of chronic disease, refusal of transfusion) [1].

The combination of acute normovolemic hemodilution with preoperative erythropoietin has been found to be effective, because acute normovolemic hemodilution is more successful when there is a higher hemoglobin before beginning hemodilution. The use of recombinant human erythropoietin and/or iron therapy is effective for increasing RBC mass preoperatively.

Current research focuses on alternatives to blood transfusion, namely, blood substitutes. Blood substitutes are volume-expanding, oxygen-carrying solutions. The two types of blood substitutes in development are hemoglobin-based oxygen carriers and perfluorocarbon emulsions. Hemoglobin-based oxygen carriers have shown some promising results but must be modified in some way to prolong vascular retention, decrease renal toxicity, and decrease vasoconstriction. Perfluorocarbon emulsions can increase the amount of oxygen carried in blood, but their particulate nature can lead to adverse effects including thrombocytopenia and influenza-like symptoms [28].

TRANSFUSION OF NON–RED BLOOD CELL COMPONENTS
During elective surgery, replacement of blood loss up to half the blood volume (equivalent to five units of packed red blood cells to restore red cell mass to control levels) will not substantially affect hemostasis in most patients, and clotting functions, platelet counts, and clotting factor assays will not reach to abnormal levels. Numerous studies suggest that between 6 and 10 units of blood loss, replaced with packed RBCs and crystalloid solution only, a gradual prolongation of the prothrombin time (PT) and partial thromboplastin time (PTT) can be detected, before signs of microvascular bleeding indicate the onset of early coagulopathy [29]. Factor assays at this time in elective cases, somewhere around one blood volume lost and replaced, will reveal significant decreases in fibrinogen, which may contribute to the generalized ooze on the surgical field [30]. In elective cases with significant ongoing blood loss, platelets decrease to abnormal levels relatively late. In trauma cases, however, thrombocytopenia may occur more rapidly, sometimes at less than one blood volume, so that defects in primary hemostasis (quantitative platelet function) may be the cause of the earliest microvascular bleeding. Maintenance of body temperature with fluid warming and forced air heating may prevent physiologic depression of clotting factor and platelet function, but in patients losing blood, a threshold eventually will be reached where blood components will be required, in addition to packed red cells and buffered salt solutions, to reverse the trend toward coagulopathy.

Although the primary focus of this discussion is on slow blood loss in elective surgical patients, it should be noted that the onset of coagulopathy occurs consistently earlier in the trauma patient, and that many of these cases show laboratory and clinical signs of ongoing coagulopathy on arrival in the emergency room. Therefore, there is a growing preference in trauma care favoring early prophylaxis for coagulopathy from the first units of blood given to emergency patients who have continuing blood loss [31]. With heavy blood loss, whether the situation is elective or emergent, it appears easier to control coagulopathy with early blood component use, rather than to regain control when coagulopathy is present.

Blood components used in massive transfusion situations are fresh-frozen plasma (FFP), platelets, cryoprecipitate, recombinant factor VIIa, and prothrombin complex concentrate (descending order of frequency of use). Component indications, major complications, and methods for monitoring hemostasis are essential knowledge for the anesthesiologist for managing the bleeding patient.

PLASMA—FRESH-FROZEN PLASMA, FRESH-THAWED PLASMA
Plasma is removed from centrifuged units of blood and frozen for later use. It contains albumin, immune globulins, and clotting factors, some of which retain

much of their activity after thawing and transfusion. In some hospitals where large amounts of plasma are used, units are thawed in advance of request, so that warm thawed plasma is ready at all times for use, hence the use of the term fresh-thawed rather than fresh-frozen in some centers. Because the indications and usages for both FTP and FFP are identical, the two terms are used interchangeably in this discussion.

Most cases of early coagulopathy can be corrected by transfusion of FFP, usually in a volume of 10 to 15 cc/kg [29]. Because most of the citrate added to blood during donation is removed with the plasma during preparation of Adsol packed red cells, transfusion of plasma rapidly often results in hypocalcemia and transient hypotension. Rapid infusion of FFP should be considered an indication for small bolus doses of calcium chloride, 3 to 5 mg/kg, infused slowly to antagonize the citrate in the plasma. Slow infusion of plasma should not affect the serum calcium.

FFP provides excellent colloid volume support, and is similar to albumin in its ability to acutely support intravascular volume. It contains some active clotting factors, but fibrinogen supplementation from a single unit is limited, so that when fibrinogen levels are inadequate, cryoprecipitate would be preferred to FFP for correction. The amount of fresh-thawed plasma (FTP) required to normalize the prothrombin time in patients taking coumadin may produce fluid overload in patients at risk of congestive heart failure. Standard FTP therapy in this situation should be avoided in high-risk patients, and correction in emergencies should be managed with prothrombin complex concentrate.

The labile clotting factors, VIII, IX, and vWF (von Willebrand factor), already may have decreased in plasma during processing before freezing, so deficiency in these factors should be corrected with specific factor concentrates, or in mild cases, treated with desmopressin. Noncellular factors in FFP also may be responsible for TRALI, which has been reported following single-unit FFP transfusions.

During rapid exsanguination in trauma, FTP may be indicated from the beginning of fluid resuscitation for prophylaxis or therapy of coagulopathy. The amount of FTP recommended ranges from 0.4 to 1 units of FTP for every unit of packed red cells, with some evidence favoring the higher dose based on computer simulation studies [32]. Such early FFP therapy is supported by reported observation in many trauma units, but no class I evidence supports this from randomized clinical trials, which would be difficult if not impossible to perform in the emergency setting [33].

PLATELETS

Murray and colleagues [29] noted that the rare patient with coagulopathy that was not corrected by FFP usually would have microvascular bleeding controlled after infusion of platelets. A platelet concentration target of 100,000/mm^3 usually is considered the threshold for thrombocytopenia and associated quantitative deficiency in primary hemostasis, in patients with ongoing blood loss requiring replacement with blood components. A lower threshold for coagulopathy, of half this level, 50,000/mm^3, generally is considered appropriate for patients with more stable blood volumes who are assumed to be maintaining an equilibrium between platelet consumption and release from reservoirs in the reticuloendothelial system.

Platelets are supplied either in pooled packs separated from five or six units of whole blood during processing, or in apheresis units from single donors. A platelet pack from either source should increase the platelet count by $50,000/mm^3$ in a nonbleeding and nonconsuming patient. Thrombocytopenia can result from dilution or consumption, and in clinical practice, the treatment is usually the same. If disseminated intravascular coagulation is suspected, however, the determination and treatment of the inciting cause should be a major focus of therapy.

Platelet sepsis and TRALI have been the two leading causes of death from blood component therapy for the last decade. Although the incidence of platelet-related sepsis is very low, from bacterial growth in the platelet packs during storage at room temperature, the mortality risk is significant. Both TRALI and platelet sepsis account for 35 to 50 deaths each per year in the United States, more than the mortality from incompatible blood transfusion.

CRYOPRECIPITATE

Cryoprecipitate is fractionated from cooled and thawed plasma, and it is given in pooled units from 10 separate donors, thawed and prepared for each patient in the blood bank. There may be some delay in preparation, and cryoprecipitate is relatively expensive. It must be given immediately when received, because it expires 4 hours after preparation. In addition to large amounts of fibrinogen in each pool, significant factor VIII, XIII, and von Willebrand factor are preserved in the processing, and are active on infusion. Cryoprecipitate is the best replacement for fibrinogen deficiency complicating moderate-to-severe blood loss, and it is included in most massive transfusion protocols.

RECOMBINANT FACTOR VIIA

Recombinant FVIIa (NovoSeven, Novo Nordisk Pharmaceuticals, Princeton, New Jersey) works through several points on the coagulation cascade to produce a thrombin burst to promote coagulation. It replaces endogenous FVII, which is the earliest clotting factor affected by dilution in vivo, and which also decreases most rapidly in vitro during storage of blood or plasma. It is very expensive, with the price of a 4.8 mg dose over $4000. Use of NovoSeven in trauma is off-label, because the factor is only approved for use in hemophilia A or B with FVIII or FIX inhibitors. The procoagulant activity of NovoSeven is inhibited by acidosis, but not by hypothermia. It requires adequate amounts of substrate to function properly, so prothrombin and other clotting factors must be present before it will slow or control coagulopathic bleeding. Loading of FFP and possibly cryoprecipitate is encouraged before its use, to provide adequate procoagulant concentrations in the circulation.

Enthusiasm for its procoagulant actions has been decreased by recent reports of possible thrombotic complications, as reported in the press, but not currently documented in the medical literature in peer-reviewed publications [34]. As a result of anecdotal experience in several trauma centers, and the military experience in Iraq, use of Novoseven in initial care of bleeding trauma patients, which was being advocated until quite recently, has been stopped in many trauma centers, or has been restricted to a lower dose (2.4 mg dose) when used treating coagulopathy. If NovoSeven does promote thrombotic complications, whether dose restriction will prevent such problems has not been proven. Retrospective review of clinical experience in several medical centers, including the authors', has not confirmed any thrombotic complications in patients who have received FVIIa, although these are admittedly not carefully conducted prospective studies. Until the potential for thrombotic events following NovoSeven therapy is either confirmed or rejected, this expensive therapy is questionable in any dose range. The authors continue to use the high dose in their massive transfusion protocol for lack of any local evidence to substantiate complications associated with its use.

PROTHROMBIN COMPLEX CONCENTRATE

This new clotting factor preparation is derived from pooled plasma, and it includes very concentrated factor II, factor VII, factor IX, and factor X, all lipid-soluble factors that are decreased by the anticoagulant coumadin. It is used in reversal of coumadin effect with correction of the prothrombin time to normal, in clinical situations when rapid reversal of coumadin is needed such as emergent surgery or when internal bleeding in patients taking coumadin requires rapid control. Prothrombin complex concentrate (PCC) only recently has been supplied to transfusion medicine services, and experience with it has been limited. There are early indications that it occasionally may reverse coumadin inadequately, because the content of factor VII may be reduced during processing. When the prothrombin time does not return to normal following its use, a half dose of FVIIa (2.4 mg) may be administered intravenously to boost inadequate FVII activity in the PCC (Ravinder Sarode, MD, personal communication, 2007). A tendency toward arterial thrombosis in a very small percentage of patients (less than 10%) has been noted following PCC in some centers, but this has not been studied prospectively in a well-designed series, probably because the preparation is new and not widely used in any center at this time.

MASSIVE TRANSFUSION PROTOCOLS

As defined by the American Association of Blood Banks, massive transfusion is the replacement of one blood volume (10 units of blood) in any 24-hour period, or of one-half of the blood volume (five units of blood) in any 4-hour period. Hospitals with busy trauma services will treat injured patients whose transfusion needs exceed these limits on an almost daily basis. In addition, occasional elective surgery and other patients with coagulopathies also meet these simple criteria. Most patients needing massive transfusion support have blunt or penetrating trauma, and already will be rapidly exsanguinating because of their injuries on arrival at the emergency room. Such patients who are hypovolemic and hypotensive on arrival usually have received large volumes of crystalloid (balanced salt solution) during initial stabilization and transport, and they may need transfusion immediately.

The decision for immediate transfusion and volume replacement with packed red cells is based on assessment of vital signs and acid–base status as reflected in arterial blood gas determinations. Blood loss may result in anemia and coagulation abnormalities, but specific coagulation assays, even performed at the bedside, may take too long to perform to reflect rapidly changing conditions in the trauma patient. Such testing will serve to confirm the effects of ongoing therapy, rather than to guide future therapy in the acute situation. Coagulation factor therapy therefore is based on empiric assumptions related to estimated blood volume loss.

Under these circumstances, trauma services in North America and Europe have set up massive transfusion protocols, designed to support rapid transfusion with regular shipments of blood products released automatically on a timed basis. These products are organized in five-unit increments of packed red cells, with varied other blood products as typically needed at that level of blood loss. Once triggered by the request of the anesthesiologist or surgeon, the blood shipments would continue uninterrupted under the protocol until the bleeding was controlled or the patient expired.

The massive transfusion protocol (MTP) at Parkland Memorial Hospital has been operational for 2.5 years (Fig. 1). During the first 10 units of blood loss, the primary need is for volume support with packed RBCs and crystalloid. Levels of specific clotting factors are maintained, but FTP usually is given to support blood volume and to attempt to control coagulopathy in its early phases. Between 10 and 15 units of blood loss, platelet levels and fibrinogen levels decrease rapidly, and replacement with platelet packs and cryoprecipitate may be necessary to support coagulation. By roughly one blood volume of blood loss, factor VII and other procoagulants may be reaching marginal levels, and early use of high-dose NovoSeven (4.8 mg) is included in the protocol at that time.

Early experience with the protocol has shown that blood products can be provided at a maximum rate of 20 units of packed red blood cells (PRBCs) per hour, with the various other components given on schedule. Under most circumstances, it has been possible to maintain blood volume and arterial pressure satisfactorily using the blood products delivered automatically according to schedule, and most patients on the protocol are maintaining their clotting functions at near normal values until their transfer to the ICU.

Patient survival does not seem to be improving using the protocol. In a group of 100 consecutive patients meeting MTP criteria, prior to beginning the protocol and treated with blood products at the direction of the anesthesiologist and trauma surgeon, patient survival at 30 days was 50%. In the first two years

Shipment	RBC	TP	5PLT/APH	CR	rFVIIa
1a	5 (O-Neg)	2 (AB)			
1b	5	2			
2	5	2	1		
3	5	2		10	rFVIIa
4	5	2	1		
5	5	2			
6	5	2	1	10	
7	5	2			
8	5	2	1		
9	5	2		10	
10	5	2	1		

Fig. 1. The current Parkland Hospital massive transfusion protocol. Each shipment takes roughly 30 minutes to prepare, and shipments may be doubled during massive transfusion as needed, to a maximum delivery rate of 20 units of PRBCs per hour. *Abbreviations:* CR: cryoprecipitate, pooled 10-unit bag (in cooler);PLT/APH, platelet pool (five-pack) or apheresis single-donor unit equivalent to five pooled transported at room temperature; RBC, packed Adsol-1 or Adsol-5 red cells (in cooler); rFVIIa, recombinant factor VIIa (lyophilized powder with diluent); TP, thawed fresh plasma (in cooler).

of the protocol, 30-day survival each year remained in the 50% range, which was no better than the control group. The amount of PRBC units transfused, as a marker of the number of blood shipments sent out on the protocol, appears to be reduced by 25% compared with the total PRBC units used for the control group. It would appear that patients are clotting better and bleeding less, assuming a homogeneous trauma population over the past 5 years. NovoSeven was introduced into wider clinical use after the control group was studied, however, so the reduction in total blood products might be due partly or solely to the use of rFVIIa, rather than to the greater use of procoagulants on schedule in the MTP. The number of patients on the MTP each year is roughly the size of the control group, (around 100), and ongoing analysis of variables within the survivor and nonsurvivor groups may yield further information (Ravinder Sarode, MD, personal communication, January 2007).

The implementation of the MTP has produced a general improvement in the delivery of blood products to operating rooms for trauma resuscitation. Relieving the anesthesia and nursing personnel of continual worry about blood supplies during urgent trauma surgery has been of great benefit in the opinion of most involved staff. Outcome data to prove that the MTP is of benefit to the patients will be more difficult to produce, and benefit in terms of better clotting functions and improved survival may be several years away. Just the savings in blood products could be cited as an advantage, if further data analysis suggests that the roughly 25% decrease in blood product usage in massive transfusion using the protocol actually persists in the future data. It appears that the MTP has proven its worth in more convenience to medical and nursing personnel, even if patient benefit and cost savings are not entirely proven benefits at this time.

References

[1] Lankin PN, Hanson CW, Manaker S. The intensive care unit manual. Philadelphia: WB Saunders; 2001. p. 185.

[2] Hebert PC, Wells G, Blaichman MA, et al. A multicenter randomized controlled clinical trial of transfusion requirements in critical care. N Engl J Med 1999;340:409–17.

[3] Stoelting RK, Hillier SC. Pharmacology and physiology in anesthetic practice. 4th edition. Philadelphia: Lippincott Williams and Wilkins; 2006. p. 849.

[4] Guyton AC, Hall J. Textbook of medical physiology. 11th edition. Philadelphia: W.B. Saunders; 2006.

[5] Marino PI. The ICU book. 2nd edition. Philadelphia: JB Lippincott; 1998. p. 22.

[6] Morgan GE Jr, Mikhail MS, Murray MJ, editors. Clinical anesthesiology. 3rd edition. New York: McGraw-Hill; 2002. p. 632, 639.

[7] Spahn D, Casutt M. Eliminating blood transfusion; new aspects and perspectives. Anesthesiology 2000;93:242–4.

[8] Miller R, Cucchiara R, Miller ED, editors. Miller's anesthesia. 6th edition. New York: Churchill Livingstone; 2002. p. 1801–2.

[9] Speiss BD, Spence RK, Shander A, editors. Perioperative transfusion medicine. 2nd edition. Philadelphia: Lippincott Williams and Wilkins; 2006.

[10] Benson K, Chapin J, Despotis G, et al. Q & A about transfusion practice. 3rd edition. Park Ridge (IL): American Society of Anesthesiologists; 1997.

[11] Surgenor SD, DeFoe GR, Fillinger MP, et al. Intraoperative red blood cell transfusion during coronary artery bypass grafting increases low output heart failure. Circulation 2006;114(Suppl):I43–8.

[12] Varmvakas EC. Transfusion-associated cancer recurrent and postoperative infection: meta-analysis of randomized, controlled clinical trials. Transfusion 1996;36:175–86.

[13] Blumberg N, Heal JM. Immunomodulation in blood transfusion: an evolving scientific and clinical challenge. The science of medical care. Am J Med 1996;101:299–308.

[14] Opel G, Terasaki P. Improvement of kidney graft survival with increased number of transfusions. N Engl J Med 1978;299:799.

[15] Klein H. Immunomodulatory aspects of transfusion: a once and future risk? Anesthesiology 1999;91:861–5.

[16] Harmening DM. Modern blood banking and transfusion practices. 5th edition. Philadelphia: FA Davis; 2005. p. 340, 346.

[17] Goodnough LT, Brecher ME, Kanter MH, et al. Transfusion medicine, blood transfusion. N Engl J Med 1999;340:438–47.

[18] Dellinger RP, Carlet JM, Masur H, et al. Surviving sepsis campaign guidelines for management of severe sepsis and septic shock. Crit Care Med 2004;32:858–72.

[19] Murray M, Coursin D, Pearl R, et al. Critical care medicine: perioperative management. 2nd edition. Philadelphia: Lippincott Williams and Wilkins; 2002. p. 569.

[20] Wall M, Surgenor S. Concepts of transfusion triggers. American Society of Anesthesiologists Newsletter 2006;70:17.

[21] Monk T. Acute normovolemic hemodilution. Anesthesiol Clin North America 2005;23:271–81.

[22] Mungai M, Tegtmeier G, Chamberland M, et al. Transfusion transmitted malaria in the United States 1963–1999. N Engl J Med 2001;344:1973–8.

[23] Goodnough LT. Autologous blood donation. Anesthesiol Clin North America 2005;23:263–70.

[24] Jones S, Whitten C, Despotis G, et al. The influence of crystalloid and colloid replacement solutions in acute normovolemic hemodilution: a preliminary survey of hemodynamic markers. Anesth Analg 2003;96:363–8.

[25] Standards for blood banks and transfusion services. American Association of Blood Banks, AABB Bulletin; 2002.

[26] Goodnough LT, Shander A, Spence R. Bloodless medicine: clinical care without allogeneic blood transfusion. Transfusion 2003;43:668–73.

[27] Handin RI, Lux SE, Stoessel TP. Blood—principles and practice of hematology. 2nd edition. Philadelphia: Lippincott Williams and Wilkins; 2002. p. 2014–15.

[28] Winslow RM. Current status of blood substitute research: towards a new paradigm. J Intern Med 2003;253:508–17.

[29] Murray DJ, Pennell BJ, Weinstein SL, et al. Packed red cells in acute blood loss: dilutional coagulopathy as a cause of surgical bleeding. Anesth Analg 1995;80:336–42.

[30] Hiippala ST, Myllyla GJ, Bahtera EM. Hemostatic factors and replacement of major blood loss with plasma-poor red cell concentrates. Anesth Analg 1995;81:360–5.

[31] Ketchum L, Hess JR, Hiippala S. Indications for early fresh-frozen plasma, cryoprecipitate, and platelet transfusion in trauma. J Trauma 2006;60:S51–8.

[32] Hirshberg A, Dugas M, Banez EI, et al. Minimizing dilutional coagulopathy in exsanguinating hemorrhage: a computer simulation. J Trauma 2003;54:454–63.

[33] Malone DL, Hess JR, Fingerhut AF. Massive transfusion practices around the globe and a suggestion for a common massive transfusion protocol. J Trauma 2006;60:S91–6.

[34] Little R. Dangerous remedy. Military doctors in Iraq say that Factor VII saves wounded soldiers, but other doctors and medical research suggest that it can cause fatal clots. The Baltimore Sun. November 19, 2006.

Advances in Anesthesia 25 (2007) 59–77

ADVANCES IN ANESTHESIA

ELSEVIER
MOSBY

Perioperative Considerations for the Morbidly Obese Patient

Wanda M. Popescu, MD*, Jeffrey J. Schwartz, MD

Department of Anesthesiology, Yale University School of Medicine, 333 Cedar Street,
P.O. Box 208051, New Haven, CT 06520, USA

O besity is defined as an abnormally high percentage of body fat (greater than 20%). The most accepted measure of obesity is the body mass index (BMI), because it best correlates with the amount of adiposity and is easy to measure [1]. It is defined as the ratio of weight (in kilograms) over the height (in meters) squared (BMI = kg/m^2). Patients are considered overweight if the BMI is between 25 and 29.9, obese if the BMI is between 30 and 39.9, morbidly obese if the BMI is between 40 and 49.9 and super-morbidly obese if the BMI is 50 or greater [2].

EPIDEMIOLOGY AND PUBLIC HEALTH ISSUES

The prevalence of obesity has increased significantly over the past decades, causing this disease to be considered an epidemic. Worldwide, 1.1 billion people are overweight, and 312 million are considered obese [3]. Unfortunately, according to the International Obesity Task Force, an additional 155 million children currently are considered overweight or obese. In the United States, two thirds of the adult population is overweight or obese. It is currently estimated that 28% of men, 34% of women and 50% of African American women are obese [4].

The increasing rates of obesity have become a major health care problem and pose a significant financial burden on society. In developed countries, 2% to 7% of the health care costs are attributable to obesity alone [3]. In the United States, the current annual health care costs of obesity are approximately $70 to $100 billion [4].

It is well-established that extra body fat is associated with major comorbidities such as diabetes [5], hypertension [6], and cardiovascular disease [7], making obesity the sixth most important risk factor for disease worldwide [8]. Moreover, being obese is associated with a decrease in life expectancy. In a recently published large prospective study, Adams and colleagues [9] demonstrated a strong correlation between obesity and risk of death in both men and women. This association held valid even at moderate increases in BMI. The risk of premature death is doubled in the obese population, and the risk

*Corresponding author. E-mail address: wanda.popescu@yale.edu (W.M. Popescu).

0737-6146/07/$ – see front matter
doi:10.1016/j.aan.2007.07.004

of death because of cardiovascular disease is increased fivefold as compared with the nonobese.

PATHOPHYSIOLOGY OF OBESITY

The word *obese* derives from the Latin word for overeat. The main pathophysiologic mechanism for obesity development is an imbalance between caloric intake and energy expenditure of the body. This mechanism, however, is modulated by various genetic and environmental factors. The energy expenditure of the body is determined mainly by the basal metabolic rate (60%). It is defined as the energy required to maintain the integrated bodily functions. The rest of the energy expenditure is determined by the thermic effect of activity (20%), food digestion, absorption, and storage. Exercise not only increases the thermic effect but also raises the basal metabolic rate. Conversely, caloric restriction without exercise promotes a defense mechanism of the body and reduces energy expenditure, thus leading to a slow weight loss during the diet phase and a rapid weight gain while resuming normal caloric intake.

The difference between energy input (calories from food) and energy output (basal metabolic rate and physical activity) produces the caloric balance of the body. If the balance is negative, weight loss occurs. If the balance is positive, the extra energy is stored as body fat. The primary form of fat storage is composed of triglycerides. Because of their high caloric density and hydrophobic nature, triglycerides permit an efficient form of energy storage without significant adverse osmotic effects.

Triglycerides are stored in adipocytes. Initially, these cells increase in size until a maximum size is achieved. Subsequently the adipocytes start dividing. It is estimated that at moderate increases of BMI (up to 40), the adipocytes just increase in size, whereas in extreme forms of obesity, there is an absolute increase in the number of cells. There are two forms of fat distribution. Central fat around the abdomen is more common in men and is also known as android fat distribution. Peripheral fat around the hips, buttocks, and thighs is more common in females and is known as gynecoid fat distribution. The storage of triglycerides is regulated by lipoprotein lipase. The activity of this enzyme is different in various parts of the body, being more active in abdominal fat as opposed to hip fat. Therefore men tend to lose weight more rapidly than women.

The abdominal fat is metabolically more active then peripheral fat, leading to a higher incidence of metabolic disturbances associated with abdominal obesity [2]. It is accepted that a waist-to-hip ratio higher then 1.0 in men and 0.8 in women is a strong predictor of ischemic heart disease, stroke, diabetes, and death independent of total body fat [3].

At the cellular level, the main pathophysiologic disturbance of obesity is insulin resistance. The engorged adipocytes not only produce insulin resistance but also are considered one of the most prolific endocrine organs, secreting various cytokines such as interleukins 1 and 6 (IL-1, IL-6) and tumor necrosis factor (TNF-α). These cytokines depress the secretion of adiponectin, which is considered the most powerful insulin sensitizer, thus reducing insulin sensitivity of the tissues. Fatty infiltration of the pancreas decreases its capacity to secrete adequate amounts of insulin to withstand the high demand caused by insulin resistance [10]. In abdominal obesity, a high level of fat infiltration of the omental adipocytes (usually devoid of fat) is present. Thus, an increased influx of portal fatty acids, hormones, and cytokines is seen by the liver. In response, there is a higher production of very low density lipoprotein (VLDL) and increased secretion of insulin and pancreatic polypeptides generating gluco- and lipotoxicity [10].

Another suggested pathophysiologic mechanism of obesity is related to leptin. Leptin is secreted by the adipose tissue and acts centrally on the ventromedial hypothalamus by modulating the secretion of neuropeptides, which regulate energy expenditure and intake. Obese people have a central resistance to leptin [10]. Leptin also significantly activates monocytes, which contribute to the proinflammatory state of obesity. Neutrophils have a decreased capacity to migrate and activate. All these mechanisms create a vicious cycle that generates and promotes insulin resistance and a chronic inflammatory state [10].

COMORBIDITIES ASSOCIATED WITH OBESITY

Obesity is considered a multisystem disease with associated problems related to pressure, weight, and metabolic conditions. The systems most profoundly affected by obesity are endocrine, cardiovascular, respiratory, gastrointestinal (GI), immune, musculoskeletal, and nervous.

Many of the comorbidities related to obesity are linked in the metabolic syndrome (or syndrome X). It includes the cardiovascular, endocrine, and immunologic consequences of obesity. Many definitions have been given to this syndrome, but the currently most accepted one requires that three out of five manifestations be present: large waist circumference, high triglyceride levels, low high-density lipoprotein (HDL) cholesterol, glucose intolerance, and hypertension.

Endocrine system
Glucose intolerance and type II diabetes mellitus
Most obese patients manifest glucose intolerance. It is estimated that 90% of type II diabetes is attributable to excess weight [3]. This is consistent with the pathophysiologic mechanism of insulin resistance and resolves with weight loss. More then 75% of patients undergoing bariatric surgery experience complete resolution of their diabetes in the postoperative state [11].

Endocrinopathies causing obesity
Endocrine disease may promote the development of obesity. Hypothyroidism, hypercortisolism, and insulinoma are associated with obesity. It is important to recognize that the obese patient could be suffering from these diseases.

Cardiovascular system
Hypertension
The risk of developing hypertension is five times higher in the obese population [3], and it is estimated that two-thirds of hypertensive cases have weight

gain as a causative agent [11]. The mechanism of hypertension in obesity is multifactorial. Because of the increased body mass, obese people have a higher circulating blood volume and cardiac output, contributing to an increase in blood pressure. At the cellular level, adipocytes release angiotensinogen, which activates the renin–angiotensin pathway, leading to vasoconstriction and blood pressure increase [10]. Peripheral circulating cytokines produce damage and fibrosis of the arterial wall, thereby increasing the stiffness of the arteries. Hyperinsulinemia activates the sympathetic nervous system and promotes sodium retention and hypertension. Weight loss significantly improves or resolves hypertension. As a general rule, a decrease of 1% body weight will decrease systolic blood pressure by 1 mm Hg and diastolic blood pressure by 2 mm Hg. Most patients undergoing bariatric procedures experience complete resolution of hypertension [12].

Coronary artery disease and heart failure
Atherosclerotic cardiovascular disease is seen very commonly in the obese population. It is more common in patients who have central distribution of fat. Manifestation of dyslipidemia (high triglycerides and low HDL cholesterol), chronic inflammatory state, hypertension and diabetes, which usually are observed in the obese population, compound the risk for coronary artery disease. Myocardial infarction is a precursor of heart failure. Obesity alone, however, is an independent risk factor for heart failure [7]. A recent study suggests that the common link between these two entities appears to be insulin resistance [13]. The pathophysiologic mechanisms implicated in the development of heart failure in the obese population are multiple. Obesity induces structural and functional modifications of the heart dependent on hemodynamic overload. Chronic volume overload produced by increased blood volume causes left ventricular (LV) hypertrophy. Hypertension, usually associated with obesity, produces a pressure overload and also causes LV hypertrophy. The LV hypertrophy renders the ventricle stiff and causes LV diastolic dysfunction followed by LV systolic dysfunction. Vasan [14] has revealed possible mechanisms for the development of obesity cardiomyopathy. These mechanisms would include cardiac steatosis, lipoapoptosis, and activation of specific cardiac genes that promote LV remodeling and cardiomyopathy. It is estimated that 11% of cases of heart failure in men and 14% of cases in women are attributable to obesity alone. It is important to mention that these changes progress with increasing duration of obesity. It is implicit that the obese person has a decreased cardiac reserve and may respond poorly in situations that increase demand, such as hemodynamic stress or exercise. The usual way by which obese patients increase their cardiac output is by increasing heart rate and not stroke volume. When assuming a supine position, there is an increase in cardiac output, pulmonary capillary wedge pressure, pulmonary artery pressure associated with a decrease in systemic vascular resistance. All these hemodynamic changes should be considered when tailoring the anesthetic plan for the obese patient.

Immune and coagulation system alterations associated with obesity

Cottam and colleagues [15] studied the effects of obesity on the function of neutrophils. In the obese person, there is a decrease in adhesion molecules rendering the neutrophils unable to activate and migrate to sites of inflammation. Therefore, the obese patient has a higher rate of infection, especially in the perioperative period.

The depressed immune system increases the risk of certain cancers in obese patients. Breast, uterine, colon, and esophageal cancers are closely linked with obesity.

Thrombogenesis is an integral part of the inflammatory syndrome present in obese patients. The mechanism of increased thrombogenicity is multifactorial. Adipocytes produce excessive plasminogen activator inhibitor (PAI), and tissues have decreased capacity of synthesis of tissue plasminogen activator, thus decreasing fibrinolysis [2]. Other implicated mechanisms for hypercoagulability are related to the increased viscosity of blood present in obese patients, increased fibrinogen, an antithrombin-III deficiency, and a very sedentary life style. All these factors render the obese patient very susceptible to the development of deep vein thrombosis (DVT) and possible fatal pulmonary embolism (PE). This phenomenon is accentuated in the intraoperative and postoperative period.

Respiratory system

The respiratory system can be affected in obesity because of the extra amount of tissue present in the upper airway (obstructive sleep apnea [OSA]) and the extra weight present around the thorax and abdomen (extrinsic restrictive lung disease).

Obstructive sleep apnea, obesity hypoventilation syndrome, and right heart failure
Approximately 5% of obese patients have OSA, defined by periodic partial or complete airflow cessation for more then 10 seconds during sleep. The apneic episodes cause repetitive arousal from sleep to restore the patency of the upper airway [16]. Occasionally, patients who have OSA may experience episodic sleep-associated oxyhemoglobin desaturation, hypercarbia, and even cardiovascular disturbances. A more advanced form of disease is obesity hypoventilation syndrome. Patients who have this disease experience central apneic episodes (apnea without respiratory efforts). These manifestations reflect the desensitization of the respiratory centers to nocturnal hypercarbia. Pickwickian syndrome represents the most extreme form of OSA. It is characterized by a constellation of signs and symptoms such as: obesity, daytime hypersomnolence, arterial hypoxemia, hypercarbia, polycythemia, respiratory acidosis, subsequent pulmonary hypertension, and eventually development of right heart failure.

Even light sedation can produce complete airway collapse. Patients who have various degrees of OSA should be thoroughly evaluated preoperatively.

Restrictive lung disease of extrinsic etiology
Obesity imposes a restrictive ventilatory defect of extrinsic etiology caused by the increased weight added to the thoracic cage and the abdomen. The obese

patient has a decrease in functional residual capacity (FRC), expiratory reserve volume (ERV), total lung capacity (TLC), and lung compliance. At the same time, because of their increased body mass, obese patients have higher oxygen consumption and carbon dioxide production. In order to maintain normocapnia, they need a higher minute ventilation. As a result, obese patients breathe rapidly and shallowly. The FRC decreases with increasing BMI and may get to the point that small airway closure occurs during normal tidal ventilation, generating a ventilation-to-perfusion mismatch, right-to-left shunting, and arterial hypoxemia. Assumption of the supine position further decreases the FRC. These factors impair the ability of obese patients to withstand long periods of apnea such as during laryngoscopy. Many obese patients experience arterial desaturation during intubation despite adequate preoxygenation.

Gastrointestinal system
Nonalcoholic steatohepatitis
Nonalcoholic steatohepatitis (NASH) is related closely to obesity. Because of the increasing prevalence of obesity, NASH has become one of the most common causes of end-stage liver disease [10]. Obesity is associated with fatty liver infiltration. In more advanced cases, this benign disease progresses to cirrhosis, portal hypertension, and hepatocellular carcinoma. It is usually asymptomatic, but some patients may manifest with tiredness and abdominal discomfort. The liver function tests may be altered. These patients, however, are not at an increased risk of developing anesthetic-induced hepatitis.

Gallbladder disease
There is a significant association between gallbladder disease, mainly cholelithiasis, and obesity. This is probably because of the abnormal cholesterol metabolism, which causes a supersaturation of bile with cholesterol. Women who have a BMI of 32 kg/m^2 have a three times higher risk of gallstones, and at a BMI of 45 kg/m^2, women have seven times higher risk of gallstones. Paradoxically, rapid weight loss, especially after bariatric surgery, increases the risk of gallstones [10].

Gastroesophageal reflux disease
Obese patients have a higher incidence of gastroesophageal reflux disease (GERD). If they have no symptoms of GERD, however, it appears that the resistance gradients between the stomach and the esophagus are similar to the nonobese patients [17]. Although obese patients have higher gastric residual volumes, they do have a faster gastric emptying. Therefore, not all obese patients are at high risk of aspiration. This is very important to consider when deciding whether to perform a rapid-sequence induction on an obese patient.

Musculoskeletal system
Degenerative joint disease
Obesity leads to degenerative joint disease (DJD) not only because of the increased weight-bearing effects, but also because of some metabolic effects.

Common joints involved by DJD in obese patients are hips, knees, and carpo-metacarpal joints of the hands. As part of the metabolic syndrome, obesity also is associated with hyperuricemia and gout. Extra care should be given in positioning patients who have DJD in the operating room.

Nervous system
Obese patients, especially those with central fat distribution, have an increased risk of stroke. Many of these patients, especially those also affected by diabetes, may manifest symptoms of peripheral neuropathy. Extra care should be given in the operating room to padding the extremities susceptible to peripheral nerve injury.

TREATMENT OF OBESITY
Nonpharmacologic treatment
Most obese patients attempt to lose weight by dieting. Caloric restriction of 500 to 1000 kcal below their regular diet promotes weight loss. More severe caloric restriction induces a faster pace of weight loss, but the rate of long-term success is low. Adding exercise to diet minimally increases weight loss in the acute phase but appears to be the key to a higher success rate for long-term maintenance of reduced weight. Adding behavioral therapy to caloric restriction and exercise promotes a higher rate of weight loss. In order to maintain results, patients need to continue their life style alterations indefinitely. Unfortunately, in most of the cases, weight loss is not maintained over time without pharmacologic or surgical interventions [18].

Medical therapy
There are two types of medications approved in the United States for treating obesity: appetite suppressants and malabsorptive agents [19]. Appetite suppressants include mixed serotonin and norepinephrine reuptake inhibitors such as sibutramine. Typical adverse effects of this drug may include increased blood pressure and pulse. Sibutramine potentially adversely interacts with fentanyl and meperidine and produce increases in blood pressure [19]. Drugs that promote a malabsorptive state act by binding to lipases in the gut and preventing the hydrolysis of dietary fat into absorbable free fatty acids. The only approved drug is orlistat. Medications that increase energy expenditure and may contain ephedrine or Ephedra alkaloids fall into a third category. They are not approved by the US Food and Drug Administration but often are found in over-the-counter drugs and in herbal supplements. These medications should be discontinued preoperatively, as they may cause cardiovascular events such as severe hypertension, cardiac arrhythmias, myocardial infarction, stroke, and even death.

Surgical therapy
Currently bariatric surgery offers the best treatment to produce sustained weight loss in patients who are morbidly obese [20]. It also provides an improved life style and a decrease in the patient's comorbidities [12,21]. It is

the most cost-effective treatment modality for patients with BMI greater than 40 kg/m^2 or with BMI 35 kg/m^2 but with other significant comorbidities.

There are three types of bariatric surgeries available: malabsorptive, restrictive, and combined operations. The malabsorptive procedures include the jejunoileal bypass, the biliopancreatic bypass, and the duodenal switch. These procedures, by promoting malabsorption, induce not only weight loss but also have a high incidence of anemia, fat-soluble vitamin deficiencies, and severe protein–caloric malnutrition in the first postoperative year. Currently, they are less preferred surgical modalities. The gastric-restrictive operations include the stapled gastroplasty and gastric banding. Gastroplasty is currently out of favor because of poor weight loss maintenance. The most recent technique of gastric banding is using an inflatable band that surrounds the stomach and can be adjusted by injecting saline into a subcutaneous reservoir. It provides similar weight loss results to gastric bypass. The preferred bariatric surgery for morbid obesity is the Roux-en-Y gastric bypass, which combines gastric restriction with some degree of malabsorption [2]. This procedure can be performed with either an open or laparoscopic technique. From a surgical standpoint, the laparoscopic approach provides significantly better outcomes, including faster postoperative recovery, fewer wound infections and a lower incidence of postoperative hernias. From the anesthesiologist's perspective, however, this type of operation may produce significant hemodynamic and respiratory compromise, especially in the patients who have altered cardiovascular status.

ANESTHETIC MANAGEMENT
Preoperative evaluation
The preoperative evaluation of the morbidly obese patient should be very thorough and particularly focused on the cardio–respiratory status of the patient and airway evaluation. These patients appear to be healthier then they actually are. They usually have a sedentary lifestyle; therefore, they are unaware of symptoms that would be triggered by exercise. The evaluation should include medical record review, patient and family interview, physical examination, review of standard laboratory work, ECG, chest radiograph, and possible request of additional investigations such as sleep studies, stress test, transthoracic echocardiogram, and room air arterial blood gas analysis.

If the patient had previous surgeries or intubations, the review of the medical record should attempt to establish whether the airway management was facile and what the weight of the patient was at that time.

During the interview, the anesthesiologist should inquire about the presence of significant symptoms of GERD and symptoms of heart disease such as chest pain, shortness of breath at rest or with minimal exertion, palpitations and the position in which the patient sleeps. Symptoms of OSA such as the presence of snoring, apneic episodes during sleep, daytime somnolence, morning headaches, and frequent sleep arousals should be sought. If a diagnosis of severe OSA or obesity hypoventilation syndrome is suspected, further evaluation may be required. There are no data to support the preoperative institution of continuous positive airway pressure (CPAP) or bilevel positive airway pressure (BIPAP) to improve postoperative outcomes. In severe cases, however, the American Society of Anesthesiologists (ASA) Practice Guidelines for the Perioperative Management of Patients with Obstructive Sleep Apnea recommend that initiation of CPAP before surgery should be considered [16]. If CPAP is ineffective, noninvasive positive pressure ventilation (NIPPV) is an alternative [16]. If the patient is already on CPAP/BIPAP, then the patient should be advised to bring his or her mask on the day of surgery to continue the therapy in the postoperative period.

A detailed examination of the airway should note the presence of a large tongue, tonsillar size, Mallampati score, and, most importantly, the neck circumference at the level of the thyroid cartilage. Brodsky and colleagues [22] demonstrated that, in morbidly obese patients, neither absolute obesity nor BMI correlated with intubation difficulties. Increased neck circumference and high Mallampati score (3 or 4) were the only predictors of possible intubation problems. A neck circumference of 40 cm was associated with a 5% risk for difficulty intubating, whereas a neck circumference of 60 cm was associated with a 35% risk of difficulty with intubation [22]. There are various risk factors for difficulty of mask ventilation including a fat and round face, presence of facial hair, presence of excessive palatal and pharyngeal soft tissue, history of OSA, and absence of teeth. Any of these findings should be noted on the preoperative evaluation to alert the anesthesiologist about possible airway complication in the operating room. If, after evaluating the airway, the clinician feels that complications during airway management are likely, the possibility of an awake intubation should be explained to the patient.

Physical examination should attempt to reveal signs and symptoms suggestive of cardiac and respiratory disease. Signs of LV or right ventricular (RV) failure such as increased jugular venous pressure, extra heart sounds, pulmonary crackles, hepatomegaly, and peripheral edema may be very difficult to elicit in the morbidly obese population because of their body habitus. Symptoms of dyspnea at rest or extreme fatigue and syncope should be investigated further, as they may suggest significant pulmonary hypertension of severe heart failure.

ECG examination may demonstrate findings suggestive of RV hypertrophy (right axis deviation, peaked P waves in V_1, presence of right bundle branch block) or LV hypertrophy and possible myocardial ischemia. Various cardiac arrhythmias also may indicate cardiorespiratory dysfunction.

Chest radiographic examination may show signs of heart failure (increased vascular markings, Kerley lines), pulmonary hypertension, chronic obstructive pulmonary disease (hyperinflated lungs), or restrictive lung disease.

A transthoracic echocardiogram will evaluate LV and RV function and, if minimal tricuspid regurgitation is present, provide a noninvasive estimation of the systolic pulmonary artery pressure.

Although not always indicated, in severe cases of OSA, a room air arterial blood gas will provide useful information for intraoperative and postoperative ventilation management.

During the preoperative evaluation, the morbidly obese patient also should be evaluated for peripheral intravenous access. If this appears to be extremely difficult, then the patient should be told about the possibility of placing a central venous catheter while awake. Consideration should be given to the possibility of placing the central catheter preoperatively in the invasive radiology suite. At the same time, if the patient is considered to be at extremely high risk for DVT, then an inferior vena cava filter should be placed before surgery.

The patient should continue taking all his or her preoperative medications with the exception of oral anticoagulants, nonsteroidal anti-inflammatory drugs (NSAIDs), oral hypoglycemics, and possibly angiotensin-converting enzyme inhibitors. The patient should be counseled to take H_2 blockers (famotidine), nonparticulate antacids (sodium bicitrate) or proton pump inhibitors (omeprazole) on the morning of surgery to decrease the risk of aspiration pneumonitis. Wound infection is twice as common in obese patients when compared with their nonobese counterparts. Preoperative antibiotic administration decreases the incidence of postoperative infections and is of utmost importance. At the same time, morbidly obese patients are at high risk of developing a hypercoagulable state during the perioperative period [23]. Thus, preoperative administration of subcutaneous heparin (5000 U) is indicated to decrease the incidence of DVT and pulmonary embolism.

Intraoperative management
Positioning
Morbidly obese patients should be placed on specially designed tables that are able to hold up to 455 kg and have extra width to accommodate the larger girth. If these tables are not available, then two regular tables joined securely together are necessary [24]. Morbidly obese patients are prone to slipping off the operating room table; therefore, they should be well-strapped at the beginning of the procedure. The Hovermatt (HoverTech International, Bethlehem, Pennsylvania) is an air transfer mattress that is a lateral transfer and repositioning device designed to eliminate injury to staff while moving heavy patients.

There are various ways of positioning these patients on the tables. The most common approach is to place a ramp behind the patient's back in such way that the head is above the chest, and a horizontal plane is formed between the sternal notch and the external auditory meatus [25]. This position not only provides better ventilatory mechanics for the patient but also aligns the mouth with the glottic opening.

Extreme care should be given to padding all pressure points (elbows, heels). Morbidly obese patients are more susceptible to brachial plexus traction, and thus efforts should be made to place the arms in a neutral position. The upper roots of the brachial plexus can be stretched by extreme rotation of the head to the opposite side [26]. Various table positions required for surgery (eg, tilting table) may induce ischemic injuries and subsequent sciatic nerve palsy [24]. Upper and lower limbs, because of their increased weight, have a higher likelihood of sliding off the table, thus producing peripheral nerve injuries. A retrospective study by Warner and colleagues [27] documented a 29% association between ulnar neuropathy and obesity versus just 1% association in the control subjects. The arms are preferably kept out on arm boards, so their position can be monitored and to prevent excess pressure from tight draping.

Choice of anesthesia
If it is reasonable to perform the surgery under local or regional anesthesia (peripheral nerve or central neuraxial blocks), this is a preferred option as opposed to general anesthesia. Placement of peripheral nerve blocks aids in managing postoperative pain by reducing the amount of narcotics used.

Regional anesthesia. The ASA Practice Guidelines for the perioperative management of patients who have obstructive sleep apnea suggest that, whenever possible, local or regional anesthesia should be the method of choice for these patients, and general anesthesia should be used only when strictly necessary [16]. It is reasonable to extend these recommendations to all morbidly obese patients. Regional anesthesia (continuous nerve blocks or epidural catheters) provides an excellent adjutant method to decrease the use of opioids in the postoperative period.

It is accepted that performance of peripheral nerve blocks is more problematic in morbidly obese patients because of the lack of visible or palpable landmarks. Nielsen and colleagues [28] performed a study on 6920 patients of various BMIs, who received a total of 9038 peripheral nerve blocks. The authors demonstrated that, in patients who had BMIs higher than 30, the risk of failed blocks was 1.62 times higher than in patients with lower BMIs and that the obese patients had a higher likelihood of complications associated with regional anesthesia. The rate of successful blocks and satisfaction, however, remained fairly high in the obese population also. In the current era of regional anesthesia, the success rate may be improved significantly by performing peripheral nerve blocks under ultrasound guidance. This technique would also decrease the complications associated with block placement. Presently, there are no studies to document this fact.

Spinal and epidural anesthesia are also technically challenging in the obese patients. Fluoroscopy can be used to facilitate placement for practitioners familiar with the technique. Local anesthetic requirements may be 20% lower then in nonobese patients, presumably because of the fatty infiltration and venous engorgement of the epidural space. Thus, a prudent approach is to decrease the initial loading dose for epidural anesthesia.

General anesthesia. Because many issues can arise with induction of general anesthesia in the morbid obese population, the anesthesiologist should create a thorough plan before commencement of any procedures. As previously discussed, obese patients have a decreased FRC and higher oxygen consumption and, therefore, a lower tolerance to apnea as compared with nonobese patients. Adequate preoxygenation becomes an important safety asset for the patient. In a randomized controlled trial by Dixon and colleagues [29] preoxygenation of morbidly obese patients in a 25° head-up position achieved a 23% higher oxygen tension than supine patients, thereby allowing a clinically significant increase in the desaturation safety period. In a recently published, randomized controlled study, Gander and colleagues [30] demonstrated that, in morbidly obese patients, 5 minutes of preoxygenation by means of CPAP at a pressure of 10 cm H_2O followed by induction of anesthesia and mechanical ventilation by means of a mask with a positive end-expiratory pressure (PEEP) of 10 cm H_2O increased the nonhypoxic apnea duration by 50%.

Rapid sequence induction versus standard induction of anesthesia in the morbidly obese patients is still a topic of debate in the anesthesiology community. Before making the final decision, one should consider the risk/benefit ratio of rapid sequence induction to this specific population. Many anesthesiologists consider morbidly obese patients at higher risk for aspiration with subsequent increase in anesthesia-related morbidity and mortality. Certainly the obese population has multiple risk factors for pulmonary aspiration: higher gastric residual volume, lower pH of gastric contents, higher intra-abdominal pressure, higher incidence of GERD and diabetes as associated comorbidities. There are no studies to document that patients with high BMIs have an increased incidence of pulmonary aspiration, however. On the other hand, multiple studies have documented that obese patients have a shorter period of apnea time before desaturation occurs. At the same time, as illustrated in the preoperative evaluation section, morbidly obese patients can be at higher risk of the "cannot intubate, cannot ventilate" scenario [31,32]. It then becomes obvious that not all morbidly obese patients should be subjected to a rapid sequence induction routinely, as the risks of committing to early paralysis outweigh the safety of a controlled induction with airway patency testing before muscle relaxation. In order to decrease the risk of pulmonary aspiration, morbidly obese patients should be fasted adequately and premedicated with nonparticulate antacids, H_2 blockers, or proton pump inhibitors. A subset of the morbidly obese patients will be at high risk of aspiration: patients with debilitating symptoms of GERD, nonfasted, pregnant, and trauma patients. If, in these particular cases, the anesthesiologist has any concerns regarding management of the airway, the safest approach is the awake fiberoptic intubation.

Airway management is a challenging part in administering general anesthesia in the morbidly obese population. As previously stated, the airway should be evaluated carefully ahead of time. An emergency airway cart should be readily available when proceeding with induction of general anesthesia in these patients. A prospective study performed on a bariatric population by Frappier and colleagues [33] demonstrated that the intubating laryngeal mask airway (ILMA) had a 96.3% success rate of tracheal intubation. A more recent study by Combes and colleagues [34] compared the airway management quality with ILMA in morbidly obese and lean patients. The most important finding was that 100% of the morbidly obese patients were ventilated through the ILMA in less than 1 minute from insertion. The authors stated that the ILMA, with its dual function allowing both ventilation and intubation, might be the rescue airway device of choice in a "cannot intubate, cannot ventilate" scenario in obese patients. The awake fiberoptic intubation technique remains the safest airway management approach for a patient who has a potentially difficult airway. In certain supermorbidly obese patients, who have extremely limited pulmonary reserve and poor anatomic landmarks of the neck, the anesthesiologist should have a back-up ear-nose-throat surgeon immediately available who could perform emergency tracheostomy.

Mechanical ventilation of the lungs during general anesthesia should attempt to decrease the formation of atelectasis and offset the lower FRC. The use of large tidal volume ventilation can induce volutrauma with subsequent development of pulmonary edema. In a study by Bardoczky and colleagues [35], large tidal volume ventilation increased peak inspiratory and end-expiratory airway pressure and did not improve arterial oxygen tension. Application of PEEP 5 to 10 cm H_2O will improve the ventilation–perfusion mismatch in morbidly obese patients and will have little adverse effect on hemodynamics. No data are available as to which ventilatory mode is optimal for the morbidly obese patient. In certain situations, such as induction of pneumoperitoneum during laparoscopic surgery or steep Trendelenburg position, there is a decrease in the pulmonary compliance with an increase in peak and plateau airway pressures at constant tidal volumes and neuromuscular blockade. At this time, pressure-controlled ventilation with a change in the inspiratory-to-expiratory ratio may help limit the maximal airway pressure transmitted to the lungs. It should be emphasized that, during this ventilatory mode, tidal volumes should be monitored constantly, as they can decline acutely with factors increasing the airway pressure (inadequate muscle relaxation, bronchospasm, abrupt increase in insufflation pressure). At the end of the procedure, when spontaneous ventilation is resumed, application of pressure support ventilation with maintenance of PEEP is helpful in decreasing the incidence of postoperative atelectasis formation.

Any combination of drugs can be used for inducing and maintaining general anesthesia in morbidly obese patients. Some recent drugs, however, appear to have a better pharmacokinetic profile for these particular patients. The choice between the newer volatile anesthetics, sevoflurane and desflurane, has little impact on wake-up times if used judiciously. Arain and colleagues [36] concluded that there was no difference in emergence and recovery profiles in morbidly obese patients receiving sevoflurane or desflurane if the inhalational agents were titrated carefully. The use of intermediate-acting muscle relaxants titrated to twitch level is optimal in achieving good surgical exposure during the case and allowing the neuromuscular block to be reversed easily at the end of the procedure. Dexmedetomidine has excellent application for the anesthesia of morbidly obese patients. It is a highly selective α_2 adrenergic agonist and has sedating, analgesic, hypnotic, and sympatholytic effects without exhibiting respiratory depressive effects. Therefore, it can be used intraoperatively and in the postoperative period as an adjunct to pain management. A case report of a 433 kg patient with severe OSA and pulmonary hypertension undergoing gastric bypass described the use of dexmedetomidine in the anesthetic management [37]. The patient was given a loading dose (1.4 µg/kg for estimated lean body mass) over 10 minutes, which was followed by a continuous infusion of 0.7 µg/kg/h. The infusion was started in the operating room and maintained through the first postoperative day for pain control in addition to morphine given as patient-controlled analgesia. Usage of morphine increased threefold after the dexmedetomidine infusion was discontinued, implying that dexmedetomidine had a significant analgesic effect. For procedures with low postoperative pain profile (ie, craniotomies), remifentanil, a short-acting narcotic, may be an excellent alternative for the intraoperative management of morbidly obese patients. Remifentanil's effects terminate shortly after infusion is discontinued, allowing excellent intraoperative analgesia with minimal risk of opioid-induced postoperative respiratory depression.

The pharmacokinetics of some anesthetic drugs are different in morbidly obese patients. As a general rule, highly lipophilic drugs show a significant increase in volume of distribution in obese patients and should be dosed based on total body weight [38,39]. These drugs include benzodiazepines, barbiturates, succinylcholine, atracurium, cisatracurium, fentanyl, and sufentanil. Drugs that are more hydrophilic have less or no change in volume of distribution and should be dosed based on the ideal body weight of the patient. These drugs include propofol, vecuronium, and rocuronium. An exception to this rule is remifentanil, which is highly lipophilic but does not have a different volume of distribution and should be dosed based on ideal body weight [24].

Emergence of the morbidly obese patients from general anesthesia should be planned long before the procedure approaches an end. It is important to note that the airway of morbidly obese patients may not be the same at the beginning and at the end of the procedure and that reintubation in an emergency setting may prove to be more difficult then the original intubation. Therefore, neuromuscular blockade should be antagonized completely, and the patient should be fully awake, following commands, and showing adequate respiratory parameters. Spontaneous ventilation should be aided by pressure support ventilation with PEEP, or at least by CPAP until extubation time. The patient should be extubated in a semiupright position or a lateral position. If the patient is on CPAP or BIPAP at home, it is important to reinstitute these measures as soon as possible after extubation occurs. If the airway was considered difficult originally, it seems prudent to extubate the patient over a tube exchanger, which usually is tolerated very well, to facilitate reintubation if necessary.

Monitoring
As with all patients undergoing anesthesia, monitoring should be tailored to the type of surgery in conjunction with the general state of health of the patient, keeping in mind that, at times, morbidly obese patients can appear healthier then they actually are. Noninvasive measurement of the blood pressure should

be performed with adequately sized cuffs. The blood pressure cuff should encircle at least 75% of the circumference of the upper arm or, ideally, the entire arm [40]. If, because of the conical shape of the arm, blood pressure cuffs cannot be placed on the arm, accurate blood pressure readings can be obtained from the wrist [41] or ankle [42] with properly fitted cuffs. An alternative to noninvasive blood pressure cuffs is the Vasotrac (Medwave, St. Paul, Minnesota), a continuous noninvasive blood pressure monitor. If this is not available or does not fit properly on the obese wrist, then an intra-arterial catheter should be placed. Invasive monitoring of the blood pressure also is recommended in morbidly obese patients with decreased cardiopulmonary reserve. An intra-arterial catheter can also be used for arterial blood sampling to provide useful information about a patient's ventilation and oxygenation status. A special continuous blood gas-monitoring system can be inserted in the arterial catheter and provide continuous values of the PaO_2, $PaCO_2$, and pH. For the morbidly obese patients, placement of arterial catheters that are kink-resistant (Cook Pressure Monitoring Catheter, Cook, Critical Care, Bloomington, Indiana) is ideal [37].

Placement of triple lumen catheters or pulmonary artery catheters may serve the dual purpose of obtaining secure large bore intravenous access and providing information on the cardiovascular status of the patient. It must be appreciated that placement of such invasive monitors can be difficult in morbidly obese patients, as palpable landmarks are masked by fat depositions. In morbidly obese patients, ultrasound guidance used for obtaining central venous access may increase the success rate and decrease the complication rate associated with blind cannulation techniques [43].

Assessment of cardiac function and volume status during anesthesia and surgery may be obtained optimally by means of transesophageal echocardiography (TEE). Continuous TEE monitoring will allow immediate detections of alterations in cardiac function and will guide fluid management adequately. TEE monitoring, however, requires expensive equipment and trained personnel and is not readily available in all hospital settings.

In cases performed under local or regional anesthesia associated with moderate intravenous sedation, the ASA Practice Guidelines recommend that continuous capnography should be performed because of the increased risk of undetected airway obstruction in these and in all morbidly obese patients [16].

Fluid management
As with all other patients, the goal for fluid management in the morbidly obese is to maintain the patient euvolemic. Achieving this goal may be very difficult in the morbidly obese population. The routine rule for calculation of maintenance fluid requirements (4-2-1) does not seem reasonable in these patients. There is a strong association between morbid obesity and diastolic dysfunction. These patients will not be able to adequately handle large volume loads and may develop pulmonary edema. TEE and central venous pressure monitoring

may be useful in guiding optimal fluid replacement. During laparoscopic cases, decreased urinary output does not necessarily reflect a hypovolemic status. In such scenarios, liberal fluid administration for morbidly obese patients may have a negative impact on outcome. As previously mentioned, many of these patients exhibit diastolic dysfunction and poorly tolerate volume overload, which can manifest as intraoperative or postoperative pulmonary edema.

Postoperative management
Postoperative pain management
The main issue of postoperative pain management in morbidly obese patients is that use of opioids can induce significant sedation, respiratory depression with potential oxygen desaturation, airway collapse, and even respiratory arrest. Therefore, the approach of pain management in these patients should be multimodal [44]. All techniques known to decrease opioid use should be employed including: nonopioid analgesics, peripheral nerve blocks, and central neuraxial blocks.

Several nonopioid drugs may be useful in this respect. NSAIDs, α_2 receptor agonists, N-methyl-D-aspartate (NMDA) receptor antagonists and sodium channel blockers are various options that can be used in the postoperative period for pain management. Ketorolac has been used successfully to reduce pain in the postoperative period. Its main adverse effects are GI and increased operative site bleeding. The drug is not indicated for use in patients who have undergone bariatric surgery, as they are at especially high risk for development of GI bleeding. Clonidine, a less selective α_2 receptor agonist, was found to reduce opioid requirements if administered as a continuous infusion of 0.3 µg/kg/h [45]. The use of postoperative dexmedetomidine has been described previously. Ketamine has been shown to enhance the analgesic effects of morphine by inhibiting the opioid activation of NMDA receptors [46]. Given in small doses postoperatively, ketamine decreases pain sensation and increases wakefulness and oxygen saturation.

Regional anesthesia, including peripheral nerve blocks and central neuraxial blocks, can be performed also in the recovery room. If the morbidly obese patient requires large doses of narcotics for adequate pain control, then attempts to place peripheral nerve blocks or epidural catheters have salutary effects.

Respiratory and cardiovascular monitoring and management
Transport of the morbidly obese patient from the operating room to the postanesthesia care unit (PACU) should be performed with oxygen. In order to aid respiratory mechanics, the patient should not be positioned supine but rather in a semiupright position. During transport, a permanent verbal contact should be maintained with the patient to assess wakefulness and adequate respiratory effort. In the PACU, the patient should be placed on oxygen therapy and monitored with continuous pulse oximetry. Oxygen therapy can be discontinued when patients are able to maintain their baseline saturation on room air. Supplemental oxygen therapy can mask significant hypoventilation if only a pulse oximeter is used for monitoring. If the patient was on CPAP or BIPAP at

home, this ventilation mode should be resumed. If the patient has not been diagnosed with OSA preoperatively but experiences frequent airway obstruction and hypoxemic episodes in the recovery room, then these ventilatory modes can be initiated. Morbidly obese patients should be monitored constantly by a nurse in the first few postoperative hours. Any sign suggestive of respiratory fatigue or cardiovascular instability should be assessed and treated immediately. Morbidly obese patients may require reintubation, which is performed best in a controlled fashion rather then in an emergency situation.

Postoperative discharge setting
There are no strong data to suggest that postoperative placement of morbidly obese patients in ICU settings, with full monitoring, decreases morbidity and mortality. The ASA Practice Guidelines conclude that continuous oximetry reduces the likelihood of perioperative complications among patients at increased perioperative risk of airway obstruction [16]. Continuous pulse oximetry can be discontinued when the patient is able to maintain a room air oxygen saturation above 90% and does not require parenteral opioids for pain management. The same guidelines mention that there are insufficient data to offer support for physicians in deciding which patients with OSA can be managed safely on an outpatient as opposed to an inpatient basis. At the same time, it is difficult to estimate when it is safe to discharge patients. This decision should be made by the anesthesiologist, surgeon, and postoperative nurse involved in the care of the patient. It is considered safe to discharge the patient to an unmonitored setting (regular hospital bed or home) when he or she is no longer at risk for postoperative respiratory depression. As a general rule, adequacy of postoperative respiratory function can be made by observing the patient in an unstimulated environment, when he or she is asleep, to establish that he or she is able to maintain baseline oxygen saturation breathing room air.

References

[1] National Institute of Health Consensus Development Conference Panel. Gastrointestinal surgery for severe obesity. Ann Intern Med 1991;115:956–61.
[2] Levi D, Goodman ER, Patel M, et al. Critical care of the obese and bariatric surgical patient. Crit Care Clin 2003;19:11–32.
[3] Hossain P, Kawar B, El Nahas M. Obesity and diabetes in the developing world—a growing challenge. N Engl J Med 2007;356(3):213–5.
[4] Olshansky SJ, Passaro DJ, Hershow RC, et al. A potential decline in life expectancy in the United States in the 21st century. N Engl J Med 2005;352(11):1138–45.
[5] Chan JM, Rimm EB, Colditz GA, et al. Obesity, fat distribution, and weight gain as risk factors for clinical diabetes in men. Diabetes Care 1994;17:961–9.
[6] Stamler J. Epidemiologic findings on body mass and blood pressure in adults. Ann Epidemiol 1991;1:347–62.
[7] Kenchaiah S, Evans JC, Levy D, et al. Obesity and the risk of heart failure. N Engl J Med 2002;347(5):305–13.
[8] Ezzati M, Lopez AD, Rodgers A, et al. Comparative Risk Assessment Collaborating Group. Selected major risk factors and global and regional burden of disease. Lancet 2002;360: 1347–60.
[9] Adams KF, Schatzkin A, Harris TB, et al. Overweight, obesity, and mortality in a large prospective cohort of persons 50 to 71 years old. N Engl J Med 2006;355(8):763–78.

[10] Haslam DW, James WPT. Obesity. Lancet 2005;366:1197–209.

[11] Cassano PA, Segal MR, Vokonas PS, et al. Body fat distribution, blood pressure, and hypertension: a prospective cohort study of men in the normative aging study. Ann Epidemiol 1990;1:33–48.

[12] Buchwald H, Avidor Y, Braunwald E, et al. Bariatric surgery a systematic review and meta-analysis. JAMA 2004;292(14):1724–37.

[13] Di Bello V, Santini F, Di Cori A, et al. Obesity cardiomyopathy: is it a reality? An ultrasonic tissue characterization study. J Am Soc Echocardiogr 2006;19(8):1063–71.

[14] Vasan RS. Cardiac function and obesity. Heart 2003;89:1127–9.

[15] Cottam DR, Schaefer PA, Fahmy D, et al. The effect of obesity on neutrophil Fc receptors and adhesion molecules (CD16, CD 11b, CD62L). Obes Surg 2001;12:230–5.

[16] Practice guidelines for the perioperative management of patients with obstructive sleep apnea. A report of the American Society of Anesthesiologists Task Force on Perioperative Management of Patients with Obstructive Sleep Apnea. Anesthesiology 2006;104(5): 1081–93.

[17] Zacchi P, Mearin F, Humbert P, et al. Effect of obesity on gastroesophageal resistance to flow in man. Dig Dis Sci 1991;36:1473–80.

[18] National Task Force on the Prevention and Treatment of Obesity. Overweight, obesity, and health risks. Arch Intern Med 2000;160:898–904.

[19] Yanovski SZ, Yanovski JA. Drug therapy; obesity. N Engl J Med 2002;346(8):591–602.

[20] Brolin RE. Bariatric surgery and long-term control of morbid obesity. JAMA 2002;288(22): 2793–6.

[21] Sjöström L, Lindroos AK, Peltonen M, et al. Lifestyle, diabetes, and cardiovascular risk factors 10 years after bariatric surgery. N Engl J Med 2004;351(26):2683–93.

[22] Brodsky JB, Lemmens HJM, Brock-Utne JG, et al. Morbid obesity and tracheal intubation. Anesth Analg 2002;94:732–6.

[23] Blaszyk H, Wollan PC, Witkiewicz AK, et al. Death from pulmonary thromboembolism in severe obesity: lack of association with genetic and clinical risk factors. Virchows Arch 1999;434:529–32.

[24] Ogunnaike BO, Jones SB, Jones DB, et al. Anesthetic considerations for bariatric surgery. Anesth Analg 2002;95:1793–805.

[25] Brodsky JB, Lemmens HJM, Brock-Utne JG, et al. Anesthetic considerations for bariatric surgery: proper positioning is important for laryngoscopy. Anesth Analg 2003;96: 1841–2.

[26] Sawyer RJ, Richmond MN, Hickey JD, et al. Peripheral nerve injuries associated with anesthesia. Anaesthesia 2000;55:980–91.

[27] Warner MA, Warner ME, Martin JT. Ulnar neuropathy: incidence, outcome, and risk factors in sedated or anesthetized patients. Anesthesiology 1994;6:1332–40.

[28] Nielsen KC, Guller U, Steele SM, et al. Influence of obesity on surgical regional anesthesia in the ambulatory setting: an analysis of 9038 blocks. Anesthesiology 2005;102(1): 181–7.

[29] Dixon BJ, Dixon JB, Carden JR, et al. Preoxygenation is more effective in the 25° head-up position than in the supine position in severely obese patients. A randomized controlled study. Anesthesiology 2005;102(6):1110–5.

[30] Gander S, Frascarolo P, Suter M, et al. Positive end-expiratory pressure during induction of general anesthesia increases duration of nonhypoxic apnea in morbidly obese patients. Anesth Analg 2005;100:580–4.

[31] Langeron O, Masso E, Huraux C, et al. Prediction of difficult mask ventilation. Anesthesiology 2000;92:1229–36.

[32] Voyagis GS, Kyriakis KP, Dimitriou V, et al. Value of oropharyngeal Mallampati classification in predicting difficult laryngoscopy among obese patients. Eur J Anaesthesiol 1998;15:330–4.

[33] Frappier J, Guenoun T, Journois D, et al. Airway management using the intubating laryngeal mask airway for the morbidly obese patient. Anesth Analg 2003;96:1510–5.
[34] Combes X, Sauvat S, Leroux B, et al. Intubating laryngeal mask airway in morbidly obese patients and lean patients. A comparative study. Anesthesiology 2005;102(6):1106–9.
[35] Bardoczky GI, Yernault JC, Houben JJ, et al. Large tidal volume ventilation does not improve oxygenation in morbidly obese patients undergoing anesthesia. Anesth Analg 1995;81: 385–8.
[36] Arain SR, Barth CD, Shankar H. Choice of volatile anesthetic for the morbidly obese patient: sevoflurane or desflurane. J Clin Anesth 2005;17:413–9.
[37] Hofer R, Sprung J, Sarr MG, et al. Anesthesia for a patient with morbid obesity using dexmedetomidine without narcotics. Can J Anaesth 2005;52(2):176–80.
[38] Jung D, Mayersohn M, Perrier D, et al. Thiopental disposition in lean and obese patients undergoing surgery. Anesthesiology 1982;56:269–74.
[39] Blouin RA, Warren GW. Pharmacokinetic considerations in obesity. J Pharm Sci 1999;88: 1–7.
[40] Mann GV. The influence of obesity on health. N Engl J Med 1974;291:178–85, 226–32.
[41] Emerick DR. An evaluation of noninvasive blood pressure (NIBP) monitoring on the wrist: comparison with upper arm NIBP monitoring. Anaesth Intensive Care 2002;30:43–7.
[42] Block FE, Schulte GT. Ankle blood pressure measurement, an acceptable alternative to arm measurements. Int J Clin Monit Comput 1996;13:167–71.
[43] El-Solh A, Sikka P, Bozkanat E, et al. Morbid obesity in the medical ICU. Chest 2001;120: 1989–97.
[44] Ebert TJ, Shankar H, Haake RA. Perioperative considerations for patients with morbid obesity. Anesthesiol Clin 2006;24:621–36.
[45] Marinangeli F, Ciccozzi A, Donatelli F, et al. Clonidine for treatment of postoperative pain: a dose-finding study. Eur J Pain 2002;6:35–42.
[46] Reuben SS, Connelly NR. Postoperative analgesic effects of celecoxib or rofecoxib following spinal fusion surgery. Anesth Analg 2000;91:1221–5.

Advances in Anesthesia 25 (2007) 79–101

ADVANCES IN ANESTHESIA

ELSEVIER
MOSBY

Impact of Obesity in Pediatric Anesthesia

Carole Lin, MD

Department of Pediatric Anesthesia, Texas Children's Hospital, 6621 Fannin Street, Houston, TX 77030, USA

Pediatric obesity is a recognized global epidemic [1]. In the United States, the National Health and Nutrition Examination Survey data as of 2003 to 2004 showed that 17.1% of the pediatric population sampled were overweight [2–4]. Minority populations such as African Americans, Hispanics, Native Americans, and people of low socioeconomic status are populations with an even higher incidence of obesity, which may reach 30% or greater [5–10]. The data also indicate that the trend of increasing prevalence and severity of obesity is unlikely to be reversed.

Obesity is a systemic disease process that alters the physiology and psychology of the pediatric patient. Obese children are a special population requiring more planning, consultations, management, and time to successfully anticipate their anesthetic needs. These children are more likely to present for certain invasive procedures related to airway management, musculoskeletal correction, and even surgical intervention for obesity. Obese children have a higher risk for airway complications, anesthesia-related adverse events, and surgical complications [11–13].

DEFINING PEDIATRIC OBESITY

Pediatric obesity is underdiagnosed by pediatricians and anesthesiologists [14,15]. From the National Ambulatory Medical care Survey and National Hospital Ambulatory Medical Care Survey 1997 to 2000, Cook found that less than 1% of the pediatric population was diagnosed with obesity [16]. Very few patients who present for surgical procedures carry the preoperative diagnosis of overweight or obese. Even though it may be obvious to the anesthesiologist, it is necessary to diagnose obesity by standardized methods.

The standardized method for classifying obesity in adults is the BMI or body mass index. BMI is defined as weight in kilograms divided by body surface area in meters; it is expected to correlate with body fat and is used to quantify obesity. As of the year 2000, the World Health Organization and the National Institutes of Health used BMI to classify adults into the categories of overweight (BMI 25 to 29.9 kg/m^2), obese (BMI 30 to 39.9 kg/m^2), morbidly obese (BMI 40 to 49.9 kg/m^2) and superobese (BMI 50 kg/m^2 or greater) [17].

E-mail address: carolelin@mac.com

0737-6146/07/$ – see front matter
doi:10.1016/j.aan.2007.07.001

The classification of obesity is different for children. In pediatrics, BMI is affected by age, gender, and puberty [18–21]. To measure this moving target, the Centers for Disease Control and Prevention place BMI in the context of the peer population [22–24]. Obesity is defined in the relative terms of percentile ranking of the respective gender of the child (Figs. 1 and 2).

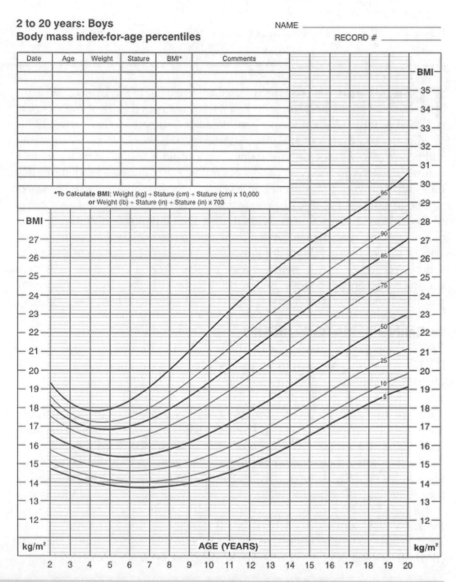

Fig. 1. Centers for Disease Control and Prevention growth curve: boys. (Developed by the National Center for Health Statistics, in collaboration with the National Center for Chronic Disease Prevention [2000]. Available at: http://cdc.gov/growthcharts.)

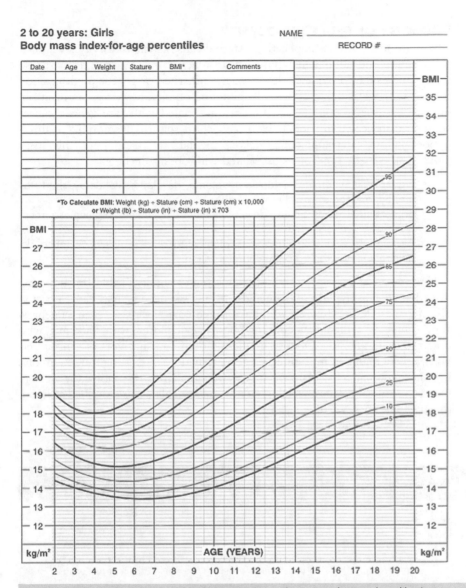

2 to 20 years: Girls
Body mass index-for-age percentiles

Fig. 2. Centers for Disease Control and Prevention growth curve: girls. (Developed by the National Center for Health Statistics, in collaboration with the National Center for Chronic Disease Prevention [2000]. Available at: http://cdc.gov/growthcharts.)

Children of 2 years to 20 years old are considered at risk for obesity if they are represented at the 80th to 95th percentile of their peers, and overweight if they are equal or greater than 95th percent of the population in BMI [23,24]. There are no standardized definitions to define superobese children yet.

ETIOLOGY OF PEDIATRIC OBESITY

There are many studies implicating external causes such as activity level, diet, social status, education, and exposure as risk factors for obesity. There are also many studies that provide evidence for the inherited or genetic predisposition of obesity. Less than 5 to 10% of all childhood obesity, however, can be attributed to a suspect etiology [25]. Obesity associated with rare genetic causes should be suspected in patients who have short stature, dysmorphic features, hypogonadism, developmental delay, mental retardation, or hirsutism [24,27,28]. Genetic syndromes associated with obesity include:

- Prader-Willi Syndrome—infantile hypotonia, developmental delay, short stature, hypogonadism psychological disturbance
- Bardet-Beidel—short stature, developmental delay, retinitis pigmentosa, renal disease
- Alstrom—nerve deafness, diabetes, pigmentary renal insufficiency, retinal degeneration, cataracts, no mental retardation

Various specific diseases predispose children to obesity (Table 1). Endocrine disorders such as hypothyroidism and Cushing's syndrome may cause obesity. Obesity is a risk for children who have psychological diseases such as depression. There is a high incidence of obesity in children with leukemia who undergo chemotherapy. Obesity frequently occurs in survivors of central nervous system injury from trauma, surgery, radiation, or existing tumors involving the hypothalamus. Damage to the hypothalamus disrupting the normal neuro–hormonal balance, which regulates energy balance, is described as hypothalamic obesity [27–30].

Table 1
Diseases associated with obesity

System	Disorder	Description
Hypothalamic obesity	Head injury	Neurological deficit hyperinsulinemia
	Central nervous system malignancy/radiation/surgery	Neurological deficit, hyperinsulinemia
Endocrine	Cushing's syndrome	Hypertension, stria hypercortisolemia
	Hypothyroidism	Constipation, lethargy, myxedema
	Growth hormone deficiency	Short stature
Cancer	Postchemotherapy	Acute lymphblastic leukemia
Psychological	Depression/anxiety	Low self-esteem, eating disorders
	Physical/sexual abuse	Low self-esteem, eating disorders

PHYSIOLOGY OF PEDIATRIC OBESITY

Pediatric obesity is a multiorgan affecting disease process. The evidence is that obese pediatric patients become obese adult patients who are more likely to suffer from the obesity-related diseases such as hypertension, hypercholesterolemia, hypertriglyceridemia, atherosclerosis, and diabetes [26,31]. The close association of obesity to these diseases has led to the definitions such as metabolic syndrome, insulin resistance syndrome, syndrome X, and the deadly quartet (upperbody obesity, glucose intolerance, hypertriglyceridemia, hypertension) [32–50]. The various obesity-described syndromes noted in the literature include:

- Metabolic syndrome—obesity, dyslipidemia, elevated blood pressure, impaired glucose tolerance, prothrombotic state, proinflammatory state
- Insulin resistance syndrome—obesity, dyslipidemia, hypertension, type 2 diabetes
- Syndrome X—central obesity, hyperinsulinemia, hyperuricemia, hypertriglyceridemia, increased risk for coronary heart disease (CHD) and stroke
- Deadly quartet—upper-body obesity, hypertension, hypertriglyceridemia, hyperinsulinemia

From the third National Health and Nutrition Examination Survey, 1988 to 1994, the prevalence of metabolic syndrome among 12- to 19-year-old children in the United States was found to be 4.2% overall. In overweight adolescents in the United States, metabolic syndrome was found to be present in 30% to 50% [35]. Unless weight loss occurs, obesity-related morbidity continues to increase as the patient ages and gains weight. Obesity-related morbidity among the pediatric population is significant and often unrecognized (Table 2) [27,28,30].

Respiratory

Obesity produces changes in the pediatric airway. The increase in fat tissues in the pharynx, tongue, and around the larynx causes anatomical narrowing of the airways. These changes increase the likelihood of an obstructed airway and the development of obstructive sleep apnea syndrome (OSAS) [51,52]. OSAS is the disease process that results from nocturnal airway obstruction, and it is highly associated with obesity [53]. Pediatric obesity is the strongest predictor of OSAS and may be present in 17% these patients [54]. It is defined as a disorder of chronic intermittent obstruction and apnea-patterned breathing during sleep. Besides apnea episodes, pediatric OSAS also has partially obstructed airway breathing that is characterized by nocturnal hypercapnea and hypoxia [55]. Polysomnography is the definitive test to determine if snoring is coupled with OSAS. Few children have a preoperative polysomnography, and parents may not be attentive to a pattern of noisy breathing, snoring, or apnea. Practice guidelines for the identification and risk assessment of pediatric OSAS have been published [56]. Clinical indicators of OSAS include: BMI greater than 95th percentile for age, increased neck circumference, snoring, congenital airway abnormalities, observed apnea, daytime hypersomnolence, inability to visualize the soft palate, and tonsillar hypertrophy. These guidelines

Table 2
Systemic disease processes in the obese pediatric population

Organ system	Specific	Description
Neurologic	Pseudotumor cerebri	Headache, vomiting, visual changes, field deficits
Pulmonary	Upper airway obstruction/ obstructive sleep apnea	Sleep disturbance, chronic tiredness, orthopnea, enuresis, learning/ developmental delay
	Asthma	Possible increased incidence, severity, occult exercise-induced asthma
Cardiovascular	Cardiomyopathy of obesity	Dyspnea on activity, left ventricular (LV) hypertrophy, decreased cardiac compliance
	Hypertension	Proteinuria, LV enlargement
	Dyslipidemia	Elevated cholesterol, triglycerides, low high-density lipoprotein cholesterol
Orthopedic	Slipped capital femoral epiphysis	Hip and knee pain, abnormal gait
	Blount disease	Tibia vara, knee pain
Gastrointestinal	Nonalcoholic fatty liver disease	Elevated transaminases, enlarged liver, liver fibrosis/cirrhosis
	Gastrointestinal reflux	Abdominal discomfort, vomiting
Endocrine	Type 2 diabetes mellitus	Elevated glucose, polyuria, polydipsia, ketoacidosis; associated infections and poor healing, acanthosis nigrans
	Polycystic ovary syndrome	Irregular menses, hirsutism, acanthosis nigrans
Psychological	Depression	Depression, poor school performance, suicidal, increased pain sensitization
	Anxiety	Anxiety, difficulty cooperating with procedures
	Poor self-esteem	Decreased activity, difficulty cooperating with procedures, low motivation

suggest that if the child has two or more positive clinical indicators for obstructive sleep apnea, then the likelihood of the presence of OSAS is high.

Respiratory physiology also is changed by obesity and may be reflected in pulmonary function tests. The weight of the fat tissue on the thorax and in the abdomen increases oxygen demand and the work of breathing. Abnormal pulmonary function tests are a common finding in adults and physiologically are similar to restrictive lung disease [57,58]. Chaussain and colleagues [59] studied pulmonary function tests on obese children who were 25% to 105% above their peers and found that in contrast to adults, most parameters (vital capacity, residual volumes, blood gases, CO_2 diffusion, dynamic lung compliance, and total resistances of the lung) were normal, while mainly the CO_2 ventilatory response was blunted. Inselma and colleagues [60] studied pulmonary function tests for children at 147% to 300% above ideal body weight with the conclusion that obese children have abnormal pulmonary tests. Decreases in expiratory reserve volume, forced expiratory volume in 1 second (FEV1), FEV 25% to 75%, diffusing capacity for carbon monoxide, and ventilatory muscle endurance were noted. Most studies involving children of moderate obesity have shown minimal abnormalities in pulmonary function tests. In contrast, children who have severe and morbid obesity have shown considerable alterations in pulmonary function tests. Ray and colleagues [61] have generalized these findings. An abnormal pulmonary function test value should be considered as caused by intrinsic lung disease and not by obesity, except in those with extreme obesity.

Extreme obesity combined with the pathology of OSAS and diminished pulmonary function can produce obesity hypoventilation syndrome (OHS), also known as Pickwickian syndrome. The source of the syndrome's name is the author Charles Dickens from his novel *Pickwick Papers*. He described a "fat and red-faced boy in a state of somnolency." By means of complex and incompletely understood mechanisms, chronic OSAS increases in severity to a state of diminished ventilatory drive, which results in hypoventilation, hypercapnea, and hypoxia [62]. Clinical OHS presents with similar findings as OSAS but with the addition of shortness of breath caused by elevated blood CO_2 pressure, dusky or cyanotic skin secondary to hypoxemia, and flushed face caused by polycythemia. Children who have OHS also may behave abnormally because of a declining mental state from chronic hypoxemia. This state can lead to pulmonary hypertension, cor pulmonale, and even congestive heart failure. These children need extensive preoperative workup and preparation before surgery.

Respiratory infections may occur with more frequency in obese infants and children [63,64]. The association between asthma and obesity is less certain, with multiple studies showing both a positive correlation and no correlation between the severity of obesity and the incidence of asthma.

Cardiac

The foundation for adult coronary artery disease, atherosclerosis, hypertension, congestive heart failure and other vascular and cardiac problems is laid during an obese childhood [65]. Cardiovascular disease is linked to obesity and diabetes [66–70]. Central or truncal weight pattern distribution of fat is more associated with these changes [71]. Hypertension is more frequent in obese children than normal-weight peers [72,73]. Hypertriglyceridemia and low levels of high-density lipoprotein (HDL) cholesterol are also present in obese children [70,71]. Obesity is a risk factor for left ventricular (LV) hypertrophy [74–76]. Significant LV hypertrophy may be present in up to 41% of obese children who have hypertension [67] and also may precede the development of hypertension [77]. Oxygen demand and cardiac output are higher. Most of these changes are occult, and it is very rare to have a severely obese pediatric patient decompensate from cardiac ischemia caused by myocardial infarction.

Diabetes

Obesity is a major risk factor for insulin resistance and diabetes mellitus type 2 independent of the other risk factors such as genetics [78]. Obesity disrupts the homeostasis of insulin sensitivity and secretion. Total body fat and visceral body fat both contribute to decreased insulin sensitivity and increased fasting insulin levels. Diabetes is characterized by high serum glucose despite a hyperinsulinemic state [66]. In 2002, 4% of screened symptomatic obese adolescents presented with type 2 diabetes mellitus. Up to 25% of this population also presented with impaired glucose tolerance [79]. Currently, the incidence is likely increased; the rise in the diagnosis of diabetes mellitus type 2 in children parallels the rise in pediatric obesity [80]. The preoperative history of polyuria, polydipsia, headaches, fatigue, acanthosis nigrans, candidal vulvovaginitis, and even recent weight loss are suspicious for diabetes [81]. Acanthosis nigricans, the hyperpigmentation of the skin under the arms, on the neck, or in the groin, is an obvious physical clinical symptom of hyperinsulinemia. In an obese child, the presence of acanthosis nigricans is a high-risk indicator for the presence of metabolic syndrome [82]. For obese children who are presenting for surgery in a state of acute illness and stress, ketoacidosis or hyperglycemic hyperosmolar nonketotic syndrome (HHNS) or coma may complicate intraoperative and postoperative management.

Hepatic

The presence of nonalcoholic fatty liver disease (NAFLD) in obese children often is underdiagnosed [15]. By international studies, sonographic evidence of hepatic steatosis is found in 2.6 % to 77% of studied obese children [81,83,84]. In the United States, 6% of overweight and 10% of obese children had elevated liver enzymes [85]. NAFLD occurs secondary to hyperinsulinemia and its inhibitory effect on the oxidation of free fatty acids that accumulate in the liver. Up to 95% of children who have the diagnosis of biopsy-proven NAFLD also meet criteria for insulin resistance [86]. Obese children who also carry the diagnosis of diabetes type 2 may have significant undiagnosed liver disease. The clinical implications of liver disease include altered drug pharmacokinetics caused by liver and renal insufficiency, coagulopathy, portal hypertension, pulmonary arteriovenous shunts, gastrointestinal varices and other sequelae of end-stage liver disease.

Endocrinology

Peripubertal obesity affects sexual development. In obese boys, sexual maturity will be delayed. Obese girls will experience precocious puberty [87]. Hyperandrogenism is associated with peripubertal obesity and is linked to polycystic ovarian syndrome and insulin resistance. Additionally, it is an independent marker of metabolic syndrome [88].

Neurology

Although the pathogenesis of idiopathic intracranial hypertension (IIH) or pseudotumor cerebri is not understood well, weight gain and obesity are definitive risk factors in case-controlled studies [89–93]. These children present with irritability, chronic headaches, diplopia or strabismus, tinnitus, or vision problems. Younger children rarely complain of these symptoms, and the physical examination may reveal papilledema with visual field defects. Brain imaging should reveal no space-occupying lesions or other pathology. Pediatric cerebrospinal fluid shunts for IIH increased by 52% in one institution from 1988 to 2002 [94]. Diagnosis, documentation, and treatment are important before cases in which visual loss is a known risk of the procedure such as scoliosis repair.

Psychology

Anesthesiologists should be aware and sensitive to the psychological issues surrounding pediatric obesity. As many as one third of obese children who are attending a weight management program report psychological maladjustment [95]. Psychological distress results from low self-esteem, poor body image, depression, school activity performance, and learning difficulties [96]. Villa and colleagues reported that general anxiety, separation anxiety, and social phobia were frequent in overweight children, with anxiety being the most frequent [97,98]. There is no clear association linking the severity of obesity to depression, although many psychosocial factors surrounding obesity could contribute to the development depression. Obesity is not a risk for other psychiatric disorders.

Musculoskeletal

Orthopedic morbidities related to being obese include scoliosis, slipped capital femoral epiphysis, Blount's disease, and fractures [99–102]. Despite obesity producing increased bone density, overweight children suffer from more fractures, experience more musculoskeletal discomfort, and develop greater lower extremity malalignment than their normal-weight peers.

ANESTHESIA CARE OF OBESE PEDIATRIC PATIENTS

Because obesity affects so many organ systems, the implications of obesity to the pediatric anesthesiologist are profound. Pediatric anesthesiologists, in the preparation and planning of the anesthetic course, play a critical role in decreasing the risk of perioperative and postoperative complications.

Preoperative workup

The preoperative visit should be tailored to the obese child. The investigative workup frequently is initiated by the anesthesiologist before major surgical procedures. Few obese children with obstructive sleep apnea have pulmonary function tests, sleep studies, or other diagnostic evaluations [56]. Thorough examination and history will help determine if more serious disease processes are present. Obtaining preoperative vital signs and routine blood workup is recommended. If a child has room air oximetry less than 96%, further investigation of pulmonary disease or OSAS is needed [103]. Laboratory testing of the complete blood count may reveal polycythemia, which is suggestive of chronic hypoxemia and possible cardiac issues. Arterial blood gas testing can reveal hypoxia, hypercapnea, and an elevated serum bicarbonate level suggestive of a chronic respiratory acidotic state. These findings are suggestive of OHS. Consultation with surgery, cardiology, endocrinology, pulmonary services, and multiple investigative studies such as arterial blood gas testing, chest radiograph, electrocardiogram, and even echocardiography should be considered for severe OSAS and OHS [104].

Preoperative management
Airway
In the period 1999 to 2000, a significant portion of closed pediatric anesthesia malpractice claims involved airway obstruction or inadequate ventilation [105]. The potential for difficult mask ventilation and intubation is greater in obese children who have coexisting diseases such as obstructive sleep apnea, craniofacial abnormalities, and neurological issues. Airway examination rarely is accomplished with cooperation. For this reason, awake fiberoptic intubations are also often not an option. Airway equipment such as the fiberoptic scope, laryngeal mask intubators, oral and nasal airways, lightwand devices, or other technologically advanced airway devices for establishing ventilation should be immediately available. Familiarity with the difficult airway algorithm is paramount. Proper positioning with adequate head elevation to produce conditions for neck flexion and the sniffing position or ramped is important [106]. Preparation for the presence of an otorhinolaryngologist and the possibility of a surgical airway may be necessary.

Aspiration risk
The risk for aspiration in obese adults is caused by increased gastric volumes, delayed gastric emptying times, and increased gastric pH. Recent studies in pediatric populations have proven the opposite [107]. In one study, morbidly obese children did not have a delay in gastric emptying time, and in a large series, no incidence of pulmonary aspiration occurred in obese children [108,109]. Many physicians, however, still prefer a rapid sequence intubation technique to prevent pulmonary aspiration and give antiparticulate antacids preoperatively. There are inconclusive data to link obesity to gastroesophageal reflux disease [110].

Peripheral access
Peripheral access is challenging in obese children. Transillumination and ultra-sound-guided technique for venous access have been described [111]. Central venous access should be considered when adequate peripheral venous access cannot be obtained [112–114].

Monitoring
All intraoperative monitoring devices are affected by obesity. Increased tissue resistance may produce falsely low voltage electrocardiogram readings. Legitimate electrocardiogram low voltage complexes are rarely present but may mask LV hypertrophy [115]. Pulse oximetry may be affected by decreased perfusion and excess tissue distance in obese fingertips [116]. Ventilation perfusion mismatching may produce falsely low end tidal CO_2 measurement. Noninvasive blood pressure monitors have to be sized appropriately; undersized cuffs produce falsely high readings. Pediatric anesthesiologists may elect invasive arterial monitoring for more accurate blood pressure readings and arterial blood gases. Neuromuscular monitoring also is affected by extreme obesity. Increased tissue resistance will diminish the evoked motor responses to external electrical stimulation. Because of the altered pharmacology, pharmacokinetics, and pharmacodynamics, the bispectral index (BIS) monitor has been a useful adjunct to intraoperative monitoring. BIS monitor application in bariatric surgery and other surgical procedures for the obese patient is becoming more established [117,118].

Drug pharmacokinetics and pharmacodynamics
The pharmacokinetics of intravenous anesthetic drugs are altered by obesity. Obesity-induced changes include the relative increase in fat over lean body mass, increased total blood volume, increased cardiac output, altered plasma protein binding, and altered regional blood flow. These change volumes of distribution and lipid solubilities [119]. Table 3 describes dosing of drugs based upon the pharmacokinetic and pharmacodynamic alterations that obesity produces [120–137]. In general, drug dosing is based upon volume of distribution and the maintenance on clearance of the drug from the body. Hydrophilic drugs should be dosed on ideal body weight, and lipophilic drugs should be dosed on total or actual body weight. NAFLD or renal disease may be present and will affect the metabolism and excretion of anesthetic drugs. The pharmacodynamics of intravenous anesthetic drugs are also altered by obesity. Obese children who have coexisting obstructive sleep apnea are more sensitive to respiratory depressant drugs.

The pharmacokinetics of inhalational drugs are affected by the altered physiology of obesity (Table 4) [120,138–142]. Table 5 lists the anesthetic considerations for the obese pediatric patient presenting for surgery. Delayed emergence may be a factor of increased central sensitivity and delayed release of agent from poorly perfused fat tissues. Emergence is faster with desflurane and sevoflurane because of low lipid accumulation and faster wash-out kinetics [142].

Table 3
Intravenous drug dosing in obese patients

Drug	Profile	Dose recommendations	Considerations
Thiopental	Lipophilic	According to total body weight	Increased sensitivity > increased of Vd[a]
Midazolam	Lipophilic	Premedication single dose according to total body weight; continuous infusion based on ideal body weight	Increased sensitivity caution with obstructive sleep apnea syndrome (OSAS)
Propofol	Lipophilic	According to actual body weight bolus and infusion	Vd correlate to total body weight
Succinylcholine	Hydrophilic	Total body weight	Increased pseudocholinesterase activity
Pancuronium	Hydrophilic	Ideal body weight	Increased requirements
Vecuronium	Hydrophilic	Ideal body weight	
Rocuronium	Hydrophilic	Ideal body weight	No change
Cisatracurium/ atracurium	Hydrophilic	Ideal body weight	Atracurium no change elimination
Morphine	Lipophilic		Increased sensitivity with OSAS
Hydromorphine	Lipophilic		Increased sensitivity with OSAS
Fentanyl	Lipophilic	Loading dose on total body weight; infusion dose at ideal body weight or less	Increased sensitivity with OSAS
Sufentanil	Lipophilic	Loading dose on total body weight; infusion dose at ideal body weight or less	Prolonged elimination, increased sensitivity
Remifentanil	Lipophilic	Ideal body weight	Ideal fast elimination and recovery
Dexmetetomidine		Ideal body weight	No change with gender or renal impairment; lower clearance with hepatic impairment; no evidence of respiratory depression
Nonsteroidal anti-inflammatory drugs			Nonsedating
Ketorolac			Nonsedating, caution with renal disease, dehydration, and gentamicin

[a]Increased sensitivity balances increased volume of distribution.

Table 4
Inhalational anesthetic agents and obesity

Inhalational agent	Profile	Differences with obesity
Halothane	High lipid solubility	Increased biotransformation, Br, Fl; hepatotoxicity; slower recovery times
Isoflurane	High lipid solubility	Slower recovery times
Desflurane	Low lipid solubility	Faster recovery times
Sevoflurane	Low lipid solubility	Increased fluoride ion; caution with renal insufficiency; faster recovery times

Preoxygenation is important before the induction of anesthesia. By providing maximal oxygen loading of functional reserve volume, more time is allowed for the safe establishment of the airway. Preoxygenation in a 25° reverse Trendelenburg or head-up position significantly increases the time before arterial desaturation occurs; this is postulated to be because of optimizing respiratory mechanics [143]. Placing the obese child in a sniffing position or lateral position improves airway patency and will assist in ease of mask ventilation and laryngeal intubation [144–147].

Positioning
Positioning an obese child correctly for surgery is important for adequate airway maintenance, ease of mask ventilation and intubation, optimization of respiratory mechanics, avoidance of nerve injury, and even cardiac hemodynamic stability. Because of the body habitus of obese children, proper positioning is difficult, and complications from various positions do occur, especially if the surgery is longer than an hour. The goal of positioning is to decrease intraabdominal pressure, decrease abdominal pressure on the diaphragm, enable adequate chest wall and lung expansion, and allow for the adequate venous return of blood volume. Without any modifications from the supine position such as a head elevating ramp or reverse Trendelenburg of at least 25° or more, respiratory mechanics will be affected adversely [144]. Lithotomy supine and Trendelenburg positions are tolerated poorly. Adequate abdominal space is necessary if a prone position is required. Pressure-point padding is necessary; it is important to distribute the weight over as much surface area as possible to avoid pressure necrosis. Shifting pressure points and movement of extremities at regular intervals are important to relieve pressure on tissues or tension on nerves in longer cases.

Regional technique
Regional anesthesia with obese children is technically challenging. Most pediatric neuraxial and peripheral blocks are placed under general anesthesia because of lack of cooperation and anxiety. Advantages of regional blocks include less respiratory depression, improved analgesia, decreased postoperative nausea, and possibly avoidance of general anesthesia or intubation.

Table 5
Anesthetic considerations for the obese pediatric patient presenting for surgery

Anesthesia	Precautions/risks	Considerations
Presedation	Increased sensitivity to opioids/benzodiazepines	Decrease dosage, appropriate monitoring, O_2, continuous positive airway pressure available
	Risk airway obstruction	Uncooperative with oral premedications, mask induction, difficult periferal intravenousaccess
	Excessive anxiety	
Mask induction	Risk airway obstruction, difficult mask ventilation	Two-handed ventilation, laryngeal mask airway, fiberoptic, oral airways available
Intravenous medication	Increased sensitivity to opioids	Decreased dose titration
	Altered pharmacokinetics and dynamics	Caution with renal or hepatic disease
Inhalational agents	Caution with hepatic disease	Sevoflurane and desflurane faster emergence times
Regional technique	Anatomy challenging	Beneficial for postoperative pain management
	Technically difficult	Less respiratory depression from systemic narcotics
Positioning	Anatomy challenging	Distribution of pressure by supplemental padding
	Increased risk of neuropathy and pressure ulcers	Head elevation preferred
	Trendelenburg, lithotomy, and supine position poorly tolerated	Free abdominal wall movement if in prone position
Extubation	Upper airway obstruction	Hypoxemia, cough, serous frothy bloody sputum, crackles on auscultation
	Postobstructive pulmonary edema	Chest radiograph: diffuse haziness bilateral
		Awake extubation
Postoperative care	Increased risk hypoxemia caused by airway obstruction, postoperative atelectasis, decreased respiratory drive	Supplemental oxygen, pulse oximetry, chest radiograph, pulmonary toilet, spirometry ambulation; CPAP or BiPAP
Pain management	Depression of respiratory drive	Cardiopulmonary monitoring, supplemental oxygen
	Psychological component	Caution with respiratory depressants; multidisciplinary approach

Technical challenges include obscure anatomical landmarks, increased depth to neurovascular site, poor patient cooperation, and positioning.

Drug doses of local anesthetics have to be adjusted to anatomical changes associated with obesity. The spinal and epidural space is decreased because of fat tissue and increased abdominal pressure. Local anesthetic spread and block height are unpredictable [148–150].

Thoracic level analgesia may help improve postoperative pulmonary function by preventing splinting of breaths, but high levels of analgesia are also likely to decrease pulmonary function in obese patients [148–152]. The decrease in pulmonary function with appropriate levels of regional anesthesia is, however, less than with opiate pain control. Postoperative pulmonary function recovery to normal values is faster with regional technique.

In a review of 9038 regional blocks on obese and non-obese patients, obese patients experienced a significantly higher block failure and complication rate [153]. The use of fluoroscopy, stimulating catheters, and ultrasound-guided regional technique may further improve block success in this anatomically challenging population [154,155].

Postoperative considerations

Extubation

Successful extubation in obese children with coexisting obstructive sleep apnea involves several factors: verification of complete reversal of paralysis agents, adequate ventilatory parameters, pain control, body position tilted upright to 25° or higher, oxygenation, and intact airway reflexes [56]. Awake extubation is the safest method and is recommended in cases involving a difficult airway. Maintaining an unobstructed airway after extubation is equally important. Postobstructive pulmonary edema has been described in children who have OSAS after airway surgery [156–158].

Postoperative respiratory care

Obese children who have other comorbidities such as obstructive sleep apnea are especially at risk for postoperative respiratory complications. Supplemental oxygenation and pulse oximetry should be provided to the patient until room air saturation remains above 92% during sleep. If the child is continuous positive airway pressure (CPAP) dependent before surgery, it should be continued afterward. Postoperative CPAP decreases pulmonary atelectasis and improves oxygenation. Pulmonary atelectasis should be suspected in major procedures and diagnostic chest radiograph, spirometry, and early ambulation are needed to avoid pneumonia [159].

If the obese child has OSAS, practice guidelines state that airway surgery such as tonsillectomy in children less than 3 years old and upper abdominal laparoscopic surgery should not be done as an outpatient [56]. Monitoring should continue in the postoperative period for a median of 7 hours after the last episode of airway obstruction or hypoxemia; this often necessitates a 23 hour observational status.

Specific surgical techniques

Laparoscopic surgery is a popular but challenging technique for abdominal surgery in obese children. Decreases in the incisional size translates into less incisional pain, faster healing, and likely improved postoperative pulmonary function and decreased overall morbidity. Because of these benefits, laparoscopic surgery is preferred for many procedures, including bariatric surgery. For obese children whose respiratory mechanics are already suboptimal in the supine position, insufflation for pneumoperitoneum will further worsen pulmonary compliance, decrease functional residual capacity, increase atelectasis, and decrease intra-abdominal organ perfusion [160]. Sprung and colleagues [162] found that maneuvers such as doubling tidal volume or respiratory rate did not decrease the amount of arterial shunting. Positive end expiratory pressure applied pre- and during induction decreases atelectasis [161]. Positive end-expiratory pressure may have a positive affect in the ventilation of laparoscopic and positionally challenged patients [162,163].

The recognized link of systemic diseases to obesity has led some authors to recommend surgical weight intervention to reverse and prevent the many comorbidities of obesity [164–166]. The surgical interventions for pediatric obesity are evolving constantly. Adolescent pediatric patients undergoing surgical weight loss procedures must have a multidisciplinary adolescent obesity health care team to screen patients and ensure that health interests of the patient are priority [167–172].

SUMMARY

Pediatric obesity is a recognized epidemic, and its impact on pediatric anesthesiology practice is pervasive. Obese children are not healthy children. These patients are a challenge that anesthesiologists are facing with increasing frequency. As literature and research continue to focus on the issues of pediatric obesity, the care and management of this special and now common population will continue to improve.

References

[1] Cheng TO. Obesity is a global challenge. Am J Med 2006;119(6):e11.
[2] Hedley AA, Ogden CL, Johnson CL, et al. Prevalence of overweight and obesity among US children, adolescents, and adults, 1999–2002. JAMA 2004;291(23):2847–50.
[3] Ogden CL, Carroll MD, Flegal KM. Epidemiologic trends in overweight and obesity. Endocrinol Metab Clin North Am 2003;32(4):741–60, vii.
[4] Ogden CL, et al. Prevalence of overweight and obesity in the United States, 1999–2004. JAMA 2006;295(13):1549–55.
[5] Cossrow N, Falkner B. Race/ethnic issues in obesity and obesity-related comorbidities. J Clin Endocrinol Metab 2004;89(6):2590–4.
[6] Crawford PB, et al. Ethnic issues in the epidemiology of childhood obesity. Pediatr Clin North Am 2001;48(4):855–78.
[7] Freedman DS, et al. Racial and ethnic differences in secular trends for childhood BMI, weight, and height. Obesity (Silver Spring) 2006;14(2):301–8.
[8] Gordon-Larsen P, Adair LS, Popkin BM. The relationship of ethnicity, socioeconomic factors, and overweight in US adolescents. Obes Res 2003;11(1):121–9.

[9] Kimm SY, et al. Racial divergence in adiposity during adolescence: the NHLBI Growth and Health Study. Pediatrics 2001;107(3):E34.

[10] Laron Z. Increasing incidence of childhood obesity. Pediatr Endocrinol Rev 2004;1(Suppl 3):443–7.

[11] Leet AI, Pichard CP, Ain MC. Surgical treatment of femoral fractures in obese children: does excessive body weight increase the rate of complications? J Bone Joint Surg Am 2005;87(12):2609–13.

[12] Reber A. [Airways and respiratory function in obese patients. anaesthetic and intensive care aspects and recommendations]. Anaesthesist 2005;54(7):715–25 [in German].

[13] Smith HL, Meldrum DJ, Brennan LJ. Childhood obesity: a challenge for the anaesthetist? Paediatr Anaesth 2002;12(9):750–61.

[14] Barlow SE, et al. Medical evaluation of overweight children and adolescents: reports from pediatricians, pediatric nurse practitioners, and registered dietitians. Pediatrics 2002;110(1 Pt 2):222–8.

[15] Riley MR, et al. Underdiagnosis of pediatric obesity and underscreening for fatty liver disease and metabolic syndrome by pediatricians and pediatric subspecialists. J Pediatr 2005;147(6):839–42.

[16] Cook S, et al. Screening and counseling associated with obesity diagnosis in a national survey of ambulatory pediatric visits. Pediatrics 2005;116(1):112–6.

[17] Obesity: preventing and managing the global epidemic. Report of a WHO consultation. World Health Organ Tech Rep Ser 2000;894:i-xii, 1–253.

[18] Daniels SR, Khoury PR, Morrison JA. The utility of body mass index as a measure of body fatness in children and adolescents: differences by race and gender. Pediatrics 1997;99(6):804–7.

[19] Maynard LM, et al. Childhood body composition in relation to body mass index. Pediatrics 2001;107(2):344–50.

[20] Pietrobelli A, et al. Body mass index as a measure of adiposity among children and adolescents: a validation study. J Pediatr 1998;132(2):204–10.

[21] Travers SH, et al. Gender and tanner stage differences in body composition and insulin sensitivity in early pubertal children. J Clin Endocrinol Metab 1995;80(1): 172–8.

[22] Ogden CL. Defining overweight in children using growth charts. Md Med 2004;5(3): 19–21.

[23] Kuczmarski RJ, Ogden CL, Guo SS, et al. 2000 CDC growth charts for the United States: methods and development. Vital Health Stat 11 2002;(246):1–190.

[24] Kuczmarski RJ, et al. CDC growth charts: United States. Adv Data 2000;(314):1–27.

[25] Speiser PW, Rudolf MD, Anhalt H, et al. Consensus statement: childhood obesity. J Clin Endocrinol Metab 2005;90(3):1871–87.

[26] Thompson DR, Obarzanek E, Franko DL, et al. Childhood overweight and cardiovascular disease risk factors: the National Heart, Lung, and Blood Institute Growth and Health Study. J Pediatr 2007;150(1):18–25.

[27] Baum VC, O'Flaherty J. Anesthesia for genetic metabolic and dysmorphic syndromes of childhood. 1st edition. Philadelphia: Lippincott, Williams & Wilkins; 1999.

[28] Hassink S. Problems in childhood obesity. Prim Care 2003;30(2):357–74.

[29] Rodin J. Obesity. Why the losing battle? In: Wolman BB, editor. Psychological aspects of obesity: a handbook. New York: Van Nostrand Reinholdt; 1982.

[30] Nathan PC, et al. The prevalence of overweight and obesity in pediatric survivors of cancer. J Pediatr 2006;149(4):518–25.

[31] Must A, Strauss RS. Risks and consequences of childhood and adolescent obesity. Int J Obes Relat Metab Disord 1999;23(Suppl 2):S2–11.

[32] Bacha F, et al. Obesity, regional fat distribution, and syndrome X in obese black versus white adolescents: race differential in diabetogenic and atherogenic risk factors. J Clin Endocrinol Metab 2003;88(6):2534–40.

[33] Caprio S. Definitions and pathophysiology of the metabolic syndrome in obese children and adolescents. Int J Obes (Lond) 2005;29(Suppl 2):S24–5.

[34] Chia DJ, Boston BA. Childhood obesity and the metabolic syndrome. Adv Pediatr 2006;53:23–53.

[35] Cook S, et al. Prevalence of a metabolic syndrome phenotype in adolescents: findings from the third National Health and Nutrition Examination Survey, 1988–1994. Arch Pediatr Adolesc Med 2003;157(8):821–7.

[36] Daskalopoulou SS, et al. Definitions of metabolic syndrome: where are we now? Curr Vasc Pharmacol 2006;4(3):185–97.

[37] Davis TM, Ee CK. Obesity and the metabolic syndrome in children and adolescents. N Engl J Med 2004;351(11):1146–8 [author reply 1146–48].

[38] de Ferranti SD, et al. Prevalence of the metabolic syndrome in American adolescents: findings from the Third National health and nutrition examination survey. Circulation 2004;110(16):2494–7.

[39] DeFronzo RA. Insulin resistance: a multifaceted syndrome responsible for NIDDM, obesity, hypertension, dyslipidaemia and atherosclerosis. Neth J Med 1997;50(5):191–7.

[40] Eisenmann JC. Secular trends in variables associated with the metabolic syndrome of North American children and adolescents: a review and synthesis. Am J Hum Biol 2003;15(6):786–94.

[41] Singh GK. Metabolic syndrome in children and adolescents. Curr Treat Options Cardiovasc Med 2006;8(5):403–13.

[42] Weiss R, Dzuira J, Burgert TS, et al. Obesity and the metabolic syndrome in children and adolescents. N Engl J Med 2004;350(23):2362–74.

[43] Alford FP. Syndrome X (insulin resistance metabolic syndrome): a deadly quartet or an awesome foursome? Med J Aust 1996;164(1):4–5.

[44] Brotman DJ, Girod JP. The metabolic syndrome: a tug of war with no winner. Cleve Clin J Med 2002;69(12):990–4.

[45] Deedwania PC. Mechanism of the deadly quartet. Can J Cardiol 2000;16(Suppl E):17E–20E.

[46] Gogia A, Agarwal PK. Metabolic syndrome. Indian J Med Sci 2006;60(2):72–81.

[47] Kaplan NM. The deadly quartet. Upper body obesity, glucose intolerance, hypertriglyceridemia, and hypertension. Arch Intern Med 1989;149(7):1514–20.

[48] Kaplan NM. The deadly quartet and the insulin resistance syndrome: an historical overview. Hypertens Res 1996;19(Suppl 1):S9–11.

[49] Nambi V, Hoogwerf RJ, Sprecher DL. A truly deadly quartet: obesity, hypertension, hypertriglyceridemia, and hyperinsulinemia. Cleve Clin J Med 2002;69(12):985–9.

[50] Opara JU, Levine JH. The deadly quartet—the insulin resistance syndrome. South Med J 1997;90(12):1162–8.

[51] Horner RL, et al. Sites and sizes of fat deposits around the pharynx in obese patients with obstructive sleep apnoea and weight-matched controls. Eur Respir J 1989;2(7):613–22.

[52] Suratt PM, et al. Fluoroscopic and computed tomographic features of the pharyngeal airway in obstructive sleep apnea. Am Rev Respir Dis 1983;127(4):487–92.

[53] Bandla P, et al. Obstructive sleep apnea syndrome in children. Anesthesiol Clin North America 2005;23(3):535–49, viii.

[54] Redline S, et al. Risk factors for sleep-disordered breathing in children. Associations with obesity, race, and respiratory problems. Am J Respir Crit Care Med 1999;159(5 Pt 1):1527–32.

[55] Standards and indications for cardiopulmonary sleep studies in children. American Thoracic Society. Am J Respir Crit Care Med 1996;153(2):866–78.

[56] Gross JB, et al. Practice guidelines for the perioperative management of patients with obstructive sleep apnea: a report by the American Society of Anesthesiologists task force on perioperative management of patients with obstructive sleep apnea. Anesthesiology 2006;104(5):1081–93 [quiz 1117–8].

[57] Bosisio E, et al. Ventilatory volumes, flow rates, transfer factor, and its components (membrane component, capillary volume) in obese adults and children. Respiration 1984;45(4):321–6.

[58] Ladosky W, Botelho MA, Albuquerque JP Jr. Chest mechanics in morbidly obese nonhypoventilated patients. Respir Med 2001;95(4):281–6.

[59] Chaussain M, et al. [Respiratory function at rest in obese children (author's transl)]. Bull Eur Physiopathol Respir 1977;13(5):599–609 [in French].

[60] Inselma LS, Milanese A, Deurloo A. Effect of obesity on pulmonary function in children. Pediatr Pulmonol 1993;16(2):130–7.

[61] Ray CS, et al. Effects of obesity on respiratory function. Am Rev Respir Dis 1983;128(3): 501–6.

[62] Olson AL, Zwillich C. The obesity hypoventilation syndrome. Am J Med 2005;118(9): 948–56.

[63] Somerville SM, Rona RJ, Chinn S. Obesity and respiratory symptoms in primary school. Arch Dis Child 1984;59(10):940–4.

[64] Tracey VV, De NC, Harper JR. Obesity and respiratory infection in infants and young children. Br Med J 1971;1(5739):16–8.

[65] Freedman DS, et al. The relation of childhood BMI to adult adiposity: the Bogalusa Heart Study. Pediatrics 2005;115(1):22–7.

[66] Goran MI, Ball GD, Cruz ML. Obesity and risk of type 2 diabetes and cardiovascular disease in children and adolescents. J Clin Endocrinol Metab 2003;88(4):1417–27.

[67] Gungor N, et al. Early signs of cardiovascular disease in youth with obesity and type 2 diabetes. Diabetes Care 2005;28(5):1219–21.

[68] Van Horn L, Greenland P. Prevention of coronary artery disease is a pediatric problem. JAMA 1997;278(21):1779–80.

[69] Whincup PH, Deanfield JE. Childhood obesity and cardiovascular disease: the challenge ahead. Nat Clin Pract Cardiovasc Med 2005;2(9):432–3.

[70] Zwiauer KF, et al. Cardiovascular risk factors in obese children in relation to weight and body fat distribution. J Am Coll Nutr 1992;11(Suppl):41S–50S.

[71] Freedman DS, et al. Relation of body fat patterning to lipid and lipoprotein concentrations in children and adolescents: the Bogalusa Heart Study. Am J Clin Nutr 1989;50(5):930–9.

[72] Falkner B, et al. The relationship of body mass index and blood pressure in primary care pediatric patients. J Pediatr 2006;148(2):195–200.

[73] Fuiano N, et al. Overweight and hypertension: longitudinal study in school-aged children. Minerva Pediatr 2006;58(5):451–9.

[74] Daniels SD, Meyer RA, Loggie JM. Determinants of cardiac involvement in children and adolescents with essential hypertension. Circulation 1990;82(4):1243–8.

[75] Li X, et al. Childhood adiposity as a predictor of cardiac mass in adulthood: the Bogalusa Heart Study. Circulation 2004;110(22):3488–92.

[76] Sivanandam S, et al. Relation of increase in adiposity to increase in left ventricular mass from childhood to young adulthood. Am J Cardiol 2006;98(3):411–5.

[77] Urbina EM, et al. Effect of body size, ponderosity, and blood pressure on left ventricular growth in children and young adults in the Bogalusa Heart Study. Circulation 1995;91(9):2400–6.

[78] Young TK, et al. Childhood obesity in a population at high risk for type 2 diabetes. J Pediatr 2000;136(3):365–9.

[79] Sinha R, et al. Prevalence of impaired glucose tolerance among children and adolescents with marked obesity. N Engl J Med 2002;346(11):802–10.

[80] Gungor N, et al. Type 2 diabetes mellitus in youth: the complete picture to date. Pediatr Clin North Am 2005;52(6):1579–609.

[81] Guzzaloni G, et al. Liver steatosis in juvenile obesity: correlations with lipid profile, hepatic biochemical parameters, and glycemic and insulinemic responses to an oral glucose tolerance test. Int J Obes Relat Metab Disord 2000;24(6):772–6.

[82] Kerem N, Guttmann H, Hochberg Z. The autosomal dominant trait of obesity, acanthosis nigricans, hypertension, ischemic heart disease, and diabetes type 2. Horm Res 2001;55(6):298–304.

[83] Chan DF, et al. Hepatic steatosis in obese Chinese children. Int J Obes Relat Metab Disord 2004;28(10):1257–63.

[84] Tominaga K, et al. Prevalence of fatty liver in Japanese children and relationship to obesity. An epidemiological ultrasonographic survey. Dig Dis Sci 1995;40(9):2002–9.

[85] Strauss RS, Barlow SE, Dietz WH. Prevalence of abnormal serum aminotransferase values in overweight and obese adolescents. J Pediatr 2000;136(6):727–33.

[86] Schwimmer JB, et al. Obesity, insulin resistance, and other clinicopathological correlates of pediatric nonalcoholic fatty liver disease. J Pediatr 2003;143(4):500–5.

[87] Wang Y. Is obesity associated with early sexual maturation? A comparison of the association in American boys versus girls. Pediatrics 2002;110(5):903–10.

[88] Coviello AD, Legro RS, Dunaif A. Adolescent girls with polycystic ovary syndrome have an increased risk of the metabolic syndrome associated with increasing androgen levels independent of obesity and insulin resistance. J Clin Endocrinol Metab 2006;91(2):492–7.

[89] Friedman DI. Pseudotumor cerebri. Neurol Clin 2004;22(1):99–131, vi.

[90] Giuseffi V, et al. Symptoms and disease associations in idiopathic intracranial hypertension (pseudotumor cerebri): a case–control study. Neurology 1991;41(2 (Pt 1)):239–44.

[91] Ireland B, Corbett JJ, Wallace RB. The search for causes of idiopathic intracranial hypertension. A preliminary case–control study. Arch Neurol 1990;47(3):315–20.

[92] Wall M. Idiopathic intracranial hypertension. Neurol Clin 1991;9(1):73–95.

[93] Wall M. Idiopathic intracranial hypertension. Semin Ophthalmol 1995;10(3):251–9.

[94] Curry WT Jr, Butler WE, Barker FG 2nd. Rapidly rising incidence of cerebrospinal fluid shunting procedures for idiopathic intracranial hypertension in the United States, 1988–2002. Neurosurgery 2005;57(1):97–108 [discussion: 97–108].

[95] Zeller MH, et al. Health-related quality of life and depressive symptoms in adolescents with extreme obesity presenting for bariatric surgery. Pediatrics 2006;117(4):1155–61.

[96] Tershakovec AM. Psychological considerations in pediatric weight management. Obes Res 2004;12(10):1537–8.

[97] Isnard-Mugnier P, et al. [A controlled study of food behavior and emotional manifestation in a population of obese female adolescents]. Arch Fr Pediatr 1993;50(6):479–84.

[98] Vila G, et al. Mental disorders in obese children and adolescents. Psychosom Med 2004;66(3):387–94.

[99] Taylor ED, et al. Orthopedic complications of overweight in children and adolescents. Pediatrics 2006;117(6):2167–74.

[100] Dietz WH Jr, Gross WL, Kirkpatrick JA Jr. Blount disease (tibia vara): another skeletal disorder associated with childhood obesity. J Pediatr 1982;101(5):735–7.

[101] Wills M. Orthopedic complications of childhood obesity. Pediatr Phys Ther 2004;16(4):230–5.

[102] Perron AD, Miller MD, Brady WJ. Orthopedic pitfalls in the ED: slipped capital femoral epiphysis. Am J Emerg Med 2002;20(5):484–7.

[103] Cartagena R. Preoperative evaluation of patients with obesity and obstructive sleep apnea. Anesthesiol Clin North America 2005;23(3):463–78, vi.

[104] Blum RH, McGowan FX Jr. Chronic upper airway obstruction and cardiac dysfunction: anatomy, pathophysiology, and anesthetic implications. Paediatr Anaesth 2004;14(1):75–83.

[105] Jiminez N. Trends in pediatric anesthesia malpractice claims over the last three decades. ASA Newsletter. June 6, 2005:69.

[106] Collins JS, et al. Laryngoscopy and morbid obesity: a comparison of the sniff and ramped positions. Obes Surg 2004;14(9):1171–5.

[107] Harter RL, et al. A comparison of the volume and pH of gastric contents of obese and lean surgical patients. Anesth Analg 1998;86(1):147–52.

[108] Borland LM, et al. Pulmonary aspiration in pediatric patients during general anesthesia: incidence and outcome. J Clin Anesth 1998;10(2):95–102.

[109] Chiloiro M, et al. Gastric emptying in normal weight and obese children—an ultrasound study. Int J Obes Relat Metab Disord 1999;23(12):1303–6.

[110] Freid EB. The rapid sequence induction revisited: obesity and sleep apnea syndrome. Anesthesiol Clin North America 2005;23(3):551–64, viii.

[111] Abboud PA, Kendall JL. Ultrasound guidance for vascular access. Emerg Med Clin North Am 2004;22(3):749–73.

[112] Marhofer P, Willschke H, Kettner S. Imaging techniques for regional nerve blockade and vascular cannulation in children. Curr Opin Anaesthesiol 2006;19(3):293–300.

[113] Galloway S, et al. A review of an anaesthetic-led vascular access list. Anaesthesia 2005;60(8):772–8.

[114] Hatfield A, Bodenham A. Portable ultrasound for difficult central venous access. Br J Anaesth 1999;82(6):822–6.

[115] Alpert MA, et al. The electrocardiogram in morbid obesity. Am J Cardiol 2000;85(7): 908–10, A10.

[116] Kabon B, et al. Obesity decreases perioperative tissue oxygenation. Anesthesiology 2004;100(2):274–80.

[117] Gaszynski T, et al. Reduction of a total propofol consumption in morbidly obese patients during general anesthesia due to BIS monitoring. Obes Surg 2005;15(7):1084 [author reply 1085].

[118] Lemmens HJ, Brodsky JB. General anesthesia, bariatric surgery, and the BIS monitor. Obes Surg 2005;15(1):63.

[119] Casati A, Putzu M. Anesthesia in the obese patient: pharmacokinetic considerations. J Clin Anesth 2005;17(2):134–45.

[120] Juvin P, et al. Postoperative recovery after desflurane, propofol, or isoflurane anesthesia among morbidly obese patients: a prospective, randomized study. Anesth Analg 2000;91(3):714–9.

[121] Servin F, et al. Propofol infusion for maintenance of anesthesia in morbidly obese patients receiving nitrous oxide. A clinical and pharmacokinetic study. Anesthesiology 1993;78(4):657–65.

[122] Jung D, et al. Thiopental disposition in lean and obese patients undergoing surgery. Anesthesiology 1982;56(4):269–74.

[123] Dundee JW, et al. The induction dose of thiopentone. A method of study and preliminary illustrative results. Anaesthesia 1982;37(12):1176–84.

[124] Wada DR, et al. Computer simulation of the effects of alterations in blood flows and body composition on thiopental pharmacokinetics in humans. Anesthesiology 1997;87(4): 884–99.

[125] Greenblatt DJ, et al. Effect of age, gender, and obesity on midazolam kinetics. Anesthesiology 1984;61(1):27–35.

[126] Rose JB, Theroux MC, Katz MS. The potency of succinylcholine in obese adolescents. Anesth Analg 2000;90(3):576–8.

[127] Lemmens HJ, Brodsky JB. The dose of succinylcholine in morbid obesity. Anesth Analg 2006;102(2):438–42.

[128] Brodsky JB, Foster PE. Succinylcholine and morbid obesity. Obes Surg 2003;13(1): 138–9.

[129] Feingold A. Pancuronium requirements of the morbidly obese. Anesthesiology 1979;50(3):269–70.

[130] Tsueda K, et al. Pancuronium bromide requirement during anesthesia for the morbidly obese. Anesthesiology 1978;48(6):438–9.

[131] Puhringer FK, et al. Pharmacokinetics of rocuronium bromide in obese female patients. Eur J Anaesthesiol 1999;16(8):507–10.

[132] Puhringer FK, Khuenl-Brady KS, Mitterschiffthaler G. Rocuronium bromide: time course of action in underweight, normal weight, overweight, and obese patients. Eur J Anaesthesiol 1995;11(Suppl):107–10.

[133] Schwartz AE, et al. Pharmacokinetics and pharmacodynamics of vecuronium in the obese surgical patient. Anesth Analg 1992;74(4):515–8.

[134] Varin F, et al. Influence of extreme obesity on the body disposition and neuromuscular blocking effect of atracurium. Clin Pharmacol Ther 1990;48(1):18–25.

[135] Egan TD, et al. Remifentanil pharmacokinetics in obese versus lean patients. Anesthesiology 1998;89(3):562–73.

[136] Hofer RE, et al. Anesthesia for a patient with morbid obesity using dexmedetomidine without narcotics. Can J Anaesth 2005;52(2):176–80.

[137] Alavi FK, Zawada ET, Hoff KK. Renal hemodynamic effects of chronic ketorolac tromethamine treatment in aged lean and obese Zucker rats. Clin Nephrol 1995;43(5):318–23.

[138] Bentley JB, et al. Halothane biotransformation in obese and nonobese patients. Anesthesiology 1982;57(2):94–7.

[139] Frink EJ Jr, et al. Plasma inorganic fluoride levels with sevoflurane anesthesia in morbidly obese and nonobese patients. Anesth Analg 1993;76(6):1333–7.

[140] Sollazzi L, et al. Volatile anesthesia in bariatric surgery. Obes Surg 2001;11(5):623–6.

[141] Torri G, et al. Randomized comparison of isoflurane and sevoflurane for laparoscopic gastric banding in morbidly obese patients. J Clin Anesth 2001;13(8):565–70.

[142] Torri G, et al. Wash-in and wash-out curves of sevoflurane and isoflurane in morbidly obese patients. Minerva Anestesiol 2002;68(6):523–7.

[143] Dixon BJ, et al. Preoxygenation is more effective in the 25 degrees head-up position than in the supine position in severely obese patients: a randomized controlled study. Anesthesiology 2005;102(6):1110–5 [discussion: 5A].

[144] Brodsky JB. Positioning the morbidly obese patient for anesthesia. Obes Surg 2002;12(6):751–8.

[145] Brodsky JB, et al. Anesthetic considerations for bariatric surgery: proper positioning is important for laryngoscopy. Anesth Analg 2003;96(6):1841–2 [author reply 1842].

[146] Isono S, et al. Sniffing position improves pharyngeal airway patency in anesthetized patients with obstructive sleep apnea. Anesthesiology 2005;103(3):489–94.

[147] Isono S, Tanaka A, Nishino T. Lateral position decreases collapsibility of the passive pharynx in patients with obstructive sleep apnea. Anesthesiology 2002;97(4):780–5.

[148] Hogan QH, et al. Magnetic resonance imaging of cerebrospinal fluid volume and the influence of body habitus and abdominal pressure. Anesthesiology 1996;84(6):1341–9.

[149] McCulloch WJ, Littlewood DG. Influence of obesity on spinal analgesia with isobaric 0.5% bupivacaine. Br J Anaesth 1986;58(6):610–4.

[150] Taivainen T, Tuominen M, Rosenberg PH. Influence of obesity on the spread of spinal analgesia after injection of plain 0.5% bupivacaine at the L3-4 or L4-5 interspace. Br J Anaesth 1990;64(5):542–6.

[151] Regli A, et al. Impact of spinal anaesthesia on perioperative lung volumes in obese and morbidly obese female patients. Anaesthesia 2006;61(3):215–21.

[152] von Ungern-Sternberg BS, et al. Effect of obesity and thoracic epidural analgesia on perioperative spirometry. Br J Anaesth 2005;94(1):121–7.

[153] Nielsen KC, et al. Influence of obesity on surgical regional anesthesia in the ambulatory setting: an analysis of 9038 blocks. Anesthesiology 2005;102(1):181–7.

[154] Eidelman A, Shulman MS, Novak GM. Fluoroscopic imaging for technically difficult spinal anesthesia. J Clin Anesth 2005;17(1):69–71.

[155] Schwemmer U, et al. Ultrasound-guided interscalene brachial plexus anaesthesia: differences in success between patients of normal and excessive weight. Ultraschall Med 2006;27(3):245–50.

[156] Ciavarro C, Kelly JP. Postobstructive pulmonary edema in an obese child after an oral surgery procedure under general anesthesia: a case report. J Oral Maxillofac Surg 2002;60(12):1503–5.

[157] Lorch DG, Sahn SA. Postextubation pulmonary edema following anesthesia induced by upper airway obstruction. Are certain patients at increased risk? Chest 1986;90(6): 802–5.

[158] Mantadakis E, et al. Near demise of a child with Prader-Willi syndrome during elective orchidopexy. Paediatr Anaesth 2006;16(7):790–3.

[159] Ebeo CT, et al. The effect of bilevel positive airway pressure on postoperative pulmonary function following gastric surgery for obesity. Respir Med 2002;96(9):672–6.

[160] Sprung J, et al. The impact of morbid obesity, pneumoperitoneum, and posture on respiratory system mechanics and oxygenation during laparoscopy. Anesth Analg 2002;94(5): 1345–50.

[161] Coussa M, et al. Prevention of atelectasis formation during the induction of general anesthesia in morbidly obese patients. Anesth Analg 2004;98(5):1491–5 [table of contents].

[162] Pelosi P, et al. Positive end-expiratory pressure improves respiratory function in obese but not in normal subjects during anesthesia and paralysis. Anesthesiology 1999;91(5): 1221–31.

[163] Whalen FX, et al. The effects of the alveolar recruitment maneuver and positive end-expiratory pressure on arterial oxygenation during laparoscopic bariatric surgery. Anesth Analg 2006;102(1):298–305.

[164] Bouldin MJ, et al. The effect of obesity surgery on obesity comorbidity. Am J Med Sci 2006;331(4):183–93.

[165] Lara MD, Kothari SN, Sugerman HJ. Surgical management of obesity: a review of the evidence relating to the health benefits and risks. Treat Endocrinol 2005;4(1):55–64.

[166] Sugerman HJ, et al. Bariatric surgery for severely obese adolescents. J Gastrointest Surg 2003;7(1):102–7 [discussion: 107–8].

[167] Xanthakos SA, Inge TH. Extreme pediatric obesity: weighing the health dangers. J Pediatr 2007;150(1):3–5.

[168] Inge TH, Xanthakos SA, Zeller MH. Bariatric surgery for pediatric extreme obesity: now or later? Int J Obes (Lond) 2007;31(1):1–14.

[169] Xanthakos SA, Daniels SR, Inge TH. Bariatric surgery in adolescents: an update. Adolesc Med Clin 2006;17(3):589–612 [abstract x].

[170] Inge TH, Lawson L. Treatment considerations for severe adolescent obesity. Surg Obes Relat Dis 2005;1(2):133–9.

[171] Inge TH. Bariatric surgery for morbidly obese adolescents: is there a rationale for early intervention? Growth Horm IGF Res 2006;16(Suppl A):S15–9.

[172] Helmrath MA, Brandt ML, Inge TH. Adolescent obesity and bariatric surgery. Surg Clin North Am 2006;86(2):441–54, x.

Advances in Anesthesia 25 (2007) 103–125

ADVANCES IN ANESTHESIA

Should Nonanesthesia Providers Be Administering Propofol?

Klaus Kjaer, MD[a],*, Anand Patel, MD[b]

[a]Weill Medical College of Cornell University, Weill Cornell Medical Center, Department of Anesthesiology, 525 East 68th Street, Suite M-302B, New York, NY 10021, USA
[b]Division of Pain Management, Department of Anethesiology, Weill Medical College of Cornell University, New York, NY, USA

M ost patients who undergo invasive procedures require some amount of sedation and analgesia. The American Society of Anesthesiologists (ASA) describes sedation and analgesia along a continuum of states according to the degree of purposeful movement in response to increasing levels of stimulation (Table 1) [1].

This article focuses on sedation and analgesia for gastrointestinal (GI) endoscopic procedures. It does not discuss whether emergency medicine physicians and critical care physicians should be administering propofol for procedural sedation in emergency rooms and ICUs.

In some geographic areas, propofol rapidly is becoming the drug of choice for GI endoscopy. Anesthesia providers, however, are not always available to administer propofol. This has invited new thinking about whether nonanesthesia providers may be able to administer propofol with the same level of efficacy and safety as anesthesia providers.

In the last few decades, the increasing emphasis on preventative care has led to a substantial increase in the volume of endoscopic procedures performed by gastroenterologists. In New Hampshire alone, with a state population of 1.3 million, just under 50,000 colonoscopies were performed in 2002 [2]. Although a very small percentage of these patients can tolerate such procedures without any sedation, most require some form of sedation and analgesia to make the experience tolerable [3–7]. The types of sedatives and analgesics commonly used for this purpose vary considerably in their properties. Pharmacokinetic and pharmacodynamic factors such as onset, duration, efficacy, potency, metabolism, tolerance, adverse effects, therapeutic index, and drug interactions make the selection of the ideal agent for sedation and analgesia complicated. In addition to drug factors, patient factors also should be included in the

*Corresponding author. *E-mail address*: kkjaer@hotmail.com (K. Kjaer).

0737-6146/07/$ – see front matter
doi:10.1016/j.aan.2007.07.007

Table 1

Continuum of depth of sedation: definition of general anesthesia and levels of sedation/analgesia

	Minimal sedation (anxiolysis)	Moderate sedation/ analgesia (conscious sedation)	Deep sedation/analgesia	General anesthesia
Responsiveness	Normal response to verbal stimulation	Purposeful response to verbal or tactile stimulation	Purposeful response after repeated or painful stimulation	Unarousable, even with painful stimulus
Airway	Unaffected	No intervention required	Intervention may be required	Intervention often required
Spontaneous ventilation	Unaffected	Adequate	May be inadequate	Frequently inadequate
Cardiovascular function	Unaffected	Usually maintained	Usually maintained	May be impaired

drug selection process. Anxiety levels and individual differences in pain tolerance will strongly influence what drug should be given, and how much. Different patients may require different levels of sedation for the same procedure, and patients may attain varying levels of sedation during a single procedure [8]. A third factor influencing the ideal choice of sedation and analgesia is the type of procedure being performed, with each procedure having its own stimulation profile, level of difficulty, duration, and potential complications. On average, simple endoscopies such as colonoscopy and upper endoscopy are technically easier, less stimulating, and shorter in duration than complex endoscopies such as endoscopic retrograde cholangiopancreatography (ERCP) and endoscopic ultrasound (EUS) [9,10]. A fourth factor that significantly affects the requirement for sedation and analgesia is the experience and skill level of the endoscopist.

BENZODIAZEPINES AND OPIOIDS

Midazolam first became available in the early 1980s and gained rapid popularity for sedation and induction of anesthesia. Several advantages made midazolam the benzodiazepine of choice for procedural sedation:

A relatively rapid onset
A short half-life compared with other intravenous benzodiazepines such as diazepam (Valium)
An ability to provide titratable sedation
An ability to provide potent amnesia
The availability of an antagonist (flumazenil) to reverse any potential oversedation
Relatively minimal pain on injection secondary to its water-solubility

Multiple studies have demonstrated the superiority of midazolam over diazepam for endoscopic procedures, with respect to amnesia, speed of onset, pain on injection, patient satisfaction, and speed of recovery [11,12].

Various sedative–hypnotics and analgesics will have synergistic effects when administered in combination with midazolam. Even a small amount of opioid, for example, will reduce the requirement for a benzodiazepine substantially [13]. Opioids also have a reliable antagonist available (naloxone). Because of their synergy and reversibility, benzodiazepines and opioids in combination have an outstanding record of efficacy and safety, and have been used for several decades by nonanesthesia providers to provide procedural sedation and analgesia [14]. The two most commonly used combinations are midazolam/meperidine and midazolam/fentanyl.

PROPOFOL

In most patients, the combination of a benzodiazepine and an opioid reliably produces a state of moderate sedation and analgesia, which is adequate for most simple endoscopies. Sometimes, however, either moderate sedation is difficult to achieve, or the patient requires deep sedation. In these cases, gastroenterologists often have sought out the services of anesthesia providers. Anesthesia providers have met this demand largely, though not exclusively, by administering moderate-to-deep sedation with propofol. The response to the quality of sedation provided by propofol, both from gastroenterologists and patients, has been overwhelmingly favorable, so much so, in fact, that in many practices propofol has become the drug of choice for all endoscopies. The use of propofol for endoscopy unintentionally called attention to the comparative shortcomings of the traditional benzodiazepine/opioid combination, including:

A delay of several minutes after administration before the drugs begin to exert their maximal effects

Greater difficulty titrating the drugs to an appropriate level of sedation secondary to longer time to onset

Residual sedation following the procedure, a requirement for longer postprocedure monitoring and a longer time to discharge

Morbidity/mortality as a result of untreated respiratory depression [15–18]

The ideal agent, by contrast, would have immediate onset at the start of the procedure, be easy to titrate, wear off shortly after completion of the procedure with quick recovery of neuropsychiatric function and amnesia lasting only for the duration of the procedure, and have minimal adverse effects and minimal risk [19]. Propofol comes remarkably close to meeting these requirements. But is it safe in the hands of nonanesthesia providers?

THE GASTROENTEROLOGIST'S PERSPECTIVE

There is a growing trend among gastroenterologists to request the services of anesthesiologists for propofol-based sedation. In a survey conducted by Faulx and colleagues [20], routine use of propofol sedation for esophagogastroduodenoscopy, colonoscopy, and ERCP/EUS by gastroenterologists was reported at 19%, 22%, and 19%, respectively. Of those gastroenterologists not currently using propofol in their practice, 43% planned to begin doing so within a year. In the last decade, numerous papers in the gastroenterology literature have been published discussing the advantages of propofol-based sedation for endoscopy.

Propofol is appealing to gastroenterologists for multiple reasons.

Technical performance

Propofol-based sedation may improve the technical performance of various endoscopic procedures. This contention, however, remains controversial. In 2004, Hansen and colleagues [16] evaluated the technical performance of colonoscopy in patients sedated with propofol. In the retrospective portion of the study, propofol was associated with a statistically significant decrease in cecal intubation time. Although not statistically significant, the prospective portion of the study also demonstrated a trend toward faster cecal intubation. Another study demonstrated that the number of cases in which maneuvers such as changing the position of the patient and/or applying pressure to the abdomen was significantly lower in the propofol group compared with the midazolam/

fentanyl group. A concern, however, has been whether the typically deeper sedation from propofol administration may diminish the ability of a patient to indicate discomfort in the case of a complication such as bowel perforation. Some endoscopists have hypothesized that during difficult or high-risk procedures, preserving a patient's ability to indicate discomfort may allow early detection of such a complication. Another concern raised by some endoscopists has been whether deep sedation with propofol, by relaxing the abdominal and bowl wall musculature, actually can increase the technical difficulty of the procedure. So far, this has not been shown to be the case. Multiple studies have demonstrated that propofol administration does not delay, and may even shorten, procedure length for simple endoscopy [17,21].

Performance of complex procedures

Endoscopic procedures can be classified into those that are technically simple (colonoscopy and upper endoscopy) and technically complex (ERCP and EUS).

Complex endoscopic procedures are frequently longer in duration and require multiple doses of medications to achieve an adequate level of sedation and analgesia throughout the procedure. A study by Riphaus and colleagues [22] demonstrated a statistically significant improvement in patient sedation when using propofol during ERCP. This was noted both by the performing endoscopist and by an independent observer. Although propofol will not always make performance of ERCP easier for the endoscopist, on average it helps both the patient and the gastroenterologist when the patient is able to tolerate the physical stimulation of the procedure smoothly. Many studies have demonstrated a statistically significant improvement in sedation and technical performance of ERCP with the use of propofol [23–25]. In a study by Vargo and colleagues [26], however, patients who underwent ERCP and EUS had no difference in duration of procedures (propofol group 53.6 minutes plus or minus 4.3 minutes versus midazolam/meperidine group 51.8 minutes plus or minus 5.1 minutes, $P = .93$).

Recovery time

Shortened recovery times have significant implications for gastroenterologists with respect to case turnover time. Vargo and colleagues [26] demonstrated the immediate impact of propofol on recovery and turnover times. More patients receiving propofol were able to transfer independently from the procedure table to a transport gurney immediately after the procedure compared with those who received midazolam/meperidine (71.1% versus 29.7%; $P < .001$). Sipe and colleagues [19] demonstrated a shorter mean time from completion of colonoscopy to arrival in the recovery area in a group of patients receiving propofol. Several studies have demonstrated that after various GI endoscopic procedures, patients receiving propofol required less time to reach full recovery and were discharged sooner [17].

Vargo and colleagues [26] also showed that recovery room time usage is reduced significantly with propofol. Fifteen minutes after procedure completion, 76.3% of patients receiving propofol had reached discharge criteria,

compared with 8% of patients receiving midazolam/meperidine. Thirty minutes after procedure, 100% of the propofol group had reached discharge criteria, compared with only 16.2% of patients in the midazolam/meperidine
group $(P < .001)$.

Other studies have confirmed that patients who received propofol for colonoscopy could ambulate significantly sooner and were ready for discharge
more than 30 minutes faster than those who received midazolam/meperidine
$(P < .0001;$ Table 2) [19].

Cost

The use of propofol has not only medical implications, but also economic implications. The added costs of propofol sedation are related mostly to the cost
of the provider dedicated to administer the drug and monitor its effects. Some
savings occur in relation to patients spending less time in recovery. Finally,
there may be potentially increased revenue per location from faster case turnover and the ability to perform more procedures in the same amount of time.
These costs and savings, along with greater productivity, partially offset each
other. They affect the different parties involved—gastroenterologists, anesthesiologists, third-party payers, and patients—differently, however.

Vargo and colleagues [26] undertook an analysis to evaluate whether the
usage of propofol was more cost-effective than the usage of midazolam/
meperidine (Table 3). The propofol group was associated with similar costs
for medications ($27 plus or minus $14 for propofol versus $29 plus or minus
$22 for midazolam/meperidine). Recovery room costs were significantly lower
in the propofol group $(P < .001)$ because of a shorter stay in the recovery room
after the procedure. The propofol group was associated with significantly
higher personnel costs compared with the midazolam/meperidine group
($144 versus $0, $P < .001$), because of the requirement that an additional physician (in this case, a gastroenterologist rather than an anesthesiologist), be
present to administer the propofol. Overall, the total costs of the procedure
were $403 more per patient in the propofol group compared with the
midazolam/meperidine group.

Table 2
Propofol versus midazolam/meperidine for colonoscopy

Mean (SD) time to:	Propofol (min)	M/M	p value
Sedate	2.1 (1.2)	7.0 (3.4)	<.0001
Cecum	4.5 (2.8)	4.6 (2.5)	>.50
Withdraw endoscope	16.6 (5.6)	16.0 (6.7)	>.50
Recovery room	9.7 (2.5)	12.2 (7.2)	<.038
Stand	14.2 (7.1)	30.2 (19.0)	<.0001
Full recovery	14.4 (6.5)	33.0 (23.3)	<.0001
Discharge	40.5 (19.2)	71.1 (29.6)	<.0001

Abbreviation: M/M, Midazolam/meperidine.

Table 3
Cost of propofol versus midazolam/meperidine

Variable	Propofol (n = 38)	Meperidine/midazolam (n = 37)	P value
Medication	$27 ± $14	$29 ± $22	.816
Anesthesia	$144 ± $67	$0	<.001
Recovery	$9 ± $3	$38 ± $24	<.001
Total	$180 ± $75	$67 ± $33	<.001

Note: all scores are reported as mean ± SEM; data are nonparametric, and P values reflect the results of the Mann-Whitney rank sum test.

Safety

A much-publicized concern with propofol is its safety profile, given its narrow therapeutic index. Once a satisfactory level of sedation is reached, some airway support often is required, even if only a simple chin lift. Benzodiazepines and opioids in combination have well-established synergy, not only in terms of sedation and analgesia, but also in terms of respiratory and cardiovascular adverse effects. Treatment of these adverse effects is relatively easy, however, because of the availability of reversal agents: flumazenil for benzodiazepines and naloxone for opioids. Propofol, meanwhile, has no available reversal agent. This fact, along with the easy transition of sedation from a moderate to a deep level, can make the use of propofol precarious. For this reason, the drug has been administered mostly by professionals trained in advanced airway management, namely anesthesiologists and certified registered nurse anesthetists. Possible complications from propofol, other than apnea, airway obstruction, and aspiration, include hypotension and cardiac dysrhythmias. Nonetheless, multiple studies have demonstrated that propofol administration, even when performed or supervised by gastroenterologists, has resulted in minimal morbidity and mortality during endoscopic procedures [17,19,21,22,26–34].

Because of the adverse effect profile of propofol, including severe respiratory and cardiovascular depression, providers have been reluctant to use propofol in critically ill or high-risk patients (classified as ASA 3 and 4). In a study conducted by Heuss and colleagues [35], complication rates were evaluated using propofol sedation on ASA 3 and 4 patients versus ASA 1 and 2 patients. The propofol was administered by registered nurses. Complications were defined as:

> The need for intervention using artificial ventilation (usually done for SaO2 less than 85%)
> A drop in SaO2 below 90%
> A decrease in mean arterial pressure of more than 25%
> A decrease in heart rate of more than 20%

There were no major complications among the critically ill patients. There was, however, an increased risk for a short period of decreased SaO2 (3.6% for ASA 3 and 4 versus 1.7% for ASA 1 and 2, $P = .04$). There were no significant differences in arterial pressure and heart rate. It appears that even in high-risk patients, propofol sedation can be accomplished safely.

There also has been concern regarding the use of propofol in the older patient population. In 2005, Riphaus and colleagues [22] conducted a randomized trial to evaluate outcomes and complication rates for 162 consecutive patients aged 80 years or older. Areas of concern included oxygen desaturation (SaO2 less than 90%) and hemodynamic stability (heart rate less than 50 or systolic blood pressure less than 90). Overall, the mean decline in oxygen saturation was significantly greater in the propofol group than in the midazolam/meperidine group, but a potentially harmful drop in oxygen saturation lower than 90% was not observed to be more frequent with propofol. This particular study demonstrated that propofol sedation may be superior to midazolam and meperidine, even in older patient populations.

In Clarke and colleagues' [36] retrospective review of 28,472 endoscopies in Australia, 107 respiratory complications (mostly hypoventilation, but including four cases of aspiration) and 78 cardiovascular complications (mostly hypotension) occurred. Fentanyl, midazolam, and propofol were used in combination as the sedative regimen. General practitioners administered the sedation and monitored the effects. Patients identified as higher than average risk were referred to the care of an anesthesiologist.

Rex and colleagues [29] looked at 36,743 endoscopies performed with nurse-administered propofol sedation (NAPS) in Oregon, Illinois, and Switzerland. There were no significant cardiac arrhythmias other than bradycardia, which was treated successfully with atropine in all cases. Eleven patients received ephedrine for hypotension and recovered uneventfully. For colonoscopies, the rate of mask ventilation was 7 in 17,527 cases (0.04%). For procedures involving upper endoscopy, the rate of mask ventilation was 42 in 19,190 cases (0.22%).

To evaluate the safety record of propofol sedation compared with that of benzodiazepine/opioid sedation, Qadeer and colleagues [37] performed a meta-analysis of 12 published studies involving a combined total of 1161 patients. The study looked at four primary cardiopulmonary complications: hypoxia, arrhythmias, apnea, and hypotension. The patients were divided into groups based on the procedures performed: upper endoscopy group, colonoscopy group, and ERCP/EUS group. Although patients receiving propofol during colonoscopy had lower odds of cardiopulmonary complications compared with those receiving benzodiazepine/opioid, the odds were similar during upper endoscopy and ERCP/EUS. In most of these studies, propofol was administered by a gastroenterologist, not an anesthesiologist. While testing the hypothesis that complication rates are higher with propofol-based sedation, this study actually found that propofol might be safer than the traditional combination of a benzodiazepine and an opioid.

THE PATIENT'S PERSPECTIVE
Patients increasingly are presenting to gastroenterologists' offices requesting to have propofol for their endoscopy. Why?

Comfort during procedure

Patients about to undergo an uncomfortable procedure typically have several areas of concern: analgesia, sedation, amnesia, recovery, and the likelihood of complications from the procedure. Elements of recovery include postprocedure pain, nausea, vomiting, and residual sedation. Opioids, which are powerful analgesics, are associated with postprocedural nausea and vomiting. By contrast, propofol is associated with a significant decrease in postprocedure nausea and vomiting.

Sipe and colleagues [19] evaluated patient satisfaction immediately afterward and 48 hours after endoscopic procedures performed with propofol-based sedation. Eighty patients were randomized to propofol versus midazolam/meperidine . The patients receiving propofol reported statistically significant higher satisfaction (Table 4).

When asked if they received enough sedation, all of the propofol patients replied they had received "just the right amount of sedation," whereas five of the control patients felt they needed an adjustment (more or less) in the amount of sedation they received.

Weston and colleagues [31] similarly reported greater satisfaction with propofol than with midazolam/meperidine at the time of discharge. But not all studies have shown a statistically significant improvement in patient satisfaction with propofol over a benzodiazepine and an opioid [26]. In a study conducted by Ulmer and colleagues [17], patients receiving propofol and midazolam/fentanyl reported similar degrees of satisfaction with the procedure, both at the time of discharge and 48 hours after colonoscopy. No studies have shown greater patient satisfaction with the combination of a benzodiazepine and an opioid than with propofol. The data clearly suggest that patient satisfaction is at least equal, and often better, with propofol.

Quality of recovery

Multiple attempts have been made to evaluate patients' cognitive function and performance after procedural sedation. The evaluation period has ranged from immediately after the procedure up until at least 48 hours after discharge. Sipe and colleagues [19] evaluated multiple aspects of patient performance after the procedure. Immediately after the procedure, patients were rated on a scale to evaluate sedation and alertness.

Following their procedure, the patients were asked to repeat various tests to evaluate their neuropsychologic performance. At the time of discharge, all of the neuropsychological tests were repeated . The investigators subsequently contacted patients within 48 hours to further assess their overall satisfaction, subjectively rate their impairment since discharge, and report how many hours they spent sleeping in the 24 hours after the procedure. The results showed substantial statistical differences on several levels. Patients in the group that received propofol had overall faster recovery times and were discharged earlier (40.5 minutes versus 71.1 minutes, $P < .0001$). Following discharge, patients in the propofol group had higher performance scores on most neuropsychologic

Table 4
Patient satisfaction after propofol versus midazolam/meperidine

	Discharge		48 hours after procedure	
	Propofol	M/M	Propofol	M/M
Patient satisfaction[a,b]	9.3 (1.1)	8.6 (1.5)	9.4 (0.8)	8.5 (2.2)
Quality of sedation				
Excellent	37 (92.5%)	33 (82.5%)	21 (75.0%)	20 (69.0%)
Good	3 (7.5%)	6 (15.0%)	7 (25.0%)	7 (24.1%)
Fair	0 (0.0%)	0 (0.0%)	0 (0.0%)	1 (3.5%)
Poor	0 (0.0%)	1 (2.5%)	0 (0.0%)	1 (3.5%)
Adjustment in sedation[a]				
More sedation	0 (0.0%)	2 (5.0%)	0 (0.0%)	2 (S.9%)
Just right	40 (100.0%)	35 (87.5%)	28 (100.0%)	24 (82.8%)
Less sedation	0 (0.0%)	3 (7.5%)	0 (0.0%)	3 (10.3%)
Pain				
None	36 (90.0%)	33 (82.5%)	28 (100.0%)	27 (93.1%)
Mild	4 (10.0%)	4 (10.0%)	0 (0.0%)	1 (3.5%)
Moderate	0 (0.0%)	1 (2.5%)	0 (0.0%)	0 (0.0%)
Severe	0 (0.0%)	2 (5.0%)	0 (0.0%)	1 (3.5%)
Patient recall				
Insertion of colonoscope				
Yes	5 (12.5%)	8 (20.0%)	4 (14.3%)	2 (6.9%)
No	35 (87.5%)	32 (80.0%)	24 (85.7%)	27 (93.1%)
During procedure				
Yes	4 (10.0%)	8 (20.0%)	2 (7.1%)	3 (10.3%)
No	36 (90.0%)	32 (80.0%)	26 (92.9%)	26 (89.7%)
Removal of colonoscope				
Yes	10 (25.0%)	8 (20.0%)	5 (17.9%)	4 (13.8%)
No	30 (75.0%)	32 (80.0%)	23 (82.1%)	25 (86.2%)
Leaving procedure room[a]				
Yes	34 (85.0%)	17 (42.5%)	21 (75.0%)	8 (27.6%)
No	6 (15.0%)	23 (57.5%)	7 (25.0%)	21 (72.4%)
Subjective impairment[a]				
None			21 (80.8%)	15 (55.6%)
Mild			5 (19.2%)	9 (33.3%)
Moderate			0 (0.0%)	3 (11.1%)
Severe			0 (0.0%)	0 (0.0%)
Time spent sleeping over the next 24 h[a,b]			8.6 (1.4)	10.9 (2.9)

Abbreviation: M/M, midazolam/meperidine.
[a] $p < .05$.
[b] Continuous variables, mean (SD).

tests administered. There was also less subjective impairment noted by patients after discharge, with the propofol group reporting less impairment. Finally, there was a statistically significant difference in the average number of hours spent sleeping in the 24 hours after discharge (8.6 hours versus 10.9 hours, $P < .05$), with patients in the propofol group sleeping less than those in the midazolam/meperidine group.

In another study, Ulmer and colleagues [17] used midazolam and fentanyl in combination rather than midazolam and meperidine. In spite of the use of a shorter-acting opioid, this study again showed a statistically significant difference in the performance on neuropsychologic tests following the procedure, with patients in the propofol group performing better on every test. A decrease in the number of hours spent sleeping during the first 24 hours after the procedure again was demonstrated. Vargo and colleagues [26] also interviewed patients 24 hours after the procedure either in person or by phone to assess the return to normal activity level, cognitive function, and food intake. Patients receiving propofol showed earlier full recovery of both food intake and a normal activity.

From a patient standpoint, the physical and cognitive impairment from sedation ideally ends upon discharge from the endoscopy suite. Faster recovery from the effects of sedation translates into an earlier return to work and normal activities. Although patients feel alert and energized following propofol sedation, subtle neurocognitive deficits may occur and deserve further in-depth study.

Cost
In geographical areas where propofol is administered only by anesthesia providers, patients may face additional costs for propofol sedation if third-party payers do not reimburse for anesthesia services during endoscopy.

THE ANESTHESIOLOGIST'S PERSPECTIVE
Anesthesia providers are accustomed to using propofol for moderate/deep sedation and for induction/maintenance of general anesthesia. They are thus also more accustomed to seeing and treating the adverse effects of propofol at higher doses.

Effects of propofol
Some studies have suggested that propofol is associated with a subjective feeling of greater awareness after awakening, making it ideal for ambulatory procedures. Propofol also has antiemetic properties. In addition, it is associated with various excitatory behaviors, including muscle twitching, spontaneous movement, and hiccupping. Although such activity sometimes has been interpreted as seizure activity, propofol actually has anticonvulsant properties.

Propofol is a profound respiratory depressant and usually causes apnea following an induction dose. Propofol also inhibits hypoxic ventilatory drive and depresses the normal response to hypercarbia, even at the subanesthetic doses used during moderate and deep sedation. Propofol also induces a greater decrease in the cough and airway reflexes compared with thiopental [38]. The depression of airway reflexes is helpful during laryngoscopy, but may also place patients at higher risk of aspiration.

Propofol's narrow therapeutic index easily allows a patient to transition from a state of sedation where a patient is arousable and breathing (moderate sedation) to a state where a patient is unarousable and possibly apneic (deep sedation). Because there is no reversal agent available for propofol, the ability to recognize deep sedation immediately, and to support ventilation if necessary, is an essential skill for any provider to administer propofol safely. The patient might require no more than a chin lift, but also could require a jaw thrust, suctioning, mask ventilation, or intubation. The need for unplanned intubation is fortunately rare. When it is needed, however, any delay could be catastrophic.

Levels of sedation

Although a benzodiazepine and an opioid can produce a state of deep sedation, propofol is able to do so much more readily, and with a much more acceptable recovery time. Even when used only to produce a state of moderate sedation, however, propofol offers patients and gastroenterologists numerous advantages. It is important to distinguish between propofol administered with the intent of moderate sedation (low-dose propofol) and propofol administered deliberately to produce deep sedation.

When anesthesia providers administer propofol for endoscopy, they typically are targeting a state of deep sedation. Numerous endoscopists, in an effort to make propofol more readily available to their patients, and to reduce the costs associated with its administration, have supervised propofol sedation without an anesthesia provider present. Under these circumstances, some have gone to great lengths to ensure that propofol be given only in the low-dose range, thus staying within the limits of moderate sedation [33].

In a paper published by Cohen and colleagues [32] in 2003, guidelines were published in an attempt to clarify which patients were at low-risk for NAPS and what standards of care needed to be met to safely administer NAPS (Box 1).

When discussing whether nonanesthesia providers should be administering propofol, it will be necessary to clarify whether one is talking about low- or high-dose propofol. At this point, few have challenged that anesthesia providers are the most qualified to administer high-dose propofol.

Cost

In geographical areas where third-party payers reimburse for anesthesia services during endoscopy, providing propofol-based sedation for endoscopy represents an expansion of the practice of anesthesia outside the traditional locale of the operating room. As long as reimbursement continues, even when the indication for propofol is no more than endoscopist and patient preference for propofol, anesthesia providers have an incentive to make themselves available in gastroenterologists' offices. The opportunity for revenue generation is significant, as large numbers of cases may be done in a short period of time. Although this arrangement generally benefits patients, gastroenterologists, and anesthesia providers, third-party payers have faced sharply increased costs for anesthesia services. But is a preference by the patient and the gastroenterologist for propofol sedation a sufficient justification for its expense?

DESIGNING THE OPTIMAL SEDATION PLAN

How does one know what level of sedation a patient will require to tolerate his or her endoscopy? The amount of sedation required for endoscopic procedures is highly variable, and depends on procedural and patient factors.

Box 1: Protocol for administration of propofol during endoscopic procedures

Patient selection

Patients should be American Society of Anesthesiologists classes I–II. Class III patients may be included at the discretion of the endoscopist.

Patients who have a history of seizures or allergy to soybeans, eggs, or propofol are excluded.

Patients who have a history of sleep apnea; short, thick neck; inability to widely open their mouth; or a history of difficult intubation are excluded.

Patient monitoring

All patients receiving propofol should be monitored for Sao_2, heart rate, blood pressure, electrocardiogram, CO_2 levels, and respiratory rate. It is the responsibility of both the endoscopist and endoscopy nurse/assistant to monitor these physiologic parameters during the examination.

Chest excursion and respiratory effort will be monitored by the endoscopy nurse.

Supplemental oxygen is not routinely administered. If the Sao_2 drops below 90%, jaw or chin thrust should be performed. If the Sao_2 remains below 90% for 30 seconds despite these maneuvers, supplemental oxygen should be provided at 4 L/min.

Full resuscitation equipment must be available within easy reach in the endoscopy room.

Protocol for sedation

Administration of meperidine and midazolam

Age 70 years and under: meperidine 50 mg (or fentanyl 75 µg) and midazolam 1 mg intravenously

Age over 70 years: meperidine 25 mg (or fentanyl 50 µg) and midazolam 0.5 mg intravenously

Administration of propofol

Propofol (at a concentration of 10 mg/mL) should be drawn into a 5 or 10 mL syringe. In general, a 10 mL syringe is used for a healthy patient younger than 70 years, and a 5-mL syringe is used for patients 70 years or older. Initial bolus of 10 mg (1 mL) intravenously. Additional boluses of 5 to 10 mg may be given at 30- to 60-second intervals until an adequate level of sedation is achieved. In some instances, a 15 mg bolus may be given, based upon the patient's previous response to a smaller-sized bolus (5 to 10 mg).

Boluses may be given at 30- to 60-second intervals with the following parameters: SaO_2 greater than 90% and $ETCO_2$ less than 45 mm Hg

The physician is responsible for dosing decisions of all medication. The physician may request that the nurse administer medication. When this has been performed, the nurse should confirm verbally that the medication has been given by stating aloud "10 mg of propofol given."

Discharge criteria

Patient responds appropriately to questions.

Patient is able to sit upright for 5 minutes.

Patient is able to dress independently.

Procedural factors

The type of procedure that the gastroenterologist plans to perform greatly influences the level of sedation required. As noted previously, each procedure has its own stimulation profile, level of difficulty, duration, and potential complications. On average, simple endoscopies such as colonoscopy and upper endoscopy are technically easier, less stimulating, and shorter in duration than complex endoscopies such as ERCP and EUS. In addition, the experience and skill level of the endoscopist will affect the requirement for sedation and analgesia significantly.

Patient factors

Anxiety levels and individual differences in pain tolerance will strongly influence what drug should be given, and how much. Different patients may require different levels of sedation for the same procedure. In addition, different patients may not tolerate the same level of sedation equally well because of airway abnormalities or cardiovascular problems.

A patient who has a high level of preprocedure anxiety likely will require a deeper level of sedation to make the procedure possible. Similarly, a patient who has a lower threshold for tolerating pain is likely to require deeper sedation and analgesia. It can be difficult to quantify how much more drug will be a required for such patients. Also, patients with a history of substance abuse may require extremely high doses of drug to reach an adequate level of sedation. It is important to realize that the level of sedation required for a given procedure, and the amount of drug needed to produce that level, will vary greatly between individuals.

In addition to considering what level of sedation a patient will need, it is equally important to consider how much sedation a patient will tolerate. The ASA physical status of the patient may provide some guidance. According to the ASA, there is suggestive evidence that comorbidities are related to adverse outcomes in patients receiving either moderate or deep sedation. Patients who have coronary artery disease and/or impaired left ventricular function would be classified as ASA 3 or higher, as would patients with respiratory illness or morbid obesity. In such patients, hypotension and/or oxygen desaturation might be more likely to occur, and might require more prompt intervention to prevent adverse sequelae. Patients who have suspected gastroparesis, such as those with recent vomiting or long-standing diabetes, are likely to represent a higher aspiration risk, especially during upper endoscopy. If deeper levels of sedation are targeted in such patients, endotracheal intubation may be indicated.

Other conditions that may make endotracheal intubation the best strategy for managing deeper levels of sedation are sleep apnea and GI bleeding, both of which can lead to airway obstruction. Predictors of difficult intubation, such as small mouth opening, large tongue, short and/or thick neck, limited neck mobility, advanced Mallampati score, short thyromental distance, prominent incisors, stridor or hoarseness, craniofacial malformations, or a history of previous difficulty with intubation, should have a major impact on the selection of sedation plan. If such predictors were present, a reasonable approach would be either to target minimal-to-moderate sedation only, or if this is not anticipated to be adequate, perform a controlled intubation with advanced airway equipment (such as a fiberoptic scope) immediately available.

The optimal setting
Gastroenterologists often choose to perform endoscopy in high-risk patients in the hospital rather than the office setting, so that complications from the procedure and/or sedation may be handled more readily. Many high-risk patients will not be good candidates for propofol-based sedation because of a high potential for propofol-related respiratory and cardiovascular complications. They will be excellent candidates for care by anesthesia providers, however, who have a range of sedation and resuscitation techniques available to them. Some very high-risk patients, such as those expected to require invasive hemodynamic monitoring or fiberoptic intubation, may be best cared for in the highly controlled environment of the operating room.

IMPLEMENTATION
In order to ensure formulation of a reasonable plan for sedation and analgesia, and smooth and safe implementation, a reliable process needs to be set up for patient evaluation, sedation, monitoring, and recovery. In addition, the appropriate equipment and personnel need to be available. The ASA have published and revised a set of practice guidelines for sedation and analgesia, most recently in 2002.

Preprocedure evaluation
According to the ASA, appropriate preprocedure evaluation increases the likelihood of satisfactory sedation and decreases the likelihood of poor outcomes. The clinician administering the sedation should be familiar with aspects of the patient's medical history, which could interact with the sedation process. Preprocedure laboratory testing, such as ECG, should be guided both by the comorbidities of the patient and the likelihood that the results will affect the management of sedation and analgesia.

Monitoring
Standard monitoring during sedation and analgesia should include heart rate, blood pressure, respiratory rate, and oxygen saturation [39]. Monitoring of patient response to verbal commands should be routine during targeted moderate sedation, to make sure the patient has not inadvertently progressed to a state of deep sedation. Similarly, during targeted deep sedation, patient responsiveness to painful stimuli should be followed carefully, to ensure the patient has not drifted into a state of general anesthesia. Again, it is important to note that a response limited to reflex withdrawal from a painful stimulus is not a purposeful response, and may be indicative of general anesthesia. ECG should be monitored during moderate sedation if patient status warrants it, and during deep sedation in all patients. In addition to respiratory rate, adequacy of ventilatory function must be assessed continually.

If ventilation cannot be observed directly during moderate sedation because of patient position, or if deep sedation is targeted, then capnography should be used. It is recommended that an individual other than the practitioner performing the procedure administers the sedation, monitors its effects, and documents patient status.

Recovery room care

Following sedation and analgesia, patients should be observed in an appropriately staffed and equipped area until they are at or near their baseline level of consciousness and are no longer at risk for depressed cardiorespiratory function. Oxygenation should be monitored periodically until patients are no longer at risk for hypoxemia. In addition, ventilation and circulation should be monitored at regular intervals until patients are suitable for discharge. Finally, discharge criteria should be established to standardize the process and minimize the risk of complications following discharge.

WHO SHOULD ADMINISTER PROPOFOL FOR ENDOSCOPY?

Gastroenterologists have been administering sedation to their patients for over 20 years, initially with a benzodiazepines and opioids, and more recently, in the last decade, with propofol. From the guidelines issued by the ASA concerning the administration of sedation/analgesia by nonanesthesiologists, it is apparent that a very particular set of rules and requirements should be met to ensure the safety of the patient. Whether gastroenterologists should be administering propofol without the presence of an anesthesia provider has spurred much debate. Questions that have come up are:

> Should all patients, in the absence of medical contraindications, have the right to receive propofol sedation for endoscopy, given that propofol is associated with greater patient satisfaction?
> Are there enough anesthesia providers to give propofol sedation to all eligible patients undergoing endoscopy?
> Is low-dose propofol a meaningful concept? That is, is it possible to reliably administer propofol in such low doses that deep sedation has an acceptably low risk of occurring? And what is an acceptably low risk? Moreover, when, propofol is used only in this dose range, are patients and endoscopists as satisfied as when it is used in higher doses, producing deep sedation?
> If low-dose propofol is workable, should nonanesthesia providers be allowed to give it? If so, should they only be allowed to give it to low-risk patients? And what training requirements should these practitioners meet?
> What about the patients who are at high risk should unintended deep sedation occur, or who are anticipated to require deep sedation? Is it safe for nonanesthesia providers to target deep sedation with propofol?

Statements

Some guidance is provided by the following statements.

> "Because of the significant risk that patients who receive deep sedation may enter a state of general anesthesia, privileges to administer deep

sedation should be granted only to practitioners who are qualified to administer general anesthesia or to appropriately supervised anesthesia professionals. —Statement on granting privileges to nonanesthesiologist practitioners for personally administering deep sedation or supervising deep sedation by individuals who are not anesthesia professionals (ASA, October 18, 2006) [1].

"The involvement of an anesthesiologist in the care of every patient undergoing anesthesia is optimal. However, when this is not possible, nonanesthesia personnel who administer propofol should be qualified to rescue patients whose level of sedation becomes deeper than initially intended and who enter, if briefly, a state of general anesthesia." — Statement safe use of propofol (ASA, October 27, 2004) [40].

"Whenever propofol is used for sedation/analgesia, it should be administered by persons trained in the administration of general anesthesia, who are not simultaneously involved in these surgical procedures. This restriction is concordant with specific language in the propofol package insert, and failure to follow these recommendations could put patients at increased risk of significant injury or death." — Joint statement regarding propofol administration (American Association of Nurse Anesthetists [AANA]-ASA, April 14, 2004) [41].

"Propofol should be administered by persons trained in the administration of general anesthesia and not involved in the conduct of the surgical/diagnostic procedure." —Diprivan package insert (Astra-Zeneca, 2000) [42].

Note, one argument against the package insert warning is that propofol used for sedation is an off-label use that differs from its indication as an anesthesia induction agent, not a sedative. Thus, the warning only applies only to its indicated use, not to its off-label use. This has not yet been tested in the medicolegal system.

Data

There are not enough anesthesia providers to administer propofol for all endoscopy procedures. Moreover, anesthesia provider services can be costly. Thus, some gastroenterologists have ventured to make propofol more available, and at lower cost, by administering it themselves. How successful have they been?

In the last decade, multiple studies have evaluated the safety of propofol administration in the hands of gastroenterologists or gastroenterologist-supervised NAPS. In fact, many of the initial studies conducted to evaluate the superiority of propofol as a sedative for endoscopic procedures usually relied on nurse- or gastroenterologist-administered propofol without anesthesia supervision.

These are the data so far (Table 5).

SUMMARY

There is increasing evidence that propofol is the best agent available for providing sedation for most endoscopic procedures. Propofol takes the patient to the

Table 5
Safety of propofol-containing sedation regimens

First author	Sample size	Type of procedure	Sedation provider	Drugs	Depth of sedation	SaO2 <90%	SBP <90 mmHg	Apnea	AR	Cost
Carlsson [21]	45 45	EGD	Gastrointestinal (GI) physician	Prop. Midaz	—	4 4	0 0	0 0	0 0	— —
Krugliak [43]	15 17	Endoscopic retrograde cholangiopancreatography (ECRP)	Anesthesiologist	Prop. Midaz	Sleepy but arousable	0 0	0 0	0 0	0 0	— —
Koshy [27]	78 72 63 61	EGD Colonoscopy EGD Colonoscopy	CRNA CRNA GI Physician GI Physician	P/F M/M	Conscious sedation	11 3	36[a] 19[a]	0 0	— —	—
Vargo [26]	38 37	ECRP/ endoscopic ultrasound	GI physician	Prop. M/M	Spontaneous eye closure	14 21	6 7	10 16	0 0	$180 ± $75 $67 ± $33
Sipe [19]	40 40	Colonoscopy	Registered nurse	Prop. M/M	—	1 0	0 3	0 0	0 1	—
Rex [28]	2000	EGD/ Colonoscopy	Registered nurse	Prop.	Moderate[b]-Deep	16	0	5	0	—
Weston [31]	10 10	EGD	Registered nurse	Prop. M/M	Deep-GA[b] Mod-Deep[b]	0 1	1 0	0 0	0 0	— —
Ulmer [17]	50 50	Colonoscopy	Registered nurse	Prop. M/F	—	0 1	4 4	— —	1 0	— —

Study	No. of patients	Procedure	Provider	Drug	Level of sedation				
Heuss [35]	1370 ASA 3,4 / 642 ASA 1,2	EGD/Colonoscopy	Registered nurse	Prop.	Moderate[b]	23 / 11	113 / 81	4 / 1	– / –
Walker [30]	9152	EGD/Colonoscopy	Registered nurse	Prop.	–	3	–	3	–[c]
Cohen [32]	819	EGD/Colonoscopy	Registered nurse	Prop./M/M[d]	–	75	218[a]	0	0
Cohen [33]	100	EGD/Colonoscopy	Registered nurse	Prop./M/M[d]	Moderate	2	41[a]	0	–
Riphaus [22]	75 ASA ≥3 / 75 ASA ≥3	ERCP	GI physician	Prop. / M/M	Moderate–deep	8 / 7	6 / 4	– / –	– / –
Rex [29]	36,743	EGD/Colonoscopy	Registered nurse	Prop.	–	–	–	49	0
Vargo [34]	8129	Colonoscopy	Anesth.	MAC	Mild-GA	18[e]	–	–	5
	3554	Colonoscopy	GI physician	Prop.	–	4	–	–	4
	3762	EGD	Anesth.	MAC	Mild-GA	16	–	–	0
	2166	EGD	GI physician	Prop.	–	5	–	–	2

Abbreviations: AR, arrhythmia; EGD, esophagogastroduodenoscopy; GA, general anesthesia; –, not numerically noted; M/F, midazolam/fentanyl; M/M, midazolam/meperidine; P/F, propofol/fentanyl; Prop., propofol; SBP, systolic blood pressure.

[a] Decrease in SBP >20 mm Hg from baselines considered significant.
[b] Level not clearly specified, but inferred from description of target level by authors.
[c] Calculated on individual basis based on 50 patients receiving propofol and 50 patients receiving midazolam/meperidine before starting propofol protocol: propofol $42.80/case, M/M $48.36/case.
[d] Propofol/meperidine/midazolam used in combination; in 94 cases, fentanyl substituted for meperidine. MAC, monitored anesthesia care; unclear exact regimen of drug, not specifically noted.
[e] All numbers listed are for SaO2 of 95%, as selected by the authors.

desired level of sedation more quickly, provides better conditions for the endoscopist, results in fewer postprocedure sedation-related adverse effects such as nausea, and has a faster recovery profile. Some studies indicate that some combination of propofol with midazolam and/or opioids provides better sedation and analgesia and may also be safer because of a lower requirement for any of the individual drugs, most importantly propofol [33].

At this point in time, the standard for the administration of propofol is that it be administered by anesthesia providers. Anesthesia providers, when administering any level of sedation, bill for a service known as monitored anesthesia care (MAC). MAC is different from the simple provision of moderate sedation, in that the anesthesia provider makes a highly skilled assessment of which patients may be at increased risk for sedation-related complications, prepares for taking the patient to any level on the continuum of sedation that may be indicated, including general anesthesia, and anticipates any technical difficulties with airway and cardiovascular management. During MAC, the anesthesia provider may provide varying levels of sedation and analgesia, tailored to the unique considerations for each patient and procedure, and can rescue patients from any sedation-related complications by rapidly providing airway and cardiovascular support if necessary. This includes being prepared and qualified to convert to general anesthesia when indicated.

Some gastroenterologists believe that nonanesthesia providers can administer propofol to the desired level of sedation without compromising safety, in spite of the warnings from the manufacturer of propofol, the ASA, and the AANA. Studies with increasing sample sizes continue to appear in the medical literature, demonstrating a very small number of complications with gastroenterologist-directed and nurse-administered propofol sedation. Most of these studies involve low-risk patients and low-dose propofol. This represents a different level of service, requiring less expertise in managing patients along the sedation continuum, than MAC. Is it possible to provide a lower level of service using providers with less training? And if so, what criteria should be used for patient selection, and how does one ensure that protocols for low-dose propofol are reliable in not exposing patients to levels deeper than moderate sedation? Moreover, what backup systems should be in place? For example, should an anesthesia provider be immediately available? In that case, what about a hybrid model where an anesthesiologist oversees NAPS at an endoscopy center? Noncertified registered nurse anesthetists could administer propofol in 10 endoscopy rooms with 10 cases per room per day, resulting in 500 cases per week, or 25,000 cases per year. Even with this number of cases, based on published complication rates, the need for the anesthesiologist to intervene might be only a few times per year.

The question of whether an anesthesia provider needs to be present continuously at the bedside when (reliably) low-dose propofol is being administered to (appropriately assessed and risk-stratified) low-risk patients is not a simple one. The specialty of anesthesiology has the best record in all of medicine in terms of promoting patient safety. The protocols for NAPS, written with assistance from anesthesiologists, essentially propose the creation of a third tier of physician extenders in the specialty of anesthesiology, in addition to anesthesiologists and certified registered nurse anesthetists. Is this an acceptable patient care model? If so, it seems reasonable that anesthesiologists, as leaders of the specialty, should be involved closely in the training and supervision of such a third tier—for example as medical directors of endoscopy units using NAPS. In addition, reimbursement for this type of anesthesia service, essentially a step down from MAC in that it does not allow for (intentional) conversion from moderate sedation to deep sedation, would have to be negotiated with third-party payers.

In such a patient care model, there may be a temptation for endoscopists to request deep sedation during NAPS, to prevent stopping the procedure when moderate sedation is not enough. Sometimes moderate sedation, unexpectedly, is inadequate. In those cases, the appropriate response would be turning the case over to an anesthesia provider, if one is available to remain continuously at the bedside, or to reschedule the case with MAC. Gastroenterologists performing endoscopy in their offices, to avoid having to reschedule the procedures not successfully completed with NAPS, will have an incentive to use MAC rather than NAPS. Will third-party payers agree to the higher cost of MAC if they are able to save on the cost of facility fees typically charged in nonoffice settings?

Although it might be ideal to have a physician caring directly for every patient, physician extenders are taking on increasing levels of responsibility in every specialty of medicine. It is inevitable that the absolute requirement for an anesthesia provider to be present at the bedside whenever propofol is given will be questioned. Whenever that question arises, one has to respond in an evidence-based manner. At this time, there are insufficient to data to argue that propofol is equally safe when administered by nonanesthesia providers. The number of low-risk patients who have received low-dose propofol by nonanesthesia providers without complications continues to rise, however. As it gets higher and higher, the quality of the data has to be looked at very carefully. Are some complications going unreported, making the numbers falsely reassuring? And how do the numbers compare with the rate of MAC-related complications for endoscopy in similar low-risk patients? If NAPS becomes increasingly common practice, but is not implemented with the proper training, supervision, and quality control, one may see an epidemic of propofol-related morbidity and mortality. To reduce the likelihood of this happening, perhaps anesthesiologists should play an active role in regulating the practice of NAPS, setting standards, guiding policy, and overseeing safe implementation.

It is not clear that NAPS presents a serious threat to the practice of anesthesia. From a public health perspective, it could represent an opportunity for anesthesiologists to leverage their expertise, making higher quality sedation available to more patients without increasing risk. And there have been no serious challenges to the principle that an anesthesia provider should manage sedation and analgesia for GI endoscopy in high-risk patients and in patients expected to require deep sedation. If anesthesiologists choose to take on the role of providing training for and managing NAPS, it will be consistent with their role as perioperative care physicians skilled in crisis management and risk assessment.

References

[1] American Society of Anesthesiologists. Practice guidelines for sedation and analgesia by nonanesthesiologists. Anesthesiology 2002;96:1004–17.

[2] Butterly L, Olenec C, Goodrich M, et al. Colonoscopy demand and capacity in New Hampshire. Am J Prev Med 2007;32(1):25–31.

[3] Rex D, Imperiale T, Portish V. Patients willing to try colonoscopy without sedation: associated clinical factors and results of a randomized controlled trial. Gastrointest Endosc 1999;49: 554–9.

[4] Thompson DG, Lennard-Jones JE, Evans SJ, et al. Patients appreciate premedication for endoscopy. Lancet 1980;2:469–70.

[5] Daneshmend TK, Bell GD, Logan RFA. Sedation for upper endoscopy: results of a nationwide survey. Gut 1991;32:12–5.

[6] Keefe EB, O'Connor KW. 1989 ASGE survey of endoscopic sedation and monitoring practices. Gastrointest Endosc 1990;36(Suppl 3):S13–8.

[7] Keefe EB. Sedation and analgesia for endoscopy. Gastroenterology 1995;108:932–4.

[8] Faigel DO, Baron TH, Goldstein JL, et al. Guidelines for the use of deep sedation and anesthesia for GI endoscopy. Gastrointest Endosc 2002;56:613–7.

[9] Froehlich F, Thornens J, Schwizer W, et al. Sedation and analgesia for colonoscopy: patient tolerance, pain, and cardiorespiratory parameters. Gastrointest Endosc 1997;45:1–9.

[10] Mahajan RJ, Johnson JC, Marshall JB. Predictors of patient cooperation during gastrointestinal endoscopy. J Clin Gastroenterol 1997;24:220–3.

[11] Magni VC, Frost RA, Leung JW, et al. Randomized comparison of midazolam and diazepam for sedation in upper gastrointestinal endoscopy. Br J Anaesth 1983;55:1095–101.

[12] Whitwam JG, Al-Khudhairi D, McCloy RF. Comparison of midazolam and diazepam in doses of comparable potency during gastroscopy. Br J Anaesth 1983;55:773–7.

[13] Bailey P, Pace N, Ashburn M, et al. Frequent hypoxemia and apnea after sedation with midazolam and fentanyl. Anesthesiology 1990;73:826–30.

[14] Rex DK. Review article: moderate sedation for endoscopy: sedation regimens for nonanesthesiologists. Aliment Pharmacol Ther 2006;24:163–71.

[15] Gamble JA, Kawar P, Dundee JW, et al. Evaluation of midazolam as an intravenous agent. Anaesthesia 1981;36:868–73.

[16] Hansen JJ, Ulmer BJ, Rex DK. Technical performance of colonoscopy in patient sedated with nurse-administered propofol. Am J Gastroenterol 2004;99(1):52–6.

[17] Ulmer BJ, Hansen JJ, Overley CA, et al. Propofol versus midazolam/fentanyl for outpatient colonoscopy: administration by nurses supervised by endoscopists. Clin Gastroenterol Hepatol 2003;1:425–32.

[18] Bell GD. Premedication and intravenous sedation for upper gastrointestinal endoscopy. Aliment Pharmacol Ther 1990;4:103–22.

[19] Sipe BW, Rex DK, Latinovich D, et al. Propofol versus midazolam/meperidine for outpatient colonoscopy: administration by nurses supervised by endoscopists. Gastrointest Endosc 2002;55:815–25.

[20] Faulx AL, Vela S, Das A, et al. The changing landscape of practice patterns regarding unsedated endoscopy and propofol use: a national Web survey. Gastrointest Endosc 2005;62(1):9–15.

[21] Carlsson U, Grattidge P. Sedation for upper gastrointestinal endoscopy: a comparative study of propofol and midazolam. Endoscopy 1995;27:240–3.

[22] Riphaus A, Stergiou N, Wehrmann T. Sedation with propofol for routine ERCP in high-risk octogenarians: a randomized, controlled study. Am J Gastroenterol 2005;100:1957–63.

[23] Jung M, Hofmann C, Kiesslich R, et al. Improved sedation in diagnostic and therapeutic ERCP: propofol is an alternative to midazolam. Endoscopy 2000;32:233–8.

[24] Wehrmann T, Kokabpick S, Lembcke B, et al. Efficacy and safety of intravenous propofol sedation during routine ERCP: a prospective, controlled study. Gastrointest Endosc 1999;49:677–83.

[25] Krugliak P, Ziff B, Rusabrov Y, et al. Propofol versus midazolam for conscious sedation guided by processed EEG during ERCP: a prospective, randomized, double-blind study. Endoscopy 2002;32:677–82.

[26] Vargo JJ, Zucarro G, Dumot JA, et al. Gastroenterologist-administered propofol versus meperidine and midazolam for advanced upper endoscopy: a prospective, randomized trial. Gastroenterology 2002;123:8–16.

[27] Koshy G, Nair S, Norkus EP, et al. Propofol versus midazolam and meperidine for conscious sedation in GI endoscopy. Am J Gastroenterol 2000;95:1476–9.

[28] Rex DK, Overley C, Kinser K, et al. Safety of propofol administered by registered nurses with gastroenterologist supervision in 2000 endoscopic cases. Am J Gastroenterol 2002;97:1159–63.

[29] Rex DK, Heuss LT, Walker JA, et al. Trained registered nurses/endoscopy teams can administer propofol safely for endoscopy. Gastroenterology 2005;129:1384–91.

[30] Walker JA, McIntyre RD, Schleinitz PF, et al. Nurse-administered propofol sedation without anesthesia specialists in 9152 endoscopic cases in an ambulatory surgery center. Am J Gastroenterol 2003;98:1744–50.

[31] Weston BR, Chadalawada V, Chalasani N, et al. Nurse-administered propofol versus midazolam and meperidine for upper endoscopy in cirrhotic patients. Am J Gastroenterol 2003;98:2440–7.

[32] Cohen LB, Dubovsky AN, Aisenberg J, et al. Propofol for endoscopic sedation: a protocol for safe and effective administration by the gastroenterologist. Gastrointest Endosc 2003;58:725–32.

[33] Cohen LB, Hightower CD, Wood DA, et al. Moderate-level sedation during endoscopy: a prospective study using low-dose propofol, meperidine/fentanyl, and midazolam. Gastrointest Endosc 2004;59(7):795–803.

[34] Vargo JJ, Holub JL, Faigel DO, et al. Risk factors for cardiopulmonary events during propofol-mediated upper endoscopy and colonoscopy. Aliment Pharmacol Ther 2006;24:955–63.

[35] Heuss LT, Schnieper P, Drewe J, et al. Safety of propofol for conscious sedation during endoscopic procedures in high-risk patients—a prospective, controlled study. Am J Gastroenterol 2003;98:1751–7.

[36] Clarke AC, Chiragakis L, Hillman LC, et al. Sedation for endoscopy: the safe use of propofol by general practitioner sedationists. Med J Aust 2002;176(4):158–61.

[37] Qadeer MA, Vargo JJ, Khandwala F, et al. Propofol versus traditional sedative agents for gastrointestinal endoscopy: a meta-analysis. Clin Gastroenterol Hepatol 2005;3:1049–56.

[38] Brown GW, Patel N, Ellis FR. Comparison of propofol and thiopentone for laryngeal mask insertion. Anaesthesia 1991;46:771–2.

[39] American Society for Gastrointestinal Endoscopy. Guidelines for conscious sedation and monitoring during gastrointestinal endoscopy. Gastrointest Endosc 2003;58:317–20.

[40] American Society of Anesthesiologists statement on safe use of propofol. 2004. Available at: http://www.asahq.org/publicationsAndServices/standards/37.pdf. Accessed October 27, 2004.

[41] AANA-ASA joint statement regarding propofol administration. Available at: http://www.asahq.org/news/propofolstatement.htm. Accessed April 14, 2004.

[42] Diprivan 1% [package insert]. Wilmington (DE): Astra-Zeneca; 2000.

[43] Krugliak P, Ziff B, Rusabrov Y, et al. Propofol versus midazolam for consious sedation guided by processed EEG during endoscopic retrograde cholangiopancreatography: a prospective, randomized, double-blind study. Endoscopy 2000;32(9):677–82.

Advances in Anesthesia 25 (2007) 127–142

ELSEVIER
MOSBY

ADVANCES IN ANESTHESIA

Challenges in Practice Management

Joanne Conroy, MD[a],*, Kevin Barry, MD[b]

[a]Morristown Memorial Hospital/Atlantic Health, 100 Madison Avenue,
Box 112, Morristown, NJ 07962-1956, USA
[b]Morristown Memorial Hospital, 100 Madison Avenue, Box 1,
Morristown, NJ 07962-1956, USA

A new era is beginning that will test the skill and expertise of anesthesia leadership in practice management. All components of the not-for-profit health care systems are experiencing workforce shortages, decreasing operating margins, and greater degrees of governmental regulation. Survival requires adept financial leadership and the ability to partner. Porter and Teisberg [1] emphasize in their book *Redefining Health Care*, that "the US health care system is on a dangerous path with a toxic combination of high costs, uneven quality, frequent errors, and limited access to care." The magnitude of the problem seems overwhelming without a quick fix using traditional solutions of consolidation and cost shifting. Anesthesia practices fortunately are well positioned to address these challenges proactively. Challenges fall into four broad categories: (1) understanding and delivering value, (2) mastering throughput and customer service, (3) competing on quality, and (4) partnering. Attention to basic business principles in each of these categories by anesthesia leadership will allow anesthesiologists to maximize success in the market place.

UNDERSTANDING AND DELIVERING VALUE

As defined by Porter and Teisberg [1] in *Redefining Health Care*, "Patient value is the compass that must guide the strategic and operational choices of every provider group, hospital, clinic, and physician practice." Value is defined as the health outcomes achieved per dollar of cost to peers. This view is a change from the historical perspective, where "practitioners, hospitals researchers, and medical schools enjoyed a broad grant of authority to run their own affairs" [2] and where physician compensation was protected from both competition and cost controls. Providers in health care have been very effective in resisting change and homogenizing breakthrough ideas and practices. Regulatory, economic and consumer-driven demand are driving a value proposition that will change everyone practices, however.

*Corresponding author. *E-mail address*: joanne.conroy@atlantichealth.org (J. Conroy).

0737-6146/07/$ – see front matter
doi:10.1016/j.aan.2007.07.003

This article reviews the approaches to creating value, how to be competitive in the marketplace and maintain margin in the value economy through realigning compensation systems, incentives, and billing compliance.

Creating value in anesthesia

Group practices in anesthesia traditionally reward dedicated service time rather than measuring and rewarding productivity. This is a natural consequence of governmental and payer procedures that pay for service delivery without any attention to value. The focus on isolated aspects of care is the perspective of many advocacy groups, medical societies, and credentialing organizations, which because of their charge, consider the needs of their specialty before the needs of the health care system as a whole. Negotiating change with the multiple stakeholder silos has slowed the progress of change. Future challenges will include defining the anesthesiologist's contribution according to medical conditions, organizing into Porter's IPUs (integrated practice units) [1], and developing information systems that will allow anesthesiologists to record, evaluate, improve and then demonstrate to payers added value. Anesthesiologists will have to participate in accurate cost accounting of the entire continuum of care, to understand and then deliver the highest value and best outcomes. This will require both hospital and physician commitment to understanding and controlling combined costs.

Getting a seat at the table

Longnecker [3] identified in his 1996 editorial that many economic arguments do not consider the value of anesthesiologists in the health care system. He points out that the future of the practice will depend on demonstrating value back to the hospital and/or patients, involving anesthesiologists in preoperative preparation and postoperative care of patients, administering the operating room, and taking a lead in critical care management and acute and chronic pain management. Although anesthesiologists have been asked by hospital partners to select their intraoperative medications judiciously, they must be included in administrative teams that focus on controlling the overall cost of care [4]. Unfortunately, present regulations and reimbursement systems have served to drive hospitals and practitioners apart rather than create collaborative teams. The challenge will be to address today's practice management issues while positioning anesthesiologist groups to adapt to and take the lead in new integrated approaches to care. This requires an understanding of future economic trends and the development of group governance, clinical processes, and internal compensation plans that will encourage collaborative behaviors.

Understanding one's competitiveness

In order for a group to compete in the market place, one must maximize value (ie, the ratio of quality delivered/market price/cost of care delivery [Q/P/C]) [1]. Quality is an elusive measurement that is affected by multiple variables. The American Society of Anesthesiologists (ASA) has been involved with the National Quality Forum (NQF) to ensure the validity of the quality measurements developed by the NQF. Market practice prices will become more transparent as anesthesiologists participate in developing risk-adjusted cost profiles of providers. Finally, costs will be tracked, adjusted for productivity, and made specific to the practice setting. Tracking capability is and will be very important in negotiating third-party payer contracts. The public demand for transparency in all medical costs will include anesthesia fees. This process, already underway, will be implemented over the next 5 years.

This trend toward some form of transparency in the cost of health care services is not unique to United States. Health care systems throughout the world are grappling with continually rising health care expenditures. In an article by Dahmen and Albrecht [5], the authors describe a fee-per-capita system in Germany that was introduced in 2003 to keep the budgets for hospital care within limits. On August 22, 2006, President George W. Bush signed an executive order to help create transparency in health care costs. This order directs federal agencies that administer or sponsor federal health insurance programs to share with beneficiaries information about prices paid to health care providers for procedures, quality of services, to develop and identify approaches that facilitate high quality and efficient care, and to release Medicare payment information for individual health care providers. There will be a move to single bills for episodes of care replacing a system of separate reimbursement for each doctor and hospital unit of service. Stanford University has experimented with this, resulting in over $1 million dollars per month reduction in bad debt write-offs, a 14% decrease in billing costs, and improved Press Ganey scores [6]. The focus is now on overall cost rather than one specific segment of cost, and care is being integrated across facilities and specialists. The transparency of costs will serve as a stepping stone for the growth of health savings accounts (HSAs) [7]. The higher deductibles and copays will create greater patient awareness of cost and quality.

Until the Q/P/C ratio can be standardized and calculated, less precise benchmarks must be used. A useful resource for private practice groups is the Medical Group Management Association's "Cost survey for anesthesia practices: 2005 report based on 2004 data" [8]. For academic centers, the authors recommend the work of Amr Abouleish and colleagues [9–11]. He provides numerous methods for measuring productivity. Although an in-depth discussion of the topic of benchmarking is beyond the scope of this article, a few cautions are worth noting. The validity of the data should be verified. Confirm that the benchmark is specific to the group's practice. Finally, remember that an individual's productivity and the group's productivity are different; therefore, do not compare individual practitioner benchmarks to the group's productivity or vice versa.

Current compensation formulas and future compensation formulas to reward value

The three most common mechanisms of reimbursement for anesthesia practices today are fee-for-service/productivity, capitation, and salary. None of these create group or individual incentives for a value-driven system. The quality of anesthesia care being delivered today is not because of a system of compensation, but it reflects the personal ethics and commitment to quality of individual practitioners and the specialty. Group practice and compensation plans will need to change to reward value. This creates a unique opportunity for anesthesiologists to become the facilitators of a P4P model in their institution.

Designing a compensation system that rewards value and measuring individual and group contribution is a challenge [12]. A value-added compensation system will need to include rewards for patient safety, clinical effectiveness, efficiency, research, and the performance of administrative responsibilities and duties. These rewards can be in the traditional forms of time, (vacation and nonclinical) money (salary, benefits, and bonuses for goals achieved), academic rank, job security. The formulas created by various practices need to be reevaluated and adjusted to meet the changing needs of both the external and internal economic forces.

There are economic challenges if one does not balance the change process while maintaining institutional margins. A recent Wall Street Journal article described an example at the Virginia Mason Medical Center (VMMC) in Seattle. The VMMC had made aggressive measures to cut health care costs to deliver a better value at the request of its largest insurers. Unfortunately for the institution, although the employers and health care plans saved money, Virginia Mason's losses started accumulating rapidly. Their chief of medicine described the situation as right "between the trapezes" [13].

Incentives

In his 2005 article on academic anesthesia faculty salaries, incentives, availability, and productivity in anesthesia and analgesia, Miller [14] reviewed historical compensation plans based on rank or clinical time. Academic practices have moved to clinical incentives and/or productivity-based incentives, but find it difficult to recruit and retain faculty where there are competitive private practice salaries and a need for anesthesiologists in the community. A 2005 survey of over 80 academic departments [15] found that nearly 70% had some type of incentive by which faculty could earn extra money. These incentives come in many forms and can be divided into those based on availability versus those based on productivity [15]. An anesthesiologist's ability to be clinically productive in the time assigned to an operating room is often a function of the external workload, the speed with which the surgical staff works, and other nonanesthetic factors. Productivity-based incentives often are dependent on the total amount of clinical care delivered. At the University of San Francisco, Miller [14] allocates extra nonclinical time rather than direct financial incentives to advance research and educational initiatives. The solutions are not easy.

The success of incentives in academic departments and private practices lies in identifying the correct clinical productivity measure that results in additional faculty compensation, without disincentivizing young investigators. The result should be better alignment of anesthesiologists, surgeons, and hospital administrators around systems and cost efficiency. Abouleish and colleagues [15] goes into great detail in his review of these systems of performance-based compensation based on productivity measurements. He identifies that anesthesiologists rarely control the number of patient visits, procedures, productivity of surgeons, or operating room schedule use. Despite many of these obstacles, most departments have implemented, drafted, or considered incentive plans. The most common incentive plan is based on charges. Net charges were used by six groups. Some use time as a basis for incentive programs. He emphasizes that most academic and private practice groups still do not measure clinical productivity. In a 2005 survey [16] performed by the AAA (Anesthesia Administrator Assembly of the Medical Group Management Association).

> "two-thirds of private practice groups use equal share compensation plans in which the revenue (is) split equally among partners regardless of any individual productivity management" [15].

These salary models do not measure continued productivity, but assume that the work will be distributed equally.

How does one create a value-based system in this environment? The most important consideration for a department is to determine which clinical activities should be incentivized. Any measurement of productivity will value and devalue specific clinical services and activities. The integration of pain management services and critical care services are often difficult to incorporate in these systems, but provide great value to the institution. In his review of incentive plans, Lubarsky [17] identified that people always act "in a rational self interest, therefore, incentives almost always work perfectly to provide behavior that's rewarded, assuming the incentive is large enough." The challenge is to define those behaviors that truly deliver value.

Total compensation beyond salary. . .keeping the workforce

In addition to considering incentives, practice leaders have to examine total compensation packages, including wages, health benefits, pretax flexible spending accounts for health and child care, retirement, expense accounts, and administrative support to pursue managerial, research, and scholarly activities. Anesthesia groups with over 50 employees must meet additional expectations of paid time off and adhere to the regulations of the Federal Family Leave Act (FMLA). They must create pension plans and vesting formulas that are applied fairly to all employees, with employer and employee contributions that comply with the Employee Retirement Income Security Act of 1974 (ERISA).

Anesthesiologists, like those in many other hospital-based subspecialties, have tried to anticipate shifts in their work force. Most anesthesiologists dedicate between 50 and 60 hours per week to their practice. Another hospital-based specialty, radiology, is trying to assess their future workforce issues. Although there is a subsegment of practitioners who indicate that they would like to work forever, in a large survey of radiologists [18], 9% indicated that they would like to make a career change at some future point; 41% answered that they plan to work part time, and 46% intended to retire at a specific age.

For those who plan a career change, the mean age for change was 53. Those who plan to work part time indicated an intention to work part time at age 57. Those who intended to retire at a specific age indicated a mean retirement age of 61 years, although 10% of this group indicated they would like to work to 68 years or older. The authors believe that there are many parallel workforce trends in anethesiology.

An article by Katz [19] identifies similar career transitions for anesthesiologists with comparable age triggers for considering retirement. He identified that physicians in general tend to deny issues involving their own aging and delay retirement planning until late in their professional lives. Anesthesiologists as a group are relatively proactive compared with other physicians. A growing number of anesthesia practices are establishing phased retirement plans. As Katz [19] describes, "this type of arrangement, (which) is essentially a shared or part-time position, has proved to be practical and effective among anesthesia residents. Formal agreements permit senior members of the group to slow down by eliminating certain aspects of their practice" [19]. The agreement can be advantageous to the group by continuing to engage the senior partner in an environment where he or she feels most vibrant, but also allow some additional income to flow to younger members of the department. The most challenging aspect, of course, is creating a formula that equitably values an individual's time. Katz [19] points out that "financing for retirement also depends on resources available, including social security, pension, deferred income, and personal savings. Most retiring anesthesiologists indicate that the majority of their retirement income will come from pension" [19]. In terms of health care after retirement, many anesthesiologists choose to participate in their health plan at a negotiated rate for up to 18 months after leaving practice under COBRA (The Consolidated Omnibus Budget Reconciliation Act of 1986). After termination of this benefit, they will be covered by Medicare Part A, need to seek coverage under Medicare Part B, and often require supplemental commercial policies. Anesthesiologists, like other physicians, are not methodical in considering long-term care in their retirement planning. In general, private health insurance covers very little toward long-term care, and Medicare pays little toward prolonged hospitalization beyond 90 days or confinement in a skilled nursing facility. These are some aspects of the total compensation plan that large anesthesia groups may have to address in more detail in the future.

Core benefits in academic or hospital employment models are generally more robust and include a medical plan, vision plan, prescription plan, dental plan, basic life and disability plan, flexible spending account, short-term disability coverage, tuition reimbursement, paid time off, and cash balance pension plans. Many also offer supplemental life, 403Bs, and 529 college savings plans. There are some other unique benefits such as child and elder care resources, legal services, financial services, adoption resources, concierge, college planning, health and wellness programs, family and life workshops, savings bonds, credit unions, homeowner's insurance, on-site fitness and day care centers, and direct deposit. In negotiating benefits and managing one's back office costs, bigger is better. Aligning with a consortium of anesthesia groups or a hospital provider can offer a tremendous advantage.

Practice structure and alignment around value

There are certain basic models of anesthesia practice:

- Private practice in alignment with a hospital, which may or may not support the group with stipends and/or employment of anesthesia extenders
- Academic practice, where the department is in a separate physician practice association that may be an exclusive provider of service to the institution
- Office-based practice with little association with a hospital
- Hospital-employed practice

The future delivery of health care will become more dependent on the interaction and collaboration between hospitals and physician providers. This will require sharing of information, creation of integrated care processes, and even pooling of payments. This will result in an evolution of practice models. Regardless of the practice type, it is essential that anesthesiologists develop solid business principles and a political strategy [20]. The success of anesthesiologists' future in a P4P arena requires practitioners to develop political and business strategies on a professional society level that shape the future rather than react to it. Anesthesiologists need to simultaneously develop adaptive strategies that can be quickly executed in the face of change [21].

Billing compliance

In an article of the American College of Physicians, Gesenway [22] reviewed lessons learned by Philadelphia institutions that underwent an Office of the Inspector General investigation. She emphasized that "documentation in the medical record that is sufficient for clinical purposes was not necessarily sufficient for billing purposes." Those that were fined were subject to institutional compliance agreements in which they agreed to a complete system overhaul of current billing practices; mandated attendance at educational programs on billing, coding, and compliance on a yearly basis; creation of a practice compliance office; and annual audits with significant additional fines for inadequate documentation. Additionally, a teaching physician had documentation that a supervising physician was present when the service was performed by a resident. For anesthesia, the requirements are physical presence for all critical portions of the case, the preoperative, and the postoperative assessment. Many academic institutions complain that this is difficult to enforce and that changing tenured physician behavior while grappling with medical staff due process is impossible. Some institutions have implemented rules that physicians cannot bill for their services if they fail to attend annual billing compliance sessions. The development of compliance standards is not only essential to have in place before any external government audit, but is simply a good business practice. The internal auditing of these standards should lead to the immediate correction of any deficiencies. Internal auditing and immediate correction of deficiencies are extremely important and protect the group and institution from penalties and ensure a group's future financial stability.

CUSTOMER SERVICE AND THROUGHPUT

Legislation and payment methodologies have served to separate hospitals and physicians in the past. Fortunately, there are many more forces now at work that are driving collaboration and shared incentives over throughput efficiencies, pricing transparencies, and quality. Market factors over the past decade have created financial challenges for teaching hospitals, community hospitals, and their affiliated anesthesia groups. Factors include the growth in complexity of cases, poor reimbursement for hospital based care, increased competition with ambulatory surgery centers for low risk, short duration cases, and decreasing numbers of anesthesiologists entering the workforce. Professional revenues for anesthesiologists are often insufficient to support rising salaries and costs associated with maintaining a healthy practice. The Clinical Advisory Board in 2004 [23] published a comprehensive abstract that described ways in which the shortage of anesthesiologists eventually could limit hospital growth. Board members identified the multiple flash points of conflict with the hospital and said that working through a formal anesthesia contractual relationship was a way to discuss the impact of these issues. The exclusive contract should address the group's desire to practice in neighboring hospitals or freestanding ambulatory surgery centers and expected performance standards on quality and throughput. There should be explicit agreement on benchmarks, a termination clause that defines the length of the agreement, an obligation for giving notice, and finally, a service provision, which is the specific amount and type of anesthesia coverage. These contractual relationships often leave nothing to the imagination and may build in work week requirements, work load expectations for anesthesiologists, and incentives. In managing the work day for anesthesiologists, there are shared responsibilities including management of the operating room, the efficiency of the preoperative evaluation process, the management of emergent cases, how the hospital deals with case delays and cancellations, and whether ancillary services in the hospital contribute to this. Inefficient turnover time in the operating room creates down time and loss of revenue for the anesthesiologists, all of which result in lower hourly rate for the anesthesiology group providing services. The authors assume maximum productivity would include offloading noncore activities, using down time strategically, and improving operating room efficiency.

COMPETING ON QUALITY

Anesthesiologists traditionally have participated in specialty-specific national efforts in patient safety and decreasing liability. The ASA Closed Claims project frequently is identified as an example of medical quality improvement at its best—changing the practice patterns nationally and aligning hospitals and physicians in a standards-based effort to decrease death and injuries associated with surgical anesthesia. In his 2000 article, Glance [24] went over market forces and legislative mandates that are shaping the face of health care. He pointed out that changing the proportion of physician to nonphysician anesthesia providers could achieve the lower cost, but could result in compromised patient outcomes. He described each of four care team models that vary according to the participation and role of physicians and nurse anesthetists. The first team model is physician-intensive. In the second team, model physicians anesthetize all high- risk patients. Intermediate-risk patients are anesthetized by an anesthesia care team with a physician-to-certified registered nurse anesthetist ratio of one to two. Low-risk patients are anesthetized by an anesthesia care team with a physician-to-certified registered nurse anesthetist ratio of one to four. Glance [24] concluded that the second team model and the physician-intensive (first team model) model have equivalent outcomes. All other models have higher mortalities. The second team model is the least expensive. This example only serves to emphasize the importance of examining data and outcomes and working as a team on new paradigms that deliver greater value.

Anesthesia information systems will be a critical factor in determining the impact of anesthesia practices on surgical outcomes. These systems also will allow costs to be managed better. This will require participation in a shared network of anesthesia and hospital information systems, where statistical analyses of large populations can be performed. Any system needs to have six critical success factors:

- The quality of the system
- The quality of information
- The frequency of system use
- User satisfaction
- An impact on the individual in terms of ability to perform his or her job,
- A positive organizational impact [25]

Organizational culture can interfere with the development of group best practices and the effective use of anesthesia information systems. The authors anticipate there will be government mandates for physician reporting by 2010 and an expansion of practice-based electronic medical record systems. Although specifics are being debated, hospitals can share in the software cost for the development of office-based patient health records until 2013. Hospital-based anesthesia systems that are owned by the institution will not have this limitation. Electronic anesthesia record system quality is improving dramatically, as is the ability to interface with equipment and various hospital system platforms. These information systems will help define cohorts of patients, compare the outcomes under different anesthesia variables, evaluate patient hemodynamics, and factor in comorbidities. Contributing aspects of the anesthetic to patient outcome also will be able to be identified. These systems will also allow anesthesiologists to better evaluate the total cost of providing such care in the system as a whole.

In a European study, Arbous and colleagues [26] reviewed records of those who died within 24 hours or remained comatose 24 hours after the anesthetic in search of a relationship of anesthesia with the patient condition. Of the anesthesia-related deaths, most were associated with cardiovascular management, ventilatory management, patient monitoring, or inadequate preparation of patient. These variables contributed to nearly 75% of the deaths. It is just one of the many papers that emphasize the importance of retrospective analysis of outcomes and the use of information to prospectively change how anesthesiologists care for patients.

In an 2003 article in *Health Affairs*, Hatley and Sheridan [27] identified the additional need for medical liability and government payer reform to be truly patient-centric in the approach to preventing injury and decreasing costs. A significant obstacle to true patient transparency is a legal system that can be adversarial and has normalized hiding information about risk. He wrote, "What results is a health care culture that lives in fear—or often—denial about the ability to prevent errors completely yet is complacent about or afraid of doing what is possible to contribute to system-wide learning and injury prevention" [27]. He emphasized that "although accidents attributable to error will never be eliminated, many sectors have engineered dramatic reductions" through initiatives such as Six Sigma and continuous quality improvement.

PARTNERING

The Clinical Advisory Board in 2004 published a comprehensive abstract regarding hospital-based anesthesia challenges in the future [23]. They identified that direct subsidies may be unavoidable for hospitals with a low commercial payer mix, especially when commercial cases comprise less than 40% of inpatient surgery. In completely clinical environments, the most effective subsidy models encourage anesthesiologists' productivity and provide additional incentive for each incremental case an anesthesiologist covers. The abstract provides numerous formulas by which to examine commercial-to-noncommercial volume ratio, weekly operating room volume, additional revenue from activities like pain management, and additional expense for obstetric and preanesthesia assessment services. There are multiple subsidy models covered in the research including:

- A productivity-based subsidy (provides escalating subsidies based on clinical research and teaching hours)
- A performance-based subsidy (identifies certain performance metrics)
- A conversion factor subsidy (maintains competitive hourly rates with neighboring hospitals)
- An operating room use subsidy
- An income guarantee
- A flat fee subsidy (identifies the delta between the market compensation and the revenue generated from services)
- A recruiting subsidy (allows anesthesia groups to offer more attractive recruitment packages)
- A certified registered nurse anesthetist subsidy (to cover the cost of employing certified registered nurse anesthetists)

This type of methodical analysis is necessary to support quality anesthesia practices, considering the tremendous hospital revenues and profits at stake.

In this abstract, the Advisory Board group identified one small hospital where the revenue generated by a single operating room was in excess of $6 million dollars a year [23]. Important additional initiatives include creating a more effective use of operating room capacity, which should result in easier scheduling and greater convenience for surgeons and patients. The key is to recruit talented nursing and physician staffs to run the operating rooms as collaborative teams and create more effective ways of delivering care.

There has been an increasing demand for institutional leadership, operating room management, and a nondegree education in business administration for anesthesiologists. In many areas, business experience has become much more relevant. Two areas that should be core management skills for anesthesia physician leaders are the ability to build consensus and a win–win approach to negotiations [28].

Stipends

There are many advantages to having a negotiated agreement on stipends for various services provided to the hospital. About 57% of the United States facilities provide one or more stipends to the group [16]. Facilities in the Northeast and the West are most likely to receive a stipend, and approximately three quarters of trauma centers pay stipends to the anesthesia group providing services. The stipend amount varies, with most under $1 million dollars. The most common academic stipend is between $500,000 and $1 million dollars per year. A third of the survey respondents were from private practice; these respondents reported a private practice stipend of approximately 20% to 30% of the academic mean stipend. Forty percent of stipends are intended to compensate the group for providing direct patient care services that cannot be covered by professional billing. These include general call coverage, obstetric anesthesia, trauma, acute pain management, and cardiac services. Another third of stipends are paid for medical director services. It appears, however, that the differences in support amounts are distinctly more regional than in prior surveys. Although some groups are commanding large stipends due to skyrocketing expenses and poor payer mix, others are finding themselves in a more competitive situation where they must agree to less attractive contractual terms or engage in competition within their facility to retain their practices. Greater group partnering with their hospital or facility and their support of each other during negotiations with third-party payers often lead to better terms for both the group and the facility. This ultimately improves the profitability and competitiveness of both and sets a working relationship for future improvement of quality of care requiring mutual support. It is essential that physicians partner with their institutions and jointly build an infrastructure that will allow them to practice high-quality medicine.

Exclusive contracts

The negotiation of an exclusive contract has not been viewed as an exercise in partnering by many anesthesia groups. Instead, these contracts have been viewed as a tool to force hospital-based physician groups into submission.

Enlightened administrations have realized that to attract quality specialty physicians, hospitals must provide for high-quality, hospital-based acute care services. The exclusive gives the hospital an advantage in that one group manages the department and ensures a level of service and quality outcomes. The advantage to the group is that its members can practice in an environment without competition from multiple providers of service. Exclusive contracts are used most commonly for the subspecialty services of anesthesiology, radiology, pathology, and emergency medicine. We have seen an emerging trend of exclusive agreements in areas where alignment along cost and quality control is an imperative. Although there are numerous articles identifying the potential pitfalls with exclusive contracts, the use of exclusive arrangements is still quite prevalent. Berstein [29] has authored numerous ASA newsletter articles on this issue. She notes that contract negotiations are more difficult than they were a few years ago, because "pressures on medical centers have been climbing as they have been for physician practices." About 55% of hospitals use exclusive contracts, as do many independent ambulatory surgery centers, although their contract terms are somewhat different [30]. The portion of anesthesiologists in nonexclusive settings has increased from 5% to 14% in the last 4 years. Seventy-four percent of the groups, however, are exclusive providers of services, even though only 55% of all groups have a written exclusive contract. Most of the groups have had their current arrangement for over 10 years, although 19% report that the relationship has changed in the last 2 years [16].

A good exclusive contract contains a provision requiring the hospital to offer the group the exclusive opportunity to provide anesthesia services at any of its locations such as a freestanding ambulatory surgery center. Other areas of interest that often are delineated in the contracts include in-house coverage requirements, malpractice insurance, and exclusive contracts for the pain clinic. Unfortunately, some exclusive contracts still are used to push initiatives instead of serving as written confirmation of a negotiated agreement. Most exclusive contracts have coverage obligation, which can change with new circumstances (ie, the creation of a new program, new operating room, or change in trauma level). The group should be able to temper the effect of any of these developments by obtaining additional concessions to maintain its profitability. It is not unusual for hospitals to seek the authority to insist that anesthesia groups participate in every health plan in the hospital network. Most groups try to limit their obligation to making a good faith effort or establish a floor in negotiating an agreement with payers. There are often specific causes for termination, and hospital privileges commonly are tied to the possession of the exclusive. Experience has shown that hospitals and groups mitigate this risk by delineating circumstances under which an individual's privileges will be revoked and those in which the entire group breaches the contract. The hospital also may agree to revoke privileges only when a subsequent exclusive contract with another anesthesiology group goes into effect. Increasingly, hospitals seek to commit their anesthesiology groups to practice at their facilities exclusively. Unfortunately, this creates financial consequences for the group. Preventing anesthesiologists from providing services in an ambulatory setting where reimbursement is higher, especially if the hospital's case volumes are declining, only serves to lower the group's profitability, and ultimately the level of service provided to the institution.

Hospital relationships are very different in many ways than they were even 5 years ago, and they continue to evolve. It is recommended that anesthesiology groups increase their sophistication in recognizing difficult contract provisions and develop positive working relationships with their hospitals. Crafting proposals that benefit both parties is the real win–win.

SUMMARY

Over the next 5 to 10 years, there will be many changes in the way health care is delivered. The Institute of Medicine's (IOM) latest monograph [31] is titled *Rewarding Provider Performance*, and it will be published this year. The report makes specific recommendations regarding changes to the health care delivery system. Although the report is not explicit in terms of its implications for anesthesiology, it broadly involves all providers. The report calls for the systematic and deliberate use of payment incentives. Pay-for-performance programs (P4P) are used effectively in many countries, with the greatest use in the United Kingdom, Australia, and New Zealand. United States use is currently at 30%, one of the smaller percentages of involvement in the developed world. The report calls for widespread use of an electronic medical record (EMR), which should include an anesthesia EMR, public reporting of outcomes, and incentives for beneficiaries. The IOM advisory group made 10 recommendations, many of which affect anesthesia providers. One of these recommendations was to establish a series of demonstration projects to determine the effectiveness of P4P programs. A number of these are already underway. The IOM discussed funding sources for performance incentives from the existing funds. Much of the report discussed combining funding sources across institutional silos to incentivize collaborative behaviors (ie, combining Medicare parts A and B). This would drive interdisciplinary collaboration and information sharing to produce higher-quality, patient-centered, and cost-efficient care. The report additionally calls for monitoring of outcomes focused on quality, cost, and customer service. The incentives initially will reward both high and most improved performers, but eventually will reward only high performers. The report outlines incentives for submission of physician data effective this year, which will become mandatory for all providers by 2010. They propose rewarding the coordination/coordinator of care. They support the national campaign to incentivize office-based use of the EMR until 2013 when the providers will have to bear the cost of EMR maintenance.

As Porter and Teisberg [1] discuss in their book, *Redefining Health Care*, the premise is that excellence in patient care will lead to greater access to care, greater efficiency, and higher margins. The financial viability of an institution cannot be the goal of the system redesign, but it will be an outcome. They identify eight imperatives for all providers:

- Redefine the business around medical conditions.
- Choose a range in the type of services that provided.
- Organize around medically integrative practice units.
- Create a distinct strategy for each unit.
- Measure results, experience methods, and patient attributes by the unit.
- Move to single, consolidated bills, and new approaches to pricing and pricing transparency.
- Market service based on excellence, uniqueness, and results.
- Grow locally and geographically in areas of strength.

Some of these will be challenges for anesthesia providers in that their practices are defined in terms of a specific service or a specialty rather than a medical condition. This view, however, is more doctor-centric than patient-centric. What has become evident to both payers and providers is that the real value depends on the performance of many people. A perfect example of this occurs daily in the operating room, where many participate in achieving the best outcome, including the surgeon, anesthesiologist, nurse, radiologist, and skilled technician, among others. The real value depends on everyone performing well. The entire care cycle will now be the focus and only will be as strong as the weakest component. This will not eliminate the need for large specialty-specific provider groups, but it will change how anesthesiologists operate. The constituent hospitals, clinics, and physician practices operate largely in their own silos.

"In a value-based health care system, (these) provider groups will retain a role only if they can demonstrate excellent results...and medically integrate services across the entities in the group. Rather than duplicating care and relying on bargaining power, care delivery must be radically restructured, or groups will lose market share once they have to compete on value" [1].

All providers face important strategic decisions on how to structurally align themselves with a health plan into a vertically integrated organization. Kaiser Permanente has been a commonly cited example. Other vertically integrated groups include Sentera Health care and Intermountain Health care. Vertical integration mitigates the adversarial relationship between a health plan and provider and allows the incentives to be better aligned. There are problems with the vertically integrated model, however. As Porter and Teisberg [1] point out, combining a health plan with the provider network eliminates or suppresses the competition at the provider level, where it matters most. Combining insurance and provision of services essentially creates a system of global capitation, which "creates a strong incentive to reduce costs via limiting services, because the health care system receives a fixed amount per provider." Success comes more from a process by which physicians and hospitals interact with each other than from any fixed employment or partnership model. Success is determined less by a model of care than by the execution of process that goes with it [32]. It seems that every decade brings a new model or structure promising to deliver quality, efficient care across the spectrum of providers. It was a promise of managed care; it was the promise of integrated networks, and today many argue that it is the model of consumer-driven choice and outcomes-based P4P. No matter what model ultimately prevails, however, the relationships with physicians are central to success. Physicians have many choices. They can choose to go into small private practice, large group practice, work under the umbrella of an organization like Kaiser, join an academic practice model, or be hospital employees. They can be competitors or part of the team. There are some trends pushing physicians toward employment models, including increasing costs and complexity of private practice and lifestyle considerations. There always are going to be a broad mix of physicians, however, and some subset of these will want to be in private practice. Hospitals will need to continue to have multiple ways of working with physicians, if for no other reason than physicians are perhaps by nature contradictory people. There are fewer are hassles and less paper work in multispecialty groups, but surveys show that control and autonomy are still of paramount importance to physicians. This requires a certain amount of flexibility from hospitals. More importantly, hospital systems will need to treat physicians as partners in a continuum of care. Giving them a meaningful role in decision making, building trust, and emphasizing good communication are all critical aspects. Fixed salary, regular hours, and administrative relief are important and attractive components, but the most successful models go further than that. They build strong relationships with physicians by equipping them with the infrastructure to be better at what they really want to do, practice medicine.

References

[1] Porter M, Teisberg E. Redefining health care: creating value-based competition on results. Boston (MA): Harvard Business School Press; 2006. p. 17, 98–101, 156, 157, 162, 167.

[2] Starr P. The social transformation of American medicine. New York: Basic Books, Persus Books Group; 1982. p. 379.

[3] Longnecker D. Planning the future of anesthesiology. Anesthesiology 1996;84(3):495–7.

[4] Watcha M, White P. Economics of anesthetic practice. Anesthesiology 1997;86(5): 1170–96.

[5] Dahmen K, Albrecht D. An approach to quality management in anaesthesia: a focus on perioperative care and outcome. Eur J of Anaesthesiol Suppl 2001;18(S23):4–9.

[6] Hammer DC. Adapting customer service to consumer-directed health care: by implementing new tools that provide greater transparency in billing, hospitals can decrease collection costs while improving customer satisfaction. Healthc Financ Manage 2006;60(9): 118–22.

[7] Ferman JH. Price transparency. Healthc Exec 2006;21(4):48–50.

[8] Medical Group Management Association. Cost survey for anesthesia practices: 2005 report based on 2004 data. Englewood (CO): MGMA; 2005.

[9] Abouleish AE. Designing meaningful industry metrics for clinical productivity for anesthesiology departments. Anesth Analg 2003;96:802–12.

[10] Abouleish AE, Zornow MH, Levy RS, et al. Measurements of individual clinical productivity in an academic anesthesiology department. Anesthesiology 2000;93:1509–16.

[11] Abouleish AE. Benchmarking your group's clinical productivity: survey says. ASA Newsl 2006;70(4):26–7.

[12] Weschler J. Pay for performance. Managed Healthcare Executive 2006;30–2.

[13] Fuhrmans V. A novel plan helps hospital wean itself off pricey tests. Wall Street Journal Friday, January 12, 2007. p. 1 and 11.

[14] Miller R. Academic anesthesia faculty salaries: incentives, availability, and productivity. Anesth Analg 2005;100:487–9.

[15] Abouleish A, Apfelbaum J, Prough D, et al. The prevalence and characteristics of incentive plans for clinical productivity among academic anesthesiology programs. Anesth Analg 2005;100:493–501.

[16] Blough G, Scott S. Hospital. Contracting survey update. 2005 Practice Management Conference. Available through the ASA at: www.ASAhq.org. Accessed in 2005.

[17] Lubarsky D. Incentivize everything, incentivize nothing. Anesth Analg 2005;100:490–2.

[18] Deitch C, Sunshine J, Chan W, et al. How US radiologists use their professional time: factors that affect work activity and retirement plans. Radiology 1995;194:33–40.

[19] Katz J. Issues of concern for the aging anesthesiologist. Anesth Analg 2001;92:1487–92.

[20] Souba WW, Weitekamp MR, Mahon JF. Political strategy, business strategy, and the academic medical center: linking theory and practice. J Surg Res 2001;100:1–10.

[21] Courtney H, Kirkland J, Viguerie P. Strategy under uncertainty. Harv Bus Rev 1997;75(6): 66–79.

[22] Gesensway D. American College of Physicians Observer, September 1996.

[23] Espino S, Stetzer A. Navigating the anesthesia shortage: ensuring sufficient coverage to enable procedure growth. In: Clinical advisory board flashpoint handbook. Washington DC: The Advisory Board Company; 2004. p. 2–6, 64–71.

[24] Glance L. The cost effectiveness of anesthesia workforce models: a simulation approach using decision–analysis modeling. Anesth Analg 2000;90:584–92.

[25] Van Der Meijden M, Tange H, Troost A. Determinants of success of in-patient clinical information systems: a literature review. J Am Med Inform Assoc 2003;10(3):235–43.

[26] Arbous M, Grobbee D, van Kleef J, et al. Mortality associated with anaesthesia: a qualitative analysis to identify risk factors. Anaesthesia 2001;56:1141–53.

[27] Hatlie M, Sheridan S. The medical liability crisis of 2003: must we squander the chance to put patients first? Health Aff (Millwood) 2003;22(4):37–40.

[28] Russell G. The anesthesiologist as physician executive. Curr Opin Anaesthesiol 1999; 12(4):429–31.

[29] Bierstein K. Pros and cons of exclusive contracts. ASA Newsletter 2006;70(8).

[30] Bierstein K. Hospital contracts survey: 2004 data. ASA Newsletter 2005;69(4).

[31] Institute of Medicine. Rewarding provider performance: aligning incentives in Medicare (Pathways to quality health care series). Washington DC: National Academies Press; 2007.

[32] Temes P. Physician hospital relationships. Fairfield (CT): ILO Institute On Call Research Report; 2006.

Advances in Anesthesia 25 (2007) 143–187

Advances in Pediatric Pain Management

Kim-Phuong T. Nguyen, MD[a,b], Nancy L. Glass, MD, MBA[a,b,*]

[a]Baylor College of Medicine, Houston, TX, USA
[b]Department of Pediatric Anesthesiology, Texas Children's Hospital, 6621 Fannin Street, Suite A300, MC 2-1495, Houston, TX 77030, USA

S ince the beginning of the twenty-first century, there has been a groundswell of interest in effective pain management for children, reflecting an appreciation of the psychologic and neurodevelopmental impact of unrelieved pain on our smallest patients. New understanding about the ontogeny of pain pathways in the developing brain and the importance of neural plasticity provide researchers with a sense of urgency to improve the management of perioperative pain.

At the bedside, clinicians have more experience in the use of the patient-controlled analgesia (PCA) modality, whether administered by patient or proxy. The advantages of this technique have now been extended to regional anesthesia, which now enjoys greater implementation and success with the advent of ultrasound techniques and stimulating catheters.

Finally, the acceptance of multimodal analgesia has caught on in pediatrics, because using several techniques together provides for good analgesia while minimizing the most onerous side effects of each. In this article, the authors discuss commonly used oral pain medications, nonsteroidal anti-inflammatory drugs (NSAIDs), intravenous opioids, including PCA therapy, nontraditional analgesics and adjuncts, alternative routes for analgesia, and regional analgesic techniques.

We also recognize the essential inclusion of nonpharmacologic approaches to perioperative pain. Perioperative teaching, parental presence, good positioning and physical measures, high-quality sleep, physical therapy, and Child Life interventions should all be components of the pain management plan, although we are unable to address those strategies here. Likewise, developmental and cognitive-behavioral approaches may significantly contribute to the management of anxiety, depression, and pain. The assessment and management of

*Corresponding author. Department of Pediatric Anesthesiology, Texas Children's Hospital, 6621 Fannin Street, Suite A300, MC 2-1495, Houston, TX 77030. *E-mail address:* nglass@bcm.edu (N.L. Glass).

0737-6146/07/$ – see front matter
doi:10.1016/j.aan.2007.07.002

chronic pain syndromes is also beyond the scope of this article, except as it affects the management of pain in the acute perioperative setting.

PAIN ASSESSMENT

The necessity for being able to measure pain and follow its course in children has led to a great deal of interest in pain rating scales. Developmental differences compound the difficulties of measuring pain, such that investigators have proposed many different pain-assessment tools. Self-report scales, as in adults, have been proposed as the gold standard, yet may be inapplicable for preverbal or developmentally delayed children. Other rating systems include behavioral (observational) and physiologic scales. Each type of scale has its own advantages and disadvantages, and probably measures different aspects of the child's pain experience. Self-report scales may have biases attributable to previous experiences and underlying personality. Behavioral or observational scales may measure global distress rather than pain intensity, whereas physiologic scales may measure nonspecific signs of arousal instead of pain [1].

A comprehensive discussion of pain rating scales is beyond the scope of this article, and yet a working knowledge of the most widely accepted scales is required for planning and monitoring the effectiveness of the pain treatment plan. The reader is referred to an excellent recent review of pediatric behavioral pain rating scales by von Baeyer and Spagrud [1]. The first well-developed observational scale was the CHEOPS tool, which scores six elements on a scale of 0 to 3 with a maximum score of 13; this tool has been found to have excellent interrater reliability for ages 4 months through 17 years, and has been used in many studies of brief procedural or surgical pain [2]. For the perioperative period and for brief procedural pain the FLACC tool, similarly scoring five elements on a scale of 0 to 2 with a maximum score of 10, first described by Merkel and colleagues [3], is simple to apply and also has good interrater reliability. Originally described for children 4 to 8 years of age, subsequent investigators have validated its use for children from 0 to 18 years [3]. Other scoring systems have been developed to assess parents' perception of children's pain at home after surgery, pain in ventilated or sedated children in the intensive care setting, and neonates [4–7]. Rating pain in premature and neonatal patients requires a different set of tools just for this age group; the reader is referred to a recent review of the use of neonatal pain scoring systems in the management of neonatal perioperative pain [8].

Unfortunately, there is little evidence of concordance between self-report scores of pain and behavioral measures of pain in young children. Beyer and colleagues [9] compared pain responses using two self-report tools, the Oucher and the Analog Chromatic Continuous Scale, to those obtained using the CHEOPS behavioral scale in 25 children ages 3 to 7 years undergoing surgery. The self-report scales trended together over time and demonstrated an expected course over the first 36 hours postoperatively; however, there was little relation between the self-report of pain intensity and the observable behavioral elements. For this reason, the behavioral scoring systems cannot be considered in isolation when evaluating pediatric pain, because many children do not exhibit the typical behavioral signs of stress.

INDIVIDUAL VARIATION IN REQUIREMENTS FOR PAIN MEDICATION

All clinicians have observed unexplainable variations in the amount of pain medication required for a given surgical stimulus. What determines these variations in pain perception and the subjective response to pain? Kain and colleagues [10] have demonstrated that which has been up to this point only intuitive and anecdotal: children who are anxious before a surgical procedure have a rockier recovery period and require more pain medication than those who are calm and relaxed. Logan and Rose [11] studied the relationships among patient and parent anxiety, expectations about pain for the upcoming procedure, and PCA use in a group of adolescent patients undergoing major surgery. They found that in this population, the patient's expectations for postoperative pain were more highly correlated with morphine consumption than was anxiety; the most anxious patients, perhaps hesitant of overusing the pain medication, had fewer PCA demands and a higher ratio of successful doses to demands. The same authors looked at gender differences in pain responses in a group of adolescent surgical patients [12]. Adolescent girls were more anxious and anticipated more pain before surgery than boys. Similarly, girls had higher minimum and average daily pain scores than boys, although the highest daily scores and PCA use were similar.

Crawford and colleagues [13] retrospectively examined opiate administration by PCA in two groups of children undergoing laparoscopic cholecystectomies—children who had sickle cell disease (SSD), and those who did not. For the same surgical procedure, patients who had SSD reported higher pain scores and used twice as much morphine as those without SSD; they required parenteral opiates for a longer period of time and had a longer hospital stay. The authors hypothesize that the differences in opiate use might have reflected tolerance related to previous administration of opiates, central sensitization from repeated episodes of vaso-occlusive pain, or differences in pain perception.

These studies emphasize the limitations in our understanding of how children and adolescents respond to the pain and stresses of the perioperative environment. Pain and anxiety are but two of the identified responses to the surgical experience, and measuring pain medication use is only a poor surrogate for the ability to quantify that stress.

MULTIMODAL ANALGESIA

Kehlet and Dahl [14] were the first to describe the term "multimodal" analgesia in 1993. The term refers to combining analgesic agents and techniques with different mechanisms of action, with the goal of improving analgesia and minimizing side effects. The practice has become standard in anesthetic practice for children and adults, although there are few studies critically examining the outcomes in children or defining the most appropriate combinations for specific surgical procedures.

PREEMPTIVE ANALGESIA IN CHILDREN

The potential for preemptive analgesia, specifically defined as techniques that alter the central processing of the afferent impulses, to modulate postoperative pain has been a focus of research for many years. Ong and colleagues [15] make the distinction between this definition of preemptive analgesia and interventions that occur before surgery, the effects of which may linger into the postoperative period. Most basic research has concentrated on interrupting pain signals at the spinal cord level, modulating central sensitization, or blunting the peripheral inflammatory reaction to surgical stimulus. Although it has been possible to demonstrate a beneficial effect of different interventions in laboratory animals, it has been more difficult to demonstrate an impact in the clinical arena, in which some studies show a positive effect and others show a negative or inconclusive effect.

In one meta-analysis of more than 3,000 adult patients, Ong and colleagues [15] found that epidural analgesia was the most efficacious at reducing pain scores and reducing and delaying the need for supplemental analgesia; local anesthetic wound injection before surgery and administration of NSAIDs were less effective, and the administration of opioids and systemic NMDA receptor antagonists showed an equivocal effect. In their elegant two-part article on preemptive analgesia, Kelly and colleagues [16,17] make several important clinical points about preemptive analgesia: regional blockade should be continued until significant afferent input has decreased, or else regional blockade only delays rather than prevents postoperative pain; NSAIDs may play a particularly important role in minimizing the inflammatory response and peripheral sensitization; and opioids, alpha-2 agonists, and ketamine may act synergistically rather than additively to enhance analgesia and prevent central sensitization.

In pediatric anesthesia, Langer and colleagues [18] showed early on that intraoperative ilioinguinal and iliohypogastric nerve injections with bupivacaine improved early outcome and postoperative pain at home in 99 children undergoing inguinal hernia repair; however, the block did not extend through the period of inflammatory response. Giannoni [19] showed some evidence of preemptive analgesia by injecting the tonsillar bed before tonsillectomy with a combination of ropivacaine and clonidine, because the reduction in pain and the opiate requirement outlasted the local anesthetic block. Others, however, have failed to demonstrate preemptive analgesia in regional blockade models, including greater auricular nerve block before or after tympanomastoidectomy [20], retrobulbar block for children undergoing strabismus surgery [21], and axillary block before or after hand or forearm surgery [22].

Using systemic agents, it has also been difficult to demonstrate preemptive analgesia in pediatric studies. Becke and colleagues [23] were unable to show evidence of preemptive analgesia in a blinded study comparing an infusion of S-ketamine at 5 µg/kg/min with a control group following major urologic surgery in children 1 to 12 years of age; morphine consumption was similar, although early reductions in pain scores may have reflected the sedative nature of ketamine. Similarly, Rose and colleagues [24] did not find a preemptive effect of two different doses of oral dextromethorphan on postoperative pain or opiate requirement in a group of children undergoing tonsillectomy.

Whether these studies fail to show an effect of preemptive analgesia, or whether our ability to measure protective effects is inadequate, key questions regarding preemptive analgesia in children demand rigorous study. Which interventions are most successful, and for which procedures? Can these interventions be successful in our current milieu of ever-shorter hospital stays? And perhaps most importantly, will we be able to prevent the development of prolonged or chronic pain syndromes in children by intervening in a proactive manner?

ORAL PAIN MEDICATIONS
Acetaminophen
Acetaminophen is the mainstay of pediatric care for mild pain relief and the foundation for basal analgesia in a multimodal therapy plan (Table 1). The reader is directed to a comprehensive review of acetaminophen and nonsteroidal anti-inflammatory agents used in children [25]. In the perioperative setting, acetaminophen is frequently administered by the rectal route in young children following the induction of anesthesia. Work by Coté and others has demonstrated that a rectal dose of 40 mg/kg is necessary and sufficient to achieve effective analgesic plasma levels [26]. Subsequent work by the same group led to

Table 1				
Oral analgesics for perioperative pain				
Drug	Single dose	Frequency	Daily max	Notes
Acetaminophen	10–15 mg/kg po or 40 mg/kg pr (1st dose only), then 10–15 mg/kg	q 4 h	75 mg/kg	Multiple preparations, including drops, suspension, chewable tabs, suppositories
Ibuprofen	10 mg/kg	q 6 h	40 mg/kg	Tabs, suspension
Naproxen	7 mg/kg initial, then 5 mg/kg	q 12 h	15 mg/kg	Tabs, suspension
Meloxicam	0.125–0.25 mg/kg po	Once daily	15 mg	Supplied as 7.5- and 15-mg tabs, suspension 7.5 mg/5 mL
Ketorolac	0.5 mg/kg IV, max 15 mg/dose	q 6 h	60 mg	Only for 5 days per month
Tramadol	1–2 mg/kg	q 4–6 h	8 mg/kg	Only available in po tablet form in United States, 50 mg

their recommendation that the initial dose be followed by 20 mg/kg every 6 hours to maintain plasma levels within the target range of 10 to 20 µg/mL [27].

In neonates, the effective absorption of acetaminophen after rectal or oral administration seems to be nearly the same, but both are delayed in infants less than 3 months of age when compared with older infants and children [28]. Preterm infants and neonates seem to be at a lower risk for acetaminophen toxicity because of lower activity of cytochrome P450 and other enzymes necessary for conversion of acetaminophen into toxic metabolites. For preterm infants between 30 and 60 weeks' postconceptual age, an oral loading dose of 25 mg/kg achieves the target plasma level for analgesia, but subsequent dosing depends on gestational age; rectal dosing is more variable by age and preparation. The reader is referred to a helpful reference for acetaminophen dosing in this age group [28].

Clinicians must be clear in their communications with parents about acetaminophen dosing after the surgical procedure so that the total daily dose remains well below the recognized toxic dose of 150 mg/kg/day in an otherwise healthy child. Practitioners should be ready to recognize the signs and symptoms of acute acetaminophen toxicity and to respond appropriately by administering *N*-acetylcysteine [29]. For oral therapy, limiting the total daily dose to 75 mg/kg has been advocated [30].

An intravenous form of paracetamol (acetaminophen) is now available outside the United States. Approved for use in children older than 1 year of age for the treatment of mild to moderate acute pain, it is administered every 6 hours as a 15-minute infusion [31]. Rapidity of onset and the ability to bypass the gastrointestinal tract are obvious advantages of this preparation, and its tolerability and efficacy have compared favorably with opiate therapy for children undergoing tonsillectomy [32] and dental restorations [33].

Nonsteroidal anti-inflammatory drugs

NSAIDs are useful agents that can be co-administered with opiates or regional blocks as a means of minimizing opiate requirements and opiate side effects following surgery. There are various preparations with differing profiles, and it is important to recognize that the drugs in this class are heterogeneous in structure, mechanism of action, and metabolism. Ibuprofen, for instance, is available in several formulations for pediatric use, and has antipyretic, anti-inflammatory, and analgesic actions. Oral dosing is frequently used postoperatively, although there is only one study demonstrating its efficacy in this setting in infants [34]. Rectal administration of ibuprofen 20 mg/kg following induction of anesthesia has been shown to achieve therapeutic blood levels of at least 10 µg/dL within 40 minutes, peaking at 1 to 2 hours in infants, and remaining greater than 10 µg/dL in most patients for more than 8 hours [35].

For the acute perioperative period, selecting ibuprofen as part of a multimodal analgesic plan is a practical choice, particularly for peripheral or musculoskeletal surgery. For those children who have conditions likely to result in longer-lasting pain syndromes, the convenience of using longer-acting agents may improve compliance and pain relief. Naproxen requires only twice-daily dosing but has been associated with a scarring, porphyria-like rash that occurs in as many as 10% of arthritis patients, particularly in fair-skinned individuals; to our knowledge, this has not been reported in children who do not have rheumatologic disease [36,37]. An alternative choice for a longer-acting agent that we have used for selected patients is the selective COX-2 inhibitor meloxicam, which is only given once a day and has no effect on platelet function [38]. There are no studies comparing the analgesic effects of the different NSAIDs, but naproxen and meloxicam were equivalent in efficacy and safety in a large group of children who had juvenile idiopathic arthritis [38].

Compared with adults, children have less difficulty with the recognized complications of NSAID therapy. To date, the risk for remote cardiovascular complications in children taking NSAIDs for long periods of time is unknown. Exacerbation of asthma following exposure to NSAIDs is less common in children than in adults, with a prevalence of 2% in one randomized provocation study [39]. Despite this lower risk, worsening asthma may follow a challenge with ibuprofen; consequently, such agents should be used with caution in this population, or other agents may be substituted [40]. Others have suggested that, in fact, the pediatric asthma patient may benefit from the antipyretic effects of these agents [41]. Gastrointestinal intolerance for the NSAIDs is also much less common than in adults; one study of more than 700 children found only four instances of significant gastrointestinal complications [42,43].

Likewise, renal dysfunction related to NSAIDs is less common in children than has been reported in adult patients, who may be more likely to present with intrinsic renal disease. Acute renal failure has been reported in previously healthy adolescents following NSAID consumption, however. In one series of seven adolescents, all of the affected patients took more than one type of NSAID; six of the seven reported vomiting or decreased oral intake before presentation, although only one demonstrated mild clinical dehydration at presentation [44]. All exhibited nonoliguric renal failure that presented with flank pain, and renal function returned to normal without dialysis in all of the patients within 2 weeks.

NSAIDs have a recognized effect on platelet aggregation and bleeding time, such that many clinicians limit their administration during neurosurgical, plastic, or otorhinolaryngology procedures. A recent Cochrane database review examined the issue of postoperative bleeding after tonsillectomy in children who received NSAIDs, reviewing 13 studies that included 955 patients [45]. They found no increase in post-tonsillar bleeding requiring reoperation and no increase in the number of nonsurgical bleeding events; however, there was less nausea and vomiting among those children who received NSAIDs.

There was considerable enthusiasm, if a paucity of controlled studies, concerning the early adoption of the selective COX-2 inhibitors for pediatric perioperative care. Several reports of rofecoxib's opioid-sparing effects in the absence of increased surgical bleeding suggested that this class of agent might be useful for tonsillectomies and other surgeries in which postoperative bleeding was a concern. Sheeran and colleagues [46] performed a double-blind, randomized, placebo-controlled study of rofecoxib in children undergoing outpatient adenotonsillectomies, giving either rofecoxib or placebo before the procedure. In their study of only 45 patients, the authors were unable to demonstrate lower pain scores or a morphine-sparing effect in the rofecoxib group, although no patient in either group experienced postoperative bleeding. Rofecoxib was taken off the market in 2004 following publication of evidence that it increased the risk for cardiovascular events in adults. Whether or not it would have had deleterious effects on children cannot be conjectured, but disappearance of rofecoxib from the market has had a chilling effect on the use of celecoxib in the perioperative period in children also.

Comparing the efficacy of acetaminophen and ibuprofen, a recent meta-analysis of 17 controlled trials involving at least 900 patients for each medication demonstrated equal effectiveness of the two for analgesia in children [47].

Combination agents

Fixed combinations of non-opiate analgesics with oral opiates have long been used for home therapy following surgery in children. The most commonly prescribed choices are acetaminophen combined with codeine, oxycodone, or hydrocodone. Although these agents have a long history of popular use, the clinician is advised to calculate carefully the amounts of acetaminophen provided if the patient takes all of his or her allowed as-needed doses. For older children and adolescents, there are now more choices with respect to the opiate strength, so that more of the opiate can be administered without exceeding the recommended daily dose for acetaminophen. Relatively new on the market are combinations of ibuprofen with hydrocodone and oxycodone; these preparations are significantly more expensive than similar combinations with the acetaminophen base. Neither ibuprofen-based medication is available in a suspension form for young children, and there are no pediatric studies comparing the analgesic effectiveness of these agents with the more commonly prescribed acetaminophen-based preparations.

Patients frequently complain of "allergy" to these combination agents when the reported side effect is nausea and vomiting. In our experience, there are fewer complaints of GI distress with hydrocodone or oxycodone than with codeine, although there are no data in children to suggest a difference. Taking the medication with food or switching from one preparation to another may solve these individual variations. All patients should be counseled about the constipating effects of oral opiates, which limit their suitability for long-term consumption.

Oral opiates

There are multiple preparations of oral opiates without acetaminophen or ibuprofen on the market in short-acting and long-acting forms, including morphine, hydromorphone, and methadone. Morphine and methadone are available in concentrated liquid preparations also. None of these has a role in acute perioperative pain management, except in patients who are already taking them when they present for surgery.

PARENTERAL OPIATE AND OPIOID THERAPY

Intravenous administration of opiate medications has largely replaced intramuscular administration for pediatric patients (Table 2). Opioid agents useful in perioperative pain management include morphine, fentanyl, hydromorphone, and methadone. The highly lipid-soluble agents sufentanil and alfentanil, important for intraoperative care, are less important for postoperative pain. Remifentanil is also more useful for intraoperative than postoperative pain, but may influence postoperative management.

Finally, we discourage the use of meperidine for postoperative pain in children. It has few, if any, advantages, and carries with it the risks of agitation, tremors, hallucinations, and postoperative seizures with the accumulation of its primary metabolite 3-nor-meperidine [48,49].

For a comprehensive review of opiate therapy and pharmacokinetics in infants and children, the reader is referred to an excellent review recently published by Jablonk and Davis [50].

Morphine

Morphine is the drug to which all other analgesics are compared. Injection of morphine in a dose of 0.1 to 0.2 mg/kg is followed by a remarkable calming of the young patient's cry, even though the peak effect occurs 20 to 30 minutes later. Young infants are particularly sensitive to the respiratory depressant effects of morphine, so smaller doses should be titrated to effect. By 2 months of age, clearance of morphine is similar to that in adults. For effective analgesia, intermittent doses must be available every 2 hours for older infants and children, because the serum half-life is 2.9 ± 0.5 hours [50]. For younger infants, dosing every 3 hours should be sufficient.

Fentanyl

Fentanyl is 80 to 100 times more potent than morphine. Because of its lipid solubility, fentanyl has a faster onset than morphine and a shorter duration of action, unless large or repeated doses are given. With repeated dosing or continuous infusions, fentanyl is redistributed to the peripheral compartment, from which it must be mobilized for elimination later. As is the case with morphine, neonates and preterm infants are particularly sensitive to the effects of fentanyl and are likely to exhibit prolonged elimination in the face of increased intraabdominal pressure, the application of PEEP, or cardiac instability with hypotension [50]. Doses of 3 to 5 µg/kg are appropriate for intraoperative analgesia for most routine, short pediatric procedures, followed by titration of 0.5 to 1.0 µg/kg boluses to comfort in the post-anesthesia care unit.

Hydromorphone

Hydromorphone is approximately five times more potent than morphine; a recommended starting dose is 0.015 to 0.02 mg/kg. The duration of action is

Table 2
Patient-controlled analgesia

	Concentration	Loading dose	Interval dose	Interval (min)	Continuous infusion	4-hour max
Morphine	1 mg/mL standard	0.1–0.2 mg/kg	0.01–0.03 mg/kg	6–12 min	0.01–0.15 mg/kg/h	0.35 mg/kg opiate naïve[a]
Fentanyl	10 μg/mL	0.5–1 μg/kg	0.15–0.30 μg/kg	6–10 min	0.1 μg/kg/h; titrate to effect	3 μg/kg[a]
Hydromorphone	200 μg/mL = 0.2 mg/mL	5–15 μg/kg	3–5 μg/kg	6–12 min	3–5 μg/kg/h	50–60 μg/kg[a]

[a]Patients receiving chronic opiates may have higher requirements.

similar to morphine, requiring repeat dosing at 2- to 3-hour intervals if it is not being administered by PCA pump. Hydromorphone PCA is an effective alternative to morphine PCA if the patient complains of adverse side effects from the morphine. Although some believe that hydromorphone causes less itching and nausea than morphine, a recent Cochrane database review failed to demonstrate any differences in side effects between hydromorphone and morphine [51,52]. For terminal pain it is easier to provide subcutaneous analgesia with hydromorphone because it can be more highly concentrated.

Remifentanil

The use of remifentanil in pediatric patients for total intravenous anesthesia is becoming more widespread, because rapid elimination and predictable pharmacokinetics across all pediatric age groups allow clinicians to awaken patients quickly and reliably, even after long procedures [53]. Those who use it recognize the need to provide additional analgesia as the remifentanil infusion is discontinued so that the patient awakens without pain. Because of remifentanil's brief effects, it is not an appropriate agent for PCA therapy, although it has been used to provide analgesia for brief painful procedures, such as bone marrow aspirations.

Whether using remifentanil for long procedures actually increases postoperative opiate requirements was addressed recently by Crawford and colleagues [54]. In this study, adolescents undergoing scoliosis repair received either continuous remifentanil or intermittent morphine intraoperatively. Postoperatively, all received morphine by PCA. The group who received remifentanil required nearly 30% more morphine at all time points, despite similar pain and sedation scores. The investigators concluded that this difference suggested that the remifentanil group had developed an acute tolerance to morphine during the intraoperative period. Additional work needs to be done to confirm this finding and to determine whether or not outcomes are affected.

Methadone

Although many practitioners think of methadone only in the context of treating substance abuse, methadone has a long history of use in the acute pain setting. Advantages include a long-lasting and smooth analgesia and a simple conversion from the intravenous to the oral form. The disadvantage of the long half-life is the challenge of responding to rapidly changing pain intensity before reaching a steady state with the methadone. There seems to be a resurgence of interest in methadone; clinical and animal studies clearly show an effect of methadone at the N-methyl-D-aspartate (NMDA) receptor [55,56] and there have also been clinical reports of successful management of neuropathic pain with methadone [57].

In our practice, we use methadone for perioperative pain in children who are already receiving oral methadone for a chronic pain syndrome, for children whose pain is particularly difficult to control, or in the setting in which we anticipate a perioperative transition from acute pain to a chronic pain state. Examples include major cancer surgery in a child suffering from neuropathic pain related to chemotherapy, or revision of an amputation for osteosarcoma. Converting oral methadone to intravenous, the classic conversion is 1:1, but we have found that this ratio overestimates the intravenous requirement; we begin with 50% to 75% of the daily oral dose as our loading dose intravenously. In a randomized, double-blind prospective study comparing morphine and methadone (0.2 mg/kg loading dose of each) in children 3 to 7 years of age undergoing major surgery, Berde and colleagues [58] found that children who received methadone required fewer rescue doses of analgesics and had lower pain scores.

In earlier studies, Berde and colleagues described a loading technique for methadone that we have found useful: 0.1 to 0.2 mg/kg slowly, followed by additional boluses of 0.05 mg/kg every 10 to 15 minutes until the patient is comfortable. Subsequent doses are based on a sliding scale of pain intensity [59,60]. After the first day or two, we use the previous day's requirement and divide it into two to three doses per day until the patient is tolerating oral fluids and medications.

As satisfied as our patients are with the quality of analgesia from methadone, we remain vigilant and respectful of the potential for delayed respiratory depression with this agent, and we keep most young children on respiratory monitors.

Patient-controlled analgesic therapy

Patient-controlled analgesia is now well accepted for use in children older than approximately 4 to 5 years, although there are only two studies in a 2006 Cochrane database review comparing PCA therapy to traditional intermittent dosing [61]. The advantages of PCA therapy, well documented in adult practice, are more difficult to demonstrate in children, but this modality still allows for management of episodic pain on demand, recognizing individual variation in pain tolerance and temporal and activity-based differences in perioperative pain during a 24-hour period. Unlike the early adult studies that showed a reduction in total opiate consumption with PCA compared with intermittent intramuscular dosing, pediatric studies have generally shown an increase in morphine use, probably because pain was undertreated with intermittent dosing. The fact remains that PCA therapy is associated with high patient and parent satisfaction.

Selection of agent

There is no evidence of superiority of one opioid over another in PCA therapy, although morphine is the most commonly used agent. Some practitioners switch over to, or select primarily, fentanyl or hydromorphone to address the perception of a higher incidence of itching, nausea, or vomiting with morphine. Only one study is available directly comparing the efficacy and side effects of PCA morphine and hydromorphone in pediatric patients. In this group of only 10 children who had mucositis from chemotherapy there were no differences between the two opioids [62]. Adult studies comparing the two agents suffer methodologic weaknesses, including small numbers of patients, study design, and the failure to resolve the question of relative potency of the two agents. These studies confirm the effectiveness of hydromorphone for postoperative analgesia but do not demonstrate any advantages of this drug over morphine [52,63,64].

The use of fentanyl or other lipid-soluble agents for PCA therapy has been described, but there is no evidence to suggest that these agents are more efficacious than morphine or hydromorphone. Ruggiero and colleagues [65] describe the use of a fentanyl PCA in 18 children who had cancer ranging from 6 to 15 years of age. All children received a background infusion of 1 µg/kg/h and interval doses of 1 µg/kg/dose; no child required rescue analgesia, and all reported a high degree of satisfaction with the treatment. Despite this positive report, there are still no studies directly comparing fentanyl PCA with either morphine or hydromorphone.

Standard orders for PCA therapy include choice of medication and concentration, the amount of the interval dose, the timing between doses, and the maximum amount that can be delivered within a 1- or 4-hour lockout period. Loading doses may be ordered if there is a time lag between the readiness of the pump and the patient's last dose of opioid. Intervals less than 8 to 10 minutes do not allow for the agent to reach peak effects at the receptor, so doses may "stack" if shorter intervals are ordered. Likewise, if the patient's pain is unrelieved on PCA therapy, the interval dose should be increased incrementally until pain relief is optimized; increasing the background infusion is less effective than increasing the interval dose.

Whether or not to use a continuous or background infusion is another question for the clinician. For pediatric patients who are awake and pushing the button themselves, the addition of a continuous infusion may improve nocturnal sleep but may also be accompanied by an increased incidence of itching and nausea. For patients receiving PCA therapy by proxy, accumulation of medication with a background infusion may reduce the safety of proxy therapy. It has been our practice to use continuous infusions only for patients self-administering the medication following major surgical procedures, such as thoracotomy or spine surgery. Because the continuous infusion may predispose the patient to daytime somnolence, we sometimes discontinue the background infusion during daylight hours to facilitate participation in schoolwork or to increase mobilization or cooperation with physical therapy. A recent study showed, however, that older children receiving a background infusion actually suffered more sleep disruption than those who had interval dosing alone [66].

There remains some controversy with respect to the safety of proxy or surrogate PCA, when a family member or nurse pushes the button. Most pediatric institutions have implemented proxy PCA, particularly for those children who are developmentally delayed or who, by virtue of neuromuscular disease or age, are unable to push the button for themselves. Some facilities manage the perception of increased risk by changing their protocols—eliminating continuous infusion, increasing intervals between doses—or by mandating respiratory monitoring. There are no studies to demonstrate that one or more of these strategies is effective. Anghelescu and colleagues [67] compared respiratory events in a group of children receiving PCA by proxy with self-administered PCA, and found no differences in outcome.

Continuous opioid infusions

There may still be a role for continuous infusion of opioid in institutions that are not comfortable instituting parent-controlled or nurse-controlled analgesia for young infants or cognitively-impaired youngsters. Most of the available studies on continuous infusions have used either morphine or fentanyl. Recognizing considerable interpatient variability in response, respiratory monitoring and repeated observation are recommended for this patient population.

For morphine, infusions as low as 5 to 10 µg/kg/h have been described for infants less than 1 week of age, increasing to 10 to 30 µg/kg/h for children older than 6 months of age [68]. Because elimination determines pharmacokinetics during continuous infusions, the clinician is wise to recognize those factors that may prolong elimination, predisposing the patient to accumulation of morphine and its active metabolites.

Continuous infusions of fentanyl are commonly used for analgesia and sedation in ventilated children in intensive care units. Rapid development of tolerance in neonates requiring rapidly escalating doses has been described [69]; many clinicians are familiar with the sight of the frantic infant receiving huge doses of fentanyl, no longer responding to its sedative effect. Continuous infusions or multiple doses lead to peripheral distribution of fentanyl and prolongation of its elimination. Other influences on its clearance include hepatic maturation and blood flow, intra-abdominal pressure, and cardiac output [50]. These factors together increase the potential for profound respiratory depression in the child receiving a prolonged fentanyl infusion.

Other extensions of the PCA principle—that is, analgesia on demand—can be found in new applications, including patient-controlled epidural analgesia, patient-controlled regional anesthesia with indwelling peripheral nerve catheters, and patient-controlled topical (iontophoretic) and intranasal analgesia. Just as PCA therapy was introduced to pediatric patients after its use was well established in adults, the study of these therapies in children likewise lags behind those in adult patients.

Other routes of administration for opioid agents

Intranasal

There is considerable interest in administration of opiates by novel routes. The simplest of these is the intranasal application of lipid-soluble opioids, including fentanyl, alfentanil, sufentanil, and butorphanol, using small volumes of concentrated drug; there are ongoing trials with special atomizers also. The administration of intranasal fentanyl has been described for emergency center analgesia for children [70], as a means of providing patient-controlled postoperative analgesia in adults [71], and for providing analgesia for children undergoing burn dressing changes [72]. Advantages of this route of administration include rapid onset and self-titration; in children, eliminating the need for intravenous access is a huge advantage.

Several investigators have contributed to our understanding of intranasal opioid therapy in children. Galinkin and colleagues [73] studied PACU and discharge serum concentrations of fentanyl following instillation of 2 µg/kg intranasal fentanyl after induction of anesthesia for myringotomies; serum levels obtained were higher than the minimum effective concentration of fentanyl necessary for postoperative analgesia in adults. Postoperative agitation was reduced compared with controls and there was no increase in vomiting, hypoxemia, or discharge times. Similarly studying children undergoing myringotomies, Finkel and colleagues [74] compared intranasal fentanyl, 1 or 2 µg/kg, to saline placebo in outpatients receiving sevoflurane anesthesia. Dripping half of the volume into each side of the nose, the investigators were careful to turn the head to each side so that the medication contacted the lateral nasal walls rather than dripping immediately into the posterior nasopharynx. Pain and agitation scores were significantly reduced in the children who received 2 µg/kg, whereas recovery and emergence were similar. In this study, postoperative vomiting was more common with fentanyl than with saline controls, but the overall vomiting rate was lower than in Galinkin's study.

Nasal sufentanil and alfentanil have been described for acute pain management and as components of sedation protocols, but probably have no advantage over fentanyl for perioperative pain management [75,76].

Transdermal

Although there is no role for the transdermal fentanyl patch in the management of perioperative pain for the opiate-naïve patient, the growing use of this pain modality for children who have chronic pain suggests that the practitioner will encounter patients presenting to the operating room who are wearing a fentanyl patch. Finkel and colleagues [77] have described the use of transdermal fentanyl patches in pediatric patients who had chronic pain of malignant and nonmalignant origin. Others have advocated transdermal fentanyl for children who have sickle cell disease [78]. For patients who have a history of fentanyl patch use, the practitioner should search the patient's body for the site of application. The authors are familiar with one instance in which an adult patient applied a fentanyl patch to his upper back, then lay down on a warmed waterbed and died, probably from vasodilation and enhanced absorption through the skin. If the patch is part of the child's ongoing pain management plan, the anesthetist should confirm that the patch is not applied to an area that might be affected by a warming blanket or forced-air warming device in the operating room. Removal of the patch does not immediately discontinue the absorption of fentanyl from the skin, because uptake continues for many hours following its removal. We recommend that the patch be left in situ during the perioperative phase, protecting the patient from the temperature considerations described earlier.

OTHER ANALGESIC AGENTS AND ADJUNCTS

Ketorolac

Ketorolac is the only parenteral form of NSAID currently available in the United States (see Table 1). It is extremely useful for outpatient surgical analgesia, particularly in combination with opioid agents, regional anesthetics, or field blocks. The advantages to the use of this agent include the lack of respiratory or central nervous system depression and its ability to minimize postoperative nausea and vomiting. Although this agent is only approved for use in children 2 to 16 years of age, there is growing interest and published experience with this agent in young infants [79]. Side effects of greatest concern in the perioperative period include increased surgical bleeding, gastrointestinal bleeding, and renal dysfunction.

Despite early concerns about perioperative bleeding with ketorolac administration, Moffett and colleagues [79] recently reported a retrospective review of postoperative ketorolac use in a group of 53 cardiac surgery patients less than 6 months of age, in whom the agent was administered for 3 days beginning 48 hours after surgery. They found no increase in bleeding and no change in hematologic parameters. Although serum creatinine rose in all patients following ketorolac administration, all values remained in the normal range for age. Similarly, from a cohort of 842 infants and children undergoing cardiac surgery, Gupta and colleagues [80] compared 94 children who received ketorolac postoperatively with the same number of age- and procedure-matched controls who did not receive the drug. Using the need for surgical re-exploration as their endpoint, the investigators found no differences in postoperative bleeding between the two groups.

The use of perioperative ketorolac for tonsillectomy patients has also been controversial and in the United States it has largely been abandoned following an initial report demonstrating an unexpected need for reoperation in children who received ketorolac [81]. More recently, however, a Cochrane database review of 955 patients showed no difference in postoperative bleeding or requirement to return to the operating room [45].

Renal dysfunction following administration of ketorolac has been reported in the perioperative period as described in the infant cardiac series and in other reports [82,83]. The relationship between hypovolemia, changes in renal perfusion, and other factors has not been completely elucidated but in each of these cases the clinical and laboratory findings normalized with conservative therapy. In contrast, one nonsurgical patient who had sickle cell disease developed irreversible renal failure in the absence of hypovolemia after receiving intramuscular and oral ketorolac for 3 days [84].

Finally, there has been a concern, at least in spinal surgery, that the use of ketorolac may retard or impair bone fusion [85]. That concern has not been validated in a series of 208 consecutive pediatric scoliosis patients, of whom 60 received ketorolac; there were no differences in acute blood loss or transfusion and no differences in revision surgery required [86]. Munro and colleagues [87], in a prospective, double-blinded study, confirmed that perioperative ketorolac improved analgesia and reduced morphine consumption in adolescent scoliosis patients; they also found no evidence of curve progression, hardware failure, or chronic back pain 2 years later in a subset of the original cohort.

Ketamine

The use of ketamine in clinical pediatric anesthesia is on the rise again, reflecting an increased understanding of its role in blocking the NMDA receptor. Long popular with pediatric practitioners as a way to calm the most recalcitrant patient, ketamine is now being used not only for its sedative properties but also during general anesthesia to provide preemptive analgesia, as an analgesic or coanalgesic agent, and as an adjunct for central and regional nerve blockade [88].

There continues to be controversy about whether or not ketamine is effective in preventing or modulating the pain response in adults or children, although this is an area of active investigation.

Two studies have examined the use of ketamine to prevent postoperative pain in healthy children undergoing adenotonsillectomy. In one cohort of 50 children, children received an intravenous bolus of either morphine 0.1 mg/kg or ketamine 0.5 mg/kg following the induction of anesthesia. There was no difference in the time to the patients' first request for supplemental analgesia between the groups, suggesting comparable analgesic action [89]. In a similar prospective, blinded study, 80 children received either morphine 0.10 to 0.15 mg/kg or ketamine 0.5 to 0.6 mg/kg intramuscularly after induction. In this group, the pain scores were higher 30 minutes after extubation but then declined without intervention and were similar to the morphine group thereafter [90]. In this study there were no differences in the rates of nausea or vomiting. Similarly, a single dose of ketamine was found to reduce postoperative analgesia requirements in a Brazilian study in which 90 adenotonsillectomy patients aged 5 to 7 years received no intraoperative opiates; rather, they received preoperative rectal diclofenac and a large dose of dexamethasone (2 mg/kg), and were randomized to receive no ketamine, or ketamine 0.5 mg/kg intravenously (IV) either before or after the surgical procedure itself. Those children who received a single dose of ketamine required less rescue analgesia during the first 24 hours after surgery; in fact, those who received ketamine at the end of the procedure required no morphine at all [91].

Prophylactic ketamine has been studied in several study designs in adult surgical patients. One meta-analysis of nearly 3000 patients concluded that ketamine reduced 24-hour morphine consumption, reduced visual analog scale scores, and delayed time to first analgesic request, all in modest decrements; it was not shown to reduce troublesome opiate side effects [92]. A Cochrane database review of 2240 patients concluded that a subanesthetic dose of ketamine reduced morphine requirements in the first 24 hours after surgery, and that it reduced postoperative nausea and vomiting [93].

Tramadol

Tramadol is a relatively new centrally-acting agent for the management of pain (see Table 1). A synthetic derivative of codeine, it has a low affinity for the mu opioid receptor, but no affinity for the gamma or kappa opioid receptors; its effects are partially antagonized by naloxone. In addition to effects at the opiate receptor, the isomers of tramadol also release serotonin and inhibit serotonin uptake (+ isomer) and also promote norepinephrine release and inhibit its re-uptake (− isomer) [94]. Its analgesic potency is intermediate, between that of the NSAIDs and morphine, and the major advantage of this agent is the neg-ligible respiratory depression [94].

In the United States, tramadol is only available as oral tablets and is only ap-proved for use in adults. One multi-institutional study of children between 7 and 16 years of age studied the effect of tramadol 1 or 2 mg/kg orally every 4 to 6 hours on morphine requirement in patients transitioning from PCA mor-phine; a dose of 2 mg/kg was found to be superior to the lower dose [95]. In this study, 10% of patients suffered vomiting on tramadol.

Outside the United States, intravenous tramadol has been used in PCA pumps for children following tonsillectomy [96] and as an infusion for sickle cell pain [97]. Khosravi found tramadol to be equivalent to ilioinguinal/iliohy-pogastric nerve blocks for postherniorrhaphy pain in boys 2 to 7 years of age. Recently, Hullett and colleagues [98] compared intravenous tramadol 2 mg/kg to morphine 0.1 mg/kg in children who had sleep apnea undergoing tonsillec-tomy. They found no differences in sedation or analgesia up to 6 hours post-operatively, but there were fewer desaturations in the children who received tramadol.

Gabapentin

Gabapentin has been used for chronic pain management in children who have complex regional pain syndrome and other neuropathic conditions [99–101] because early reports suggesting its efficacy in reducing neuropathic pain in adults [102]. Except for somnolence at initiation of therapy, gabapentin is easily tolerated by most children; we find that increasing the dose gradually mini-mizes the somnolence and allows the child to attend school. The manufac-turer's recommended maximum dose is 35 mg/kg/d in three divided doses, but other investigators report higher doses without adverse sequelae [100].

Lauder and White [100] reported a series of children who had cerebral palsy who developed neuropathic pain syndromes following tendon-lengthening pro-cedures; in these children, normal nociceptive pain became neuropathic after the first week. In all but one, gabapentin was part of the multimodal approach to the changing pain syndrome. Mendham [103] reported on the efficacy of ga-bapentin in a group of 35 children who had refractory itching during the heal-ing phase of burn recovery. Again, in this model of acute-to-chronic pain patients, gabapentin—at much lower doses than recommended for seizure treatment—was effective in all of the children in relieving symptoms and reducing doses of anti-histamines. Three patients developed acute disruptive behaviors, however, ne-cessitating lower doses or discontinuation of the drug.

There is also growing interest in the use of gabapentin during the acute peri-operative period for prevention and treatment of acute surgical pain. In a recent meta-analysis of adult perioperative studies, gabapentin administered preoperatively in a single dose was found to reduce 24-hour morphine consumption, reduce pain scores, and reduce nausea and vomiting [104]. The mechanism for this decrease is not well understood, but may reflect gabapentin's ability to reduce central sensitization by its action on dorsal horn cells, or a synergistic effect with the analgesic effects of morphine, or by preventing the development of tolerance to morphine [104].

To date, there are no pediatric studies that demonstrate that children would benefit from preoperative administration of gabapentin to reduce opiate requirements or to improve analgesia. Several such studies are currently under development, however (Glass, personal communication, 2006). The authors recommend that patients already taking gabapentin for neuropathic pain conditions should continue its use throughout the perioperative period, in case these patients should require surgery for a related or incidental surgical procedure.

Alpha-2 agonists

Clonidine, a semiselective alpha-2 agonist, is an old drug originally released for the treatment of hypertension. More recently, anesthesiologists have taken advantage of its most confounding side effect, sedation, and turned that into a therapeutic advantage in the perioperative period. In the United States, clonidine is available in tablet form in doses of 0.1 to 0.3 mg, as a transdermal patch containing 0.1 to 0.3 mg/d for 1 week, and as a solution for epidural administration. An intravenous form is available in Europe and other parts of the world.

In an oral dose of 4 µg/kg clonidine is an effective premedicant for children undergoing surgery, although compared with midazolam its onset is slower and its duration of effect is longer. For this reason, it is not useful for short, ambulatory procedures. At least two studies have demonstrated a reduction in postoperative analgesic requirements in patients who receive preoperative clonidine [105,106]. At this dose, the sedative effect is not accompanied by an effect on hypoxic or hypercapnic respiratory drive. Its administration is also accompanied by a reduction in doses required for induction agents and volatile anesthetics [107,108].

We find clonidine to be a particularly advantageous agent for adolescent spinal surgery because the sedative effect is largely gone by the end of the procedure, yet the stable hemodynamic profile and morphine-sparing effects allow our patients to awaken calmly and comfortably. Clonidine is even more effective as an analgesic agent for neuraxial analgesia, and is discussed again later in this article.

Dexmedetomidine, a highly selective alpha-2 agonist, is now frequently used in pediatric institutions as a component of general anesthetics [109–112], as a sedative agent for imaging or catheterization procedures [113,114], and for sedation of burned or ventilated patients in the intensive care unit [115,116]. In addition, dexmedetomidine has been described to facilitate weaning or extubation from opiate sedation when standard weaning protocols have failed

[117,118]. An initial infusion of 1 µg/kg over 10 minutes followed by a titrated infusion of 0.2 to 0.7 µg/kg/h has been described for children and adults. Bradycardia and hypotension are mild in patients who have an adequate intravascular volume, and respiratory depression is uncommon.

Zub and colleagues [119] have recently published their preliminary experience with the off-label administration of dexmedetomidine orally. Citing previous studies showing an oral bioavailability of 15% to 20% when the intravenous form is administered, they gave 3 to 4 µg/kg orally to a group of uncooperative autistic children. Adequate sedation was achieved at 20 to 30 minutes so that they could then insert an IV or proceed with inhalation anesthesia. The rapid onset they described may be attributable to buccal absorption rather than oral, because they did not dilute the medication. Prospective, randomized studies will be required to confirm the usefulness of this technique compared with more traditional approaches.

Lidocaine

Systemic lidocaine may prove to be a helpful adjunct in acute pain management, supplementing its use in regional and local anesthesia. In adult pain clinics, lidocaine, administered by various routes, has long been considered an adjunct for chronic neuropathic pain. Likewise, in pediatrics, lidocaine has been used as a component for intravenous regional blockade for complex regional pain syndrome. Although the mechanism of action is not completely understood, most investigators believe that the analgesic effects are mediated at the level of the sodium channel, preventing transmission of aberrant impulses from peripheral nerve endings [120,121], although an effect at the spinal cord level may also play a role [121].

There are several pediatric examples of the use of lidocaine infusions for acute neuropathic pain. Nathan and colleagues [122] reported successful treatment of acute neuropathic pain from erythromelalgia in an 11-year-old boy, followed by transition to the oral form, mexiletine. Similarly, Wallace and colleagues [123] described lidocaine infusion for a child suffering from severe acute peripheral neuropathy related to chemotherapy for neuroblastoma. Finally, a lidocaine infusion was successfully used to manage the rapidly escalating, morphine-resistant terminal pain in a toddler; however, blood levels were not measured [124].

Although children who have neuropathic pain may present to the operating room for surgical procedures, most clinicians are interested in whether or not lidocaine has an effect on acute, perioperative, nociceptive pain. One study of adult patients undergoing major abdominal surgery demonstrated a morphine-sparing effect of an intraoperative lidocaine infusion at 1.5 mg/kg/h [125]; another similar protocol found decreased pain scores and morphine consumption following laparoscopic colectomy, although endocrine and metabolic responses were not different from the control group [126]. Other investigators are less convinced that lidocaine has a role in nonneuropathic pain [127]. To date, there are no comparable studies in pediatric populations to suggest that intravenous lidocaine infusions are beneficial in children who have acute perioperative pain.

REGIONAL ANESTHETIC BLOCKS IN CHILDREN

A review of pediatric pain management would be incomplete without considering advances and latest innovative approaches to neuraxial and peripheral nerve blocks.

For several years, most pediatric procedures were performed solely under general anesthesia, but since the mid-1980s there has been a resurgence of interest in regional analgesia for pediatric procedures. Today, regional anesthesia has become a fundamental component of most modern pediatric anesthesia practices.

The advantages of neuraxial analgesia for thoracic and abdominal surgery in children have been studied and documented. These advantages include improved hemodynamic stability, reduced need for postoperative ventilatory support, improved analgesia without the risk for opiate-induced respiratory depression, and lower perioperative stress levels. The Collaborative Overview of Randomized Trials of Regional Anesthesia meta-analysis demonstrates that regional anesthesia alone or in combination with general anesthesia reduces postoperative complications and postoperative mortality rate by 30% [128].

The development of sophisticated and appropriately sized equipment has improved the success, safety, and efficacy of regional blocks in children. To provide high-quality analgesia to pediatric patients, the placement of regional blocks in carefully selected instances should be considered whenever possible.

Safety of regional block in children under general anesthesia

A controversial topic for most general anesthesiology practitioners is the safety of performing regional blocks in anesthetized patients. Several case reports of neurologic injury from blocks performed under anesthesia in adults led to the recommendation that central and regional nerve blocks be done awake or only lightly sedated, so that the patient can respond if the needle touches the nerve. That practice cannot be extrapolated to the placement of regional blocks in children, however.

The dictum "children are not small adults" certainly holds true here. It is now acknowledged and generally accepted that the performance of a neuraxial or peripheral nerve block in children under general anesthesia is safe. The safety of this practice was established after a large multicenter prospective study including more than 24,000 central and peripheral nerve block procedures revealed only 23 adverse events [129]. All of the adverse effects occurred after central nerve blocks; however, they were minor complications with no permanent sequelae. In fact, one could advance the argument that regional blocks in children are actually safer when they are performed under general anesthesia, because it can be so difficult to assure cooperation of a sedated child. Sudden patient movement at a time when a needle is close to vital structures could result in nerve damage or insertion of the needle into vessels or organs.

SINGLE-SHOT CAUDAL EPIDURAL BLOCK

The single-shot caudal epidural block remains the cornerstone of postoperative regional analgesia in children, offering a reliable and effective block for patients undergoing procedures involving the lower abdomen and lower extremities. The attractiveness of this regional technique lies in the simplicity of the procedure and high success rates. According to a study by Schuepfer and colleagues [130], anesthesiology residents first exposed to caudal blocks were able to achieve high success rates after performing the technique just a few times; by the time they had done 32 blocks, the success rate for residents was comparable to that of staff anesthesiologists.

The choice of needle size or type does not seem to affect the success rate or complications from caudal epidural analgesia and therefore needle selection should be based on the practitioner's preference. Newman and colleagues [131] published a randomized prospective study comparing three types of needles, 21- and 23-gauge standard cutting bevel intramuscular needles and 22-gauge short bevel regional block needle, and found no significant differences with respect to success or complications. Some prefer the use of a styletted, short-bevel, 22-gauge needle, which may reduce the risk for introducing a dermal plug into the caudal space [129]. Baris and colleagues [132] reported that the incidence of transporting nucleated epidermal cells during puncture for caudal block is low and no differences exist between 22-gauge hollow needles or 22-gauge caudal block needles. Others advocate for the use of 22-gauge intravenous catheters, believing that ease of advancement confirms correct position in the caudal space. Proponents also believe that intravenous catheters allow for easier detection of intravascular placement and may help the clinician avoid an interosseous placement [133]. Intravenous catheters should be threaded cautiously into the caudal space, because inadvertent "shearing" of the catheter may occur, leaving behind a foreign body in the space and creating a nidus for infection. Whether the resulting foreign body requires surgical intervention or not is unclear.

The most important variables determining the effectiveness of caudal analgesia for a specific local anesthetic are the volume, dose, and concentration of local anesthetic solution used (Table 3) [134].

ADJUNCTS TO CAUDAL BLOCK IN CHILDREN—TO ADD OR NOT TO ADD?

The major limitation of the single-shot caudal block is the duration of analgesia, which only extends to 6 hours, even with the use of long-acting local anesthetics at a dose and concentration that may result in an undesired motor

Table 3
Caudal epidural block

Local anesthetic	Minimum concentration	Volume for below T10 level analgesia	Max dose (mg/kg)	Duration of analgesia
Bupivacaine	0.125	0.5–1 mL/kg	2.5 mg/kg	4–6 hours
Ropivacaine	0.175	1 mL/kg	3–4 mg/kg	>6 hours
Levobupivacaine	0.2	1 mL/kg	2.5 mg/kg	4 hours

blockade (Table 4). As a result, several agents have been studied to enhance the efficacy and duration of single-injection caudal analgesia.

Opioids

Opioids have been documented to enhance and prolong the duration of analgesia. In a retrospective study of 138 patients, a third of whom were less than 6 months old, caudal morphine 70 µg/kg provided effective postoperative analgesia in most patients, with 75% of patients not requiring any supplemental analgesia for the first 10 hours after the single shot [135]. Although a meta-analysis of 18 studies conducted in adults showed that fentanyl added to local anesthetics provides safe and effective pain relief [136], the analgesic efficacy of fentanyl added to single-shot caudal remains less clear. No significant analgesic benefit was demonstrated when fentanyl 1 µg/kg was added to caudally administered bupivacaine 0.125% [137] or lidocaine 2% with epinephrine 1:200,000 [138] in children undergoing urologic surgery. Unwanted side effects, such as respiratory depression, nausea, vomiting, itching, and urinary retention, may preclude the use of opioid adjuncts in day surgery patients by potentially delaying discharge or causing inadvertent hospital admission.

Clonidine

Clonidine is an alpha-2 agonist antihypertensive agent that has sedative and analgesic effects when administered along the neuraxis. The analgesic action of intrathecal or epidural clonidine results from direct stimulation of pre- and post-synaptic alpha-2 adrenoceptors in the dorsal horn gray matter of the spinal cord, thereby inhibiting the release of nociceptive neurotransmitters [139]. De Negri and colleagues [140] demonstrated improved postoperative analgesia when clonidine 0.1 µg/kg/h was infused epidurally along with ropivacaine. Numerous other studies have consistently shown that caudal clonidine increases the duration of postoperative analgesia from a single-shot caudal block. The main side effects of caudal clonidine are hypotension, bradycardia, and sedation. In children, clonidine 1 to 5 µg/kg has been used without clinically important respiratory or hemodynamic effects [141]. The sedative effects of clonidine seem to be dose-dependent; however, many studies report no episodes of respiratory depression. The safety of clonidine in premature infants is still in

Table 4 Recommended doses for caudal additives	
Caudal adjunct	Recommend dose
Morphine	0.03–0.07 mg/kg
Fentanyl	1–3 µg/kg
Clonidine	1–2 µg/kg
Ketamine[a]	0.5 mg/kg
Midazolam[a]	0.05 mg/kg
Neostigmine[a]	0.02 mg/kg

[a]These medications are not available in the United States in preservative-free formulations.

question. Apnea has been reported in premature infants after the inclusion of clonidine in the caudal solution. It is not recommended to use this adjunct in these high-risk patients until further studies are done.

Ketamine

The analgesic effect of ketamine on the neuraxis is primarily attributable to blockage of NMDA receptors located throughout the central nervous system (CNS) and substantia gelatinosa in the spinal cord. Weber and Wulf [142] compared use of ketamine with bupivacaine versus bupivacaine alone in a randomized study of 30 children between the ages of 1 month and 9 months. They reported a significantly better quality of postoperative analgesia compared with bupivacaine alone. After circumcision, caudal ropivacaine 0.2% plus ketamine 0.25 mg/kg produced a median duration of analgesia of 12 hours compared with 3 hours for ropivacaine alone [143]. There have been no reports in literature of respiratory depression, cardiovascular changes, or major neurologic problems following the use of epidural ketamine 0.5 mg/kg in humans [143–145]. Although there have been no neurologic symptoms reported with use of ketamine with preservatives in animals, it should not be administered epidurally because of the risk for neurotoxicity from the preservative agent benzethonium chloride. Preservative free S(+)-ketamine has similar pharmacokinetic properties to the racemic mixture, but has twice the analgesic potency [146]. Marhofer and colleagues [147] showed that S(+) ketamine 1 mg/kg provided intraoperative and postoperative analgesia equivalent to bupivacaine 0.25% 0.75 mL/kg with epinephrine. Despite the lack of reported adverse effects following the use of S(+) ketamine, more randomized controlled trials are needed before it can be recommended for routine use in pediatric caudal analgesia. The S(+) preservative-free isomer is not available in the United States.

Midazolam

Epidural midazolam seems to exert its analgesic effect on binding sites in the spinal cord, particularly those within lamina II of the dorsal horn linked to the GABA receptor complex. Early studies showed that caudal midazolam produced postoperative analgesia comparable to that of bupivacaine, without motor weakness or behavioral changes; however, a more recent study by Baris and colleagues [148] failed to confirm this finding. The recommended dose is 50 μg/kg; larger doses are associated with prolonged sedation.

Neostigmine

Neostigmine is believed to act at muscarinic receptors in the dorsal horn by inhibiting the breakdown of acetylcholine. Abdulatif and El-Sanabary [149] first reported its use in children. In a randomized, double-blinded study, neostigmine alone was compared with bupivacaine. Although neostigmine produced postoperative analgesia comparable with bupivacaine, an unacceptably high incidence of vomiting may deter its routine use. In addition, the safety of neostigmine preservatives on the neuroaxial space is still unknown.

Ketamine, midazolam, and neostigmine are not approved, licensed, or marketed for epidural injection in the United States at this time. As interesting as the research is in this area, the practitioner is cautioned against the instillation of drugs into the neuraxis that have not specifically been tested for safety in this application. Further research is necessary to see how these agents may improve on our current choices.

CONTINUOUS EPIDURAL ANALGESIA

Although the feasibility of placing epidural catheters directly in the thoracic space has been demonstrated [150], many pediatric anesthesiologists are uncomfortable placing epidural catheters in small infants, preferring instead to thread the catheter from the caudal space to the thoracic or lumbar epidural space. Bosenberg and colleagues [151] first described their technique of threading an epidural catheter through the sacral hiatus to the thoracic region, which is generally easy to accomplish in infants less than 1 year of age. This technique may carry a smaller risk for dural puncture or spinal cord trauma compared with direct thoracic epidural insertion [152].

One disadvantage to caudal catheter placement is the difficulty of maintaining a dry and intact dressing in the diaper area, raising concerns about fecal contamination and bacterial colonization at the insertion site, which may in turn increase the risk for infection in the epidural space. Bacterial colonization of epidural catheters occurred more rapidly with caudal catheters compared with lumbar catheters in two studies [153,154], although the relationship between colonization and epidural abscess formation is still not clear. Because of the increased incidence of bacterial colonization with caudal catheters, the direct approach to the thoracic or lumbar epidural space should be used when possible. If a caudal epidural catheter is placed, however, steps to reduce the rate of bacterial colonization should be used. Bubeck and colleagues [155] found that subcutaneous tunneling of caudal catheters delays the rate of bacterial colonization similar to that of lumbar epidural catheters. Other studies have evaluated special dressing techniques and skin disinfection maneuvers to reduce the bacterial colonization rate [156,157].

Confirming epidural catheter placement

Although it is generally easy to advance catheters through the sacral hiatus, it is not always easy to place the tip at the desired interspace, and the success rate declines as the infant ages (Box 1). Blanco and colleagues [158] were able to reach the thoracic epidural space in only 52% of the patients less than 1 year of age by way of the caudal route. Several other authors reported success rates between 85% and 95% for infants less than 6 months of age, but had lower success rates in older infants [151,159,160].

The ease of epidural catheter advancement is not a good predictor for placement at the desired location. Valairucha and colleagues [161] reviewed the medical records of 115 infants less than 6 months old who had a thoracic or lumbar epidural catheter threaded by way of the caudal route. Radiographic

Box 1: Protocol for confirming epidural catheter position

Intraoperatively (while the patient is under general anesthesia)

Radiography with contrast

Radiography with a radio-opaque catheter

Electrical stimulation

Electrocardiogram

Ultrasonography

Postoperatively (while the patient is awake)

Radiography with contrast

Electrical stimulation

Chloroprocaine test: incremental dosing of 3% chloroprocaine solution to demonstrate analgesia and signs of segmental effect

  a. Lumbar catheter tip: at least partial sensory and motor blockage in both legs; warming of the volar surface of the toes

  b. Lower thoracic catheter tip: reduced strength in hip flexion; reduced abdominal skin reflexes; some reduction in heart rate and blood pressure

  c. Upper thoracic catheter tip: some reduction in heart rate and blood pressure; warming of the volar surface of hands; unilateral or bilateral Horner's syndrome

Dosing is given in four increments at 60-s intervals according to body weight:

0–10 kg, 0.2 mL/kg increments (0.8 mL/kg total)

10–25 kg, 0.15 mL/kg increments (0.6 mL/kg)

25–40 kg, 0.1 mL/kg increments (0.4 mL/kg)

>40 kg, 0.075 mL/kg increments (0.3 mL/kg total, to a max of 20 mL)

Adapted from Tsui BC, Berde CB. Caudal analgesia and anesthesia techniques in children. Curr Opin Anaesthesiol 2005;18(3):283–8.

studies were available for 86 of these infants, and the authors found that the position was inadequate in 32% of the cases. Ten of these catheters were located in the high thoracic or cervical region, whereas 17 were coiled in the lumbosacral area. Only 17% of the catheters were successfully placed at the correct dermatome. The authors recommend confirmation of the catheter tip location to avoid either the potential respiratory compromise that may occur when catheters are placed too high or the inadequate analgesia that may occur when the catheter coils within the lumbosacral area.

Correct positioning of the epidural catheter tip is crucial for its effectiveness and safety. Delivery of local anesthetic to the proper dermatome involved in the painful procedures is necessary for effective analgesia, and allows the practitioner to avoid excessive dosing of local anesthetic that might predispose to toxic reactions.

Confirmation by radiography

There are several ways to confirm catheter tip location (Fig. 1). If the catheter is radiopaque, the tip location may be verified by a standard radiograph or with fluoroscopy. Contrast medium may also be injected under fluoroscopy. The volume of contrast needed to fill most standard catheters is 0.2 mL, and a small amount of extra contrast, approximately 0.3 mL, is necessary to visualize the catheter on the radiograph. One disadvantage of using standard radiographs is the inability to readjust the catheter without removing the dressing and taking another film. Real-time fluoroscopy permits continuous observation and adjustment during catheter advancement, but exposure to radiation for the infant and the equipment and resources required make intraoperative fluoroscopy impractical for many clinicians.

Ultrasound-guided placement of epidural catheters

Cork and colleagues [162] were the first to describe the use of ultrasound for visualizing neuraxial structures. It has not been until recently that higher-resolution images have made the application of ultrasound to placement of epidural catheters feasible, however.

In infants less than 6 months of age, the posterior elements of the spinal canal are incompletely ossified, providing an acoustic window for sonographic

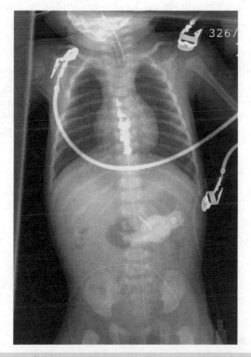

Fig. 1. Epidurogram confirming caudal catheter tip location at T7–T8.

imaging. Because of developmental calcification of the posterior vertebral bodies, Chen and colleagues [163] concluded that ultrasound could only be used to image the spinal cord in children younger than 6 months of age. Yet in a recent study of pediatric American Society of Anesthesiologists I–II patients older than 6 months scheduled for elective surgery under general anesthesia with epidural analgesia, the ligamentum flavum, dural structures, and epidural space, including the location and depth, could all be identified by ultrasound [164].

Willschke and colleagues [165] were the first to evaluate the neuraxial sonoanatomy in neonates, in a cohort of 145 infants weighing less than 4 kg. The ligamentum flavum, dura mater, and termination of the spinal cord could be identified in all patients. They found that the termination of the conus medullaris corresponded to the second lumbar vertebra with the neonate positioned in the left lateral position. This finding was different from traditional teaching, which described the spinal cord ending at L3 in infants, rising to the adult level of L1–2 by 1 year of age. There is good correlation between the skin- to-epidural space depth measured by ultrasound and the depth identified using the loss of resistance technique. The depth of the epidural space is approximately 1 mm per kg of body in children older than 6 months. One benefit of using ultrasound is the opportunity to measure the depth of the epidural space before needle insertion.

The use of ultrasound technology also allows the anesthesiologist to verify catheter tip positioning by direct visualization of the spread of local anesthetic in the epidural space. Visualizing the local anesthetic spread within the epidural space may enhance safety by reducing the dose needed for maximum therapeutic effect. Tissue expansion with the injection of fluid is used as surrogate markers for catheter tip placement.

The acoustic windows for ultrasound images in the thoracic region are narrower because of ossification; however, this impediment may be overcome by placing the probe in a paramedian position. With this technique, the thoracic dura can still be visualized in adults. The use of ultrasound for epidural catheter placement is a practical option in children weighing between 0.95 and 23 kg [166].

Electrocardiographic guidance

Tsui's practice of electrocardiographic guidance is another approach to epidural catheter placement. The catheter is adapted so it functions as an ECG lead. Vertebral level is gauged by comparing a baseline ECG at the required catheter tip level against the evolving ECG of the catheter as it is advanced [167]. One advantage of the ECG-guided technique is that it can still be used after the administration of neuromuscular blocking agents or epidural local anesthetics [168]. This technique cannot rule out subarachnoid, or intravascular placement of the catheter, however.

Tsui test

Tsui described another innovative approach to threading thoracic epidural catheters from the caudal space using the dermatomal response to electrical nerve stimulation to guide the catheter to the thoracic region. Low-voltage electrical current, conducted through saline in an electrically conducting catheter, stimulates spinal nerve roots and shows the clinician where the tip of the catheter is located as it advances [169]. After standard sterile preparation of the skin, the catheter and an adaptor are primed with sterile normal saline. The cathode lead of the nerve stimulator is connected to the epidural catheter by way of an electrode adapter and the anode lead is connected to an electrode on the patient's skin for grounding. A motor response is usually elicited between 1 mA to 10 mA. Motor responses elicited at less than 1 mA may indicate that the catheter is in the subarachnoid space or in close proximity to a nerve root. The level of the muscle twitch can be observed as it advances from the lower limb muscles to the abdominal and intercostal muscles. Confirming the catheter tip position radiographically, Tsui and colleagues [169] reported a success rate of 98.2% for threading the catheter from the caudal to the thoracic space in infants between 5 months and 1.6 years old.

Local anesthetics in epidurals

Newer local anesthetics are becoming increasingly more attractive because compared with racemic bupivacaine, these agents have a lower potential for cardiac and central nervous system toxicity.

Ropivacaine is a long-acting amide local anesthetic with single S (−) enantiomer structure. Ropivacaine has been reported to have a better safety profile than bupivacaine for children and adults. A large multicenter study of children [170] found that mean onset time and mean time to first analgesia with caudal ropivacaine 0.2% is similar to that seen with bupivacaine 0.25%. In addition, there was a less dense and briefer motor block than that seen with bupivacaine.

Levobupivacaine is the S (−) enantiomer of bupivacaine. A study by Foster [171] showed that in human volunteers, levobupivacaine produced less negative inotropic effect, less prolongation of the QT interval, and fewer CNS effects than racemic bupivacaine.

In a recent pediatric study by Ivani and colleagues [172], the authors compared caudal levobupivacaine with ropivacaine and bupivacaine in children undergoing minor surgery. They found no differences among the three with respect to time to first analgesic demand; in addition, ropivacaine was associated with less motor block than bupivacaine. Breschan and colleagues [173] also reported similar perioperative pain relief in children in comparing 0.2% of levobupivacaine, ropivacaine, and bupivacaine; similarly, they found that both ropivacaine and levobupivacaine produced less motor block during the first 2 hours postoperatively than bupivacaine. Astuto and colleagues [174] found that caudal levobupivacaine provides analgesia with a comparable onset and duration as that obtained by the same volume and concentration of ropivacaine.

Ropivacaine has the advantage of a lower toxic potential when compared with bupivacaine [175]; for this reason, some pediatric anesthesiologists have begun using ropivacaine preferentially for epidural analgesia. Bosenberg and colleagues [176] studied the pharmacokinetics and efficacy of ropivacaine for continuous epidural infusion in neonates and infants and found that the clearance of ropivacaine increased with age but remained basically unchanged across age groups regardless of the duration of the infusion. In contrast, the plasma concentration of bupivacaine increases and does not reach a steady-state level, whereas the clearance decreases proportionally with the infusion time [177]. Because it is less likely to accumulate over time, ropivacaine may offer a safer therapeutic index for continuous infusions.

For single-shot caudal blocks, levobupivacaine might offer a better therapeutic index than ropivacaine and racemic bupivacaine in infants. Additional studies are required to determine the most appropriate clinical uses of levobupivacaine in continuous epidural infusions and peripheral nerve blocks.

Studies have shown that all the amino amides, including bupivacaine, levo-bupivacaine, lidocaine, and ropivacaine, have diminished clearance in neo-nates, with maturation over the first 3 to 8 months of age [178]. Because of the neonate's lower levels of albumin and alpha glycoprotein, they are at greater risk for toxic effects of local anesthetics because of higher levels of un-bound drug. Previous work in an infant animal model, and calculations derived from that model, suggest to us that there is no infusion rate for bupivacaine or lidocaine that can assure effective analgesia while maintaining safe plasma concentrations in neonates.

Neonates and infants up to 6 months of age have half of the adult levels of plasma cholinesterases; even so, Berde [179] found that preterm neonates have sufficient plasma esterase activity to effectively clear comparatively large infusion rates of chloroprocaine. For this reason, his group routinely uses chloro-procaine infusions in neonates, avoiding concerns about toxicity from the amide local anesthetics.

Spinal analgesia in the preterm and young infant

Spinal anesthesia is one of the oldest techniques for providing pain relief for surgery below the umbilicus (Fig. 2). It offers the practitioner an alternative technique to general anesthesia, with its CNS depressant effects and requisite airway manipulation.

For many years clinicians have observed the predisposition of premature infants for postoperative apnea, defined as breath holding, hypoxemia, or brady-cardia following the induction of general anesthesia. The risk for apnea decreases between 44 and 60 weeks postconceptual age but may persist in older anemic infants. Cote and colleagues [180] analyzed the outcomes of eight studies on postoperative apnea following general anesthesia. He and his colleagues affirmed that postconceptual age is not the only risk factor, and that other factors, including a history of apnea at home, a history of chronic lung disease, central nervous system morbidity, and anemia should be considered when deciding whether or not to admit a formerly premature infant after surgery.

Most postoperative studies show that approximately 20% to 30% of otherwise healthy former preterm infants having hernia repairs under general anesthesia have one or more apneic spells in the postoperative period [181]. Because of the high incidence of postoperative apnea in preterm infants, many

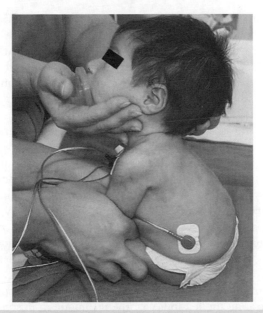

Fig. 2. Holding technique of infant spinal in sitting position.

institutions recommend that elective surgery for ex-preterm infants should be delayed until the infant is older than 44 to 60 weeks postconceptual age; if the surgery cannot be delayed, infants in this age group should be admitted for apnea monitoring for at least 12 to 24 hours after surgery.

In several small comparative trials, infant spinal anesthesia has been associated with a lower incidence of hypotension, bradycardia, and postoperative apnea compared with general anesthesia. Both Welborn and colleagues [182] and Krane and colleagues [183] have reported that spinal anesthesia may reduce the risk for postoperative apnea in preterm infants. According to the Vermont Infant Spinal Registry, the incidence of serious complications associated with spinal anesthesia in infants undergoing major surgical procedures is low [184]. Reporting prospectively acquired data on more than 1500 spinal anesthesia procedures performed on infants at the University of Vermont since 1978, Williams and colleagues reported successful spinal anesthesia in 95.4% of patients. Only 26 infants developed bradycardia to less than 100 bpm, and none had hypotension. Only 55 required oxygen supplementation during surgery, whereas in another 56 children the spinal level was higher than intended, requiring airway intervention in 10 infants. In this summary report, they did not report on the incidence of postoperative apnea [184]. In an earlier publication, however, Williams and colleagues compared the incidence of postoperative apnea under spinal anesthesia with that of general anesthesia, selecting sevoflurane and a caudal blockade to minimize residual effects from the volatile agent or opiates. In the general anesthesia group, 5 of the 14 patients developed postoperative complications, whereas none of 10 spinal anesthesia patients showed such complications [185].

Kunst and colleagues found no advantages for spinal anesthesia over general anesthesia. The Cochrane Collaboration published a meta-analysis review evaluating regional versus general anesthesia in preterm infants undergoing inguinal hernia repair in early infancy. They reported that there was no evidence that spinal anesthesia was superior to general anesthesia with respect to the incidence of postoperative apnea, bradycardia, or oxygen desaturations in ex-preterm infants undergoing hernia repair [186].

Somri and colleagues [187] evaluated spinal anesthesia as an alternative option to general anesthesia in infants undergoing pyloromyotomy. Despite correction of the systemic metabolic alkalosis before surgical intervention, the cerebrospinal fluid may still be alkalotic at the time of surgery, so that administration of opioids or hyperventilation increases the risk for central apnea. In this study, 23 patients (4 of whom were born prematurely) underwent successful pyloromyotomy under spinal anesthesia. None of the patients experienced perioperative or postoperative apnea. The Vermont Registry report also included 136 infants who underwent pyloromyotomy under spinal anesthesia, further demonstrating the feasibility of the technique in this population [184].

Unfortunately there are no large, randomized, prospective studies that test the hypothesis that regional techniques are superior to general anesthesia in these high-risk patients. Based on recent literature, the current recommendation is that most otherwise healthy formerly preterm infants at a postconceptual age greater than 60 weeks may be discharged home after simple procedures without further monitoring, provided that the anesthetic and PACU course is free from apneic events. Those infants younger than 44 to 60 weeks should be admitted for monitoring for at least 12 hours postoperatively; between 46 and 60 weeks the perioperative course must be individualized.

As long as no sedative agents or general anesthetics are administered, a practitioner may minimize the risk for postoperative apnea by using spinal anesthesia for appropriate procedures. Shenkman and colleagues [188] have described in detail their technique for spinal blockade and reported their experience with 62 infants undergoing inguinal herniorrhaphy, 55 of whom were born prematurely.

Patients should be appropriately selected based on their overall health status and the nature of the procedure. In addition, the ability of the surgeon to perform the procedure in less than 60 minutes should also be considered. Relatively larger doses of local anesthetic drugs are required in this population to achieve an adequate level because of larger volumes, faster circulation, and clearance of cerebrospinal fluid [189,190]. Cerebrospinal fluid volume is larger on an mL/kg basis in infants and neonates (4 mL/kg) compared with adults (2 mL/kg), which may also account for the higher dose requirements and shorter duration of action [189,190].

Thirty to 60 minutes before surgery, 1 mL of EMLA cream with an occlusive dressing should be applied to the midline over L4–S1. The patient is positioned at the edge of the operating table in a sitting position while a second assistant gently supports the chin to avoid obstruction of the airway (see Fig. 2). A 25-gauge Whitacre spinal needle is inserted in the midline in the interspace between L4–S1, because the conus medullaris terminates at L3 in infants. A dose of 1 mL/kg of 1% tetracaine with epinephrine provides 60 minutes of spinal analgesia. See Table 5 for recommended doses.

Use of ultrasound in peripheral nerve blocks

It is beyond the scope of this article to describe in detail all of the ultrasound approaches to upper and lower extremity nerve blocks in children. Instead, we focus on the basic concepts of ultrasound, introducing the practitioner to the future potential of ultrasound-guided regional anesthesia.

Compared with central neuraxial blocks, peripheral nerve blocks remain underused in pediatric anesthesia. Clinicians' resistance to incorporating peripheral nerve blocks into clinical practice may result from concerns about reliability of the block, perceived difficulty of block placement, time required, and lack of experience with the more proximal blocks. Too often, the anesthesiologist performs the block using a blind technique using anatomical landmarks or a nerve-stimulator technique, resulting in a high failure rate and possibly serious complications.

The success of peripheral nerve blocks depends on the practitioner's familiarity with the anatomic landmarks and insertion of the needle in close proximity to the nerve. Anatomic variations in the growing child make precise placement of the needle particularly challenging to the pediatric anesthesiologist. Techniques that rely on measurements from a fixed point clearly have limitations when applied to all age groups.

Ultrasound has been in use in other clinical arenas for several years; however, the technique was slow to catch on for regional blocks because of poor resolution of the images. In addition, the large probes initially available were not conducive to needle placement on a small child, and the bulky size of the machine in the operating room further discouraged its application. The development of new high-resolution portable ultrasound machines with smaller probes makes this imaging modality more feasible for regional anesthesia in children.

Table 5	
Spinal anesthesia for infants	
Local anesthetic	Typical dose and concentration
Bupivacaine	1 mg/kg 0.5% hyperbaric with 1:1000 epinephrine[a], provides 60 minutes of surgical anesthesia
Tetracaine	1 mg/kg 0.5% hyperbaric with 1:1000 epinephrine[a], provides 60–75 minutes of surgical anesthesia

[a] Reduce to 0.8 mg/kg in patients receiving diuretics.

The term ultrasound applies to all acoustic energy with a frequency above that of human hearing (20 kilohertz). Typical diagnostic sonography scanners operate in the frequency range of 2 to 15 MHz. Ultrasound probes are named after the geometric arrangement of their piezoelectric elements [191]. Piezoelectric elements are crystals located in the probe and undergo periodic deformation to produce sound waves when an alternating voltage is applied. Linear probes have piezoelectric elements arranged in parallel.

Most pediatric nerve blocks can be performed using a linear "hockey stick" ultrasound probe with a 25-mm active surface area, whereas for an older child a probe with a 38-mm active surface area can be used. The optimum frequency is a trade-off between the resolution of the image and the depth of the structures to be visualized: lower frequencies produce less resolution but penetrate deeper into the body. Transducers covering a bandwidth of 5 to 10 MHz or 8 to 14 MHz offer excellent resolution of superficial structures and good penetration to deeper structures [192].

In general, most standard block needles can be used for ultrasonographic techniques. An insulated stimulating needle offers the anesthesiologist additional confirmation on selected nerves being blocked, but is not necessary once mastery of ultrasound-guided nerve blocks has been achieved. Currently, manufacturers are working to develop needles with improved visibility on ultrasound.

Ultrasound techniques for peripheral nerve blocks fall into two categories depending on the needle position relative to the probe: cross-sectional and in-line techniques. With the cross-sectional technique, the needle is placed transverse to the plane of the probe and is identified by tissue displacement and the acoustic shadow that emerges at its tip. One advantage of this technique is that the image reveals the target structures and the needle position. Because the needle penetration is less than with the in-line technique, there may be less trauma and pain associated with the cross-sectional technique.

With the in-line technique, the needle enters along the longitudinal axis of the ultrasound probe. This approach facilitates visualization of the shaft of the needle in addition to the tip. Slight transverse movements away from the long axis remove the needle from the image, however. Regardless, it is crucial to visualize the spread of the local anesthetic during injection.

Before starting to perform ultrasound-guided nerve blocks in children, the practitioner should avail himself or herself of specialized training, either at hands-on workshops or under the supervision of an experienced colleague. In addition, the safety and success of ultrasound techniques depends on adequate technical specifications, the proper selection of ultrasound probes, and proper adjustment of the ultrasound unit. Randomized prospective studies with sufficient power are necessary to determine the superiority of ultrasound-guided regional blocks over other techniques. Guidelines for basic equipment requirements, along with descriptions of optimal views for appropriate imaging of nerve structures, still need to be developed before this modality is adapted for routine practice.

MANAGING SIDE EFFECTS AND COMPLICATIONS OF ANALGESIA

Side effect management

The most common and irritating side effects of any analgesic technique that includes opiates are nausea and vomiting (PONV), urinary retention, and itching, whether delivered systemically or along the neuraxis. Many strategies are available to minimize the incidence of PONV, as discussed in a recent review article [193]. One strategy that has generated interest recently is the addition of a naloxone infusion for children experiencing refractory nausea and vomiting with intravenous opiates. In a prospective, double-blind, placebo-controlled trial, Maxwell and colleagues [194] demonstrated that a low-dose naloxone infusion at 0.25 µg/kg/h was effective at aborting these effects.

A similar strategy may also be effective for the nausea and vomiting that accompanies epidural analgesia. For itching related to epidural analgesia, we administer antihistamines initially. If there is no relief, our next strategy is to administer a small dose of nalbuphine, an agonist–antagonist agent, which has been considered helpful in this situation.

Respiratory depression

Respiratory depression is the most feared complication of opiate therapy, which can occur with opiates administered by any route. Recognition of the patient's intrinsic risk factors, careful titration of appropriate opiate therapy, minimizing opiate dosing by using multimodal therapy, and vigilance are the best preventive strategies. Cardiorespiratory monitoring, which may be recommended for the youngest or most fragile patients, or for selected patients receiving neuraxial opioids, can never be a substitute for monitoring the level of consciousness or for counting and observing the patient's respiration. The goal for monitoring and observation, of course, is to intervene at the earliest sign of respiratory depression, before respiratory and cardiac arrest. Small doses of naloxone, or small doses of an agonist–antagonist agent, such as nalbuphine, can reverse respiratory depression without reversing analgesia. Subsequent management may require changing the analgesic plan, transferring the patient to a unit with higher-level nursing care, or the institution of a low-dose naloxone infusion. Each institution should develop standard protocols for prevention, recognition, and management of this dreaded complication.

Local anesthetic toxicity

The most dreaded complication from performing regional blocks is the potential for intravascular injection of the local anesthetic resulting in cardiac arrest. In the largest prospective cohort of more than 24,000 pediatric patients undergoing regional anesthesia, there were no cases of cardiac arrest secondary to local anesthetics, so the incidence of this complication was believed to be extremely low [129]. In the initial analysis of the ASA Closed Claim Study, however, local anesthetic was associated with 7 of 238 pediatric cardiac arrests, for an incidence of 0.3% [195]; in a more recent analysis of closed cases, still unpublished, 18 of 559 pediatric claims (0.3%).

Bupivacaine is considered more cardiotoxic than ropivacaine, and until recently there were few reports of successful resuscitation following inadvertent intravascular injection of bupivacaine [196]. Weinberg and colleagues [197] have demonstrated the efficacy of injecting 20% lipid emulsion in reversing the cardiotoxic effects of bupivacaine in dogs. Extrapolating from adult data, a dose of 1 mL/kg has been recommended. We believe that the increased use of safer local anesthetics and ultrasound-guided regional blocks in children will further enhance safety of regional techniques in children. Even so, we advocate the ready availability of the 20% lipid emulsion in all locations where central or peripheral blocks are performed.

SUMMARY

Effective analgesia for children begins with an age-appropriate assessment of pain and requires a sound knowledge of pharmacology and developmental physiology. Initiating analgesia before the surgical stimulus and using a multimodal approach with a combination of agents, including NSAIDs, opioids, regional analgesia techniques, and adjuncts, minimizes the pain and distress our smallest patients' experience.

Despite the advances of the last 10 years, anesthesiologists caring for children continue to face challenges and uncertainties in providing adequate analgesia to pediatric surgical patients. There is still a frustrating time lag for approval of new drugs for use in children and a delay in approval for drugs in the United States that have long enjoyed pediatric indications in other parts of the world. Techniques and equipment appropriately sized for use in children lag in development and implementation. The role of pre-emptive analgesia, and how best to provide it, remains unclear.

Our greatest challenge as pediatric specialists is not only to advance the practice of more technically sophisticated pain management with new gadgets and pumps but also to educate our pediatric colleagues on the effective use of the medications already available to us, to teach them how to respond in a timely manner to unrelieved pain, and to manage the side effects of treatment.

References

[1] von Baeyer CL, Spagrud LJ. Systematic review of observational (behavioral) measures of pain for children and adolescents aged 3 to 18 years. Pain 2007;127(1–2):140–50.

[2] McGrath PJ, Johnson G, Goodman JT, et al. CHEOPS: a behavioral scale for rating postoperative pain in children. In: Fields HL, Dubner R, Cervero F, editors, Advances in pain research and therapy, vol. 9. New York: Raven Press; 1985. p. 395–402.

[3] Merkel SI, et al. The FLACC: a behavioral scale for scoring postoperative pain in young children. Pediatr Nurs 1997;23(3):293–7.

[4] Chambers CT, et al. The parents' postoperative pain measure: replication and extension to 2-6-year-old children. Pain 2003;105(3):437–43.

[5] Ambuel B, et al. Assessing distress in pediatric intensive care environments: the COMFORT scale. J Pediatr Psychol 1992;17(1):95–109.

[6] Krechel SW, Bildner J. CRIES: a new neonatal postoperative pain measurement score. Initial testing of validity and reliability. Paediatr Anaesth 1995;5(1):53–61.

[7] Stevens B, et al. Premature infant pain profile: development and initial validation. Clin J Pain 1996;12(1):13–22.

[8] Taylor BJ, et al. Assessing postoperative pain in neonates: a multicenter observational study. Pediatrics 2006;118(4):e992–1000.

[9] Beyer JE, McGrath PJ, Berde CB. Discordance between self-report and behavioral pain measures in children aged 3–7 years after surgery. J Pain Symptom Manage 1990;5(6):350–6.

[10] Kain ZN, et al. Preoperative anxiety, postoperative pain, and behavioral recovery in young children undergoing surgery. Pediatrics 2006;118(2):651–8.

[11] Logan DE, Rose JB. Is postoperative pain a self-fulfilling prophecy? Expectancy effects on postoperative pain and patient-controlled analgesia use among adolescent surgical patients. J Pediatr Psychol 2005;30(2):187–96.

[12] Logan DE, Rose JB. Gender differences in post-operative pain and patient controlled analgesia use among adolescent surgical patients. Pain 2004;109(3):481–7.

[13] Crawford MW, Galton S, Naser B. Postoperative morphine consumption in children with sickle-cell disease. Paediatr Anaesth 2006;16(2):152–7.

[14] Kehlet H, Dahl JB. The value of "multimodal" or "balanced analgesia" in postoperative pain treatment. Anesth Analg 1993;77(5):1048–56.

[15] Ong CK, et al. The efficacy of preemptive analgesia for acute postoperative pain management: a meta-analysis. Anesth Analg 2005;100(3):757–73, Table of contents.

[16] Kelly DJ, Ahmad M, Brull SJ. Preemptive analgesia II: recent advances and current trends. Can J Anaesth 2001;48(11):1091–101.

[17] Kelly DJ, Ahmad M, Brull SJ. Preemptive analgesia I: physiological pathways and pharmacological modalities. Can J Anaesth 2001;48(10):1000–10.

[18] Langer JC, Shandling B, Rosenberg M. Intraoperative bupivacaine during outpatient hernia repair in children: a randomized double blind trial. J Pediatr Surg 1987;22(3):267–70.

[19] Giannoni C, et al. Ropivacaine with or without clonidine improves pediatric tonsillectomy pain. Arch Otolaryngol Head Neck Surg 2001;127(10):1265–70.

[20] Suresh S, et al. Does a preemptive block of the great auricular nerve improve postoperative analgesia in children undergoing tympanomastoid surgery? Anesth Analg 2004;98(2):330–3, Table of contents.

[21] Ates Y, et al. Postoperative analgesia in children using preemptive retrobulbar block and local anesthetic infiltration in strabismus surgery. Reg Anesth Pain Med 1998;23(6):569–74.

[22] Altintas F, et al. The efficacy of pre- versus postsurgical axillary block on postoperative pain in paediatric patients. Paediatr Anaesth 2000;10(1):23–8.

[23] Becke K, et al. Intraoperative low-dose S-ketamine has no preventive effects on postoperative pain and morphine consumption after major urological surgery in children. Paediatr Anaesth 2005;15(6):484–90.

[24] Rose JB, et al. Preoperative oral dextromethorphan does not reduce pain or analgesic consumption in children after adenotonsillectomy. Anesth Analg 1999;88(4):749–53.

[25] Maunuksela E-L, Olkkola K. Nonsteroidal anti-inflammatory drugs in pediatric pain management. In: Schechter N, Berde C, Yaster M, editors. Pain in infants, children, and adolescents. 2nd edition. Philadelphia: Lippincott Williams & Wilkins; 2003. p. 171–80.

[26] Birmingham PK, et al. Twenty-four-hour pharmacokinetics of rectal acetaminophen in children: an old drug with new recommendations. Anesthesiology 1997;87(2):244–52.

[27] Birmingham PK, et al. Initial and subsequent dosing of rectal acetaminophen in children: a 24-hour pharmacokinetic study of new dose recommendations. Anesthesiology 2001;94(3):385–9.

[28] Jacqz-Aigrain E, Anderson BJ. Pain control: non-steroidal anti-inflammatory agents. Semin Fetal Neonatal Med 2006;11(4):251–9.

[29] Marzullo L. An update of N-acetylcysteine treatment for acute acetaminophen toxicity in children. Curr Opin Pediatr 2005;17(2):239–45.

[30] Kozer E, et al. Repeated supratherapeutic doses of paracetamol in children—a literature review and suggested clinical approach. Acta Paediatr 2006;95(10):1165–71.

[31] Wurthwein G, et al. Pharmacokinetics of intravenous paracetamol in children and adolescents under major surgery. Eur J Clin Pharmacol 2005;60(12):883–8.

[32] Alhashemi JA, Daghistani MF. Effects of intraoperative I.V. acetaminophen vs I.M. meperidine on post-tonsillectomy pain in children. Br J Anaesth 2006;96(6):790–5.

[33] Alhashemi JA, Daghistani MF. Effect of intraoperative intravenous acetaminophen vs. intramuscular meperidine on pain and discharge time after paediatric dental restoration. Eur J Anaesthesiol 2007;24(2):128–33.

[34] Rey E, et al. Stereoselective disposition of ibuprofen enantiomers in infants. Br J Clin Pharmacol 1994;38(4):373–5.

[35] Kyllonen M, et al. Perioperative pharmacokinetics of ibuprofen enantiomers after rectal administration. Paediatr Anaesth 2005;15(7):566–73.

[36] De Silva B, et al. Pseudoporphyria and nonsteroidal antiinflammatory agents in children with juvenile idiopathic arthritis. Pediatr Dermatol 2000;17(6):480–3.

[37] Bryant P, Lachman P. Pseudoporphyria secondary to non-steroidal anti-inflammatory drugs. Arch Dis Child 2003;88(11):961.

[38] Ruperto N, et al. A randomized, double-blind clinical trial of two doses of meloxicam compared with naproxen in children with juvenile idiopathic arthritis: short- and long-term efficacy and safety results. Arthritis Rheum 2005;52(2):563–72.

[39] Debley JS, et al. The prevalence of ibuprofen-sensitive asthma in children: a randomized controlled bronchoprovocation challenge study. J Pediatr 2005;147(2):233–8.

[40] Palmer GM. A teenager with severe asthma exacerbation following ibuprofen. Anaesth Intensive Care 2005;33(2):261–5.

[41] Lesko SM, et al. Asthma morbidity after the short-term use of ibuprofen in children. Pediatrics 2002;109(2):E20.

[42] Ilowite NT. Current treatment of juvenile rheumatoid arthritis. Pediatrics 2002;109(1):109–15.

[43] Keenan GF, Giannini EH, Athreya BH. Clinically significant gastropathy associated with nonsteroidal antiinflammatory drug use in children with juvenile rheumatoid arthritis. J Rheumatol 1995;22(6):1149–51.

[44] Krause I, et al. Acute renal failure, associated with non-steroidal anti-inflammatory drugs in healthy children. Pediatr Nephrol 2005;20(9):1295–8.

[45] Cardwell M, Siviter G, Smith A. . Non-steroidal anti-inflammatory drugs and perioperative bleeding in paediatric tonsillectomy. Cochrane Database Syst Rev 2005;2:CD003591.

[46] Sheeran PW, et al. Rofecoxib administration to paediatric patients undergoing adenotonsillectomy. Paediatr Anaesth 2004;14(7):579–83.

[47] Perrott DA, et al. Efficacy and safety of acetaminophen vs ibuprofen for treating children's pain or fever: a meta-analysis. Arch Pediatr Adolesc Med 2004;158(6):521–6.

[48] Armstrong PJ, Bersten A. Normeperidine toxicity. Anesth Analg 1986;65(5):536–8.

[49] Morisy L, Platt D. Hazards of high-dose meperidine. JAMA 1986;255(4):467–8.

[50] Jablonka DH, Davis PJ. Opioids in pediatric anesthesia. Anesthesiol Clin North America 2005;23(4):621–34, viii.

[51] Quigley C. Hydromorphone for acute and chronic pain. Cochrane Database Syst Rev 2002;1:CD003447.

[52] Quigley C, Wiffen P. A systematic review of hydromorphone in acute and chronic pain. J Pain Symptom Manage 2003;25(2):169–78.

[53] Ross AK, et al. Pharmacokinetics of remifentanil in anesthetized pediatric patients undergoing elective surgery or diagnostic procedures. Anesth Analg 2001;93(6):1393–401, Table of contents.

[54] Crawford MW, et al. Development of acute opioid tolerance during infusion of remifentanil for pediatric scoliosis surgery. Anesth Analg 2006;102(6):1662–7.

[55] Zimmermann C, et al. Rotation to methadone after opioid dose escalation: how should individualization of dosing occur? J Pain Palliat Care Pharmacother 2005;19(2):25–31.

[56] Inturrisi CE. Pharmacology of methadone and its isomers. Minerva Anestesiol 2005; 71(7–8):435–7.

[57] Gagnon B, Almahrezi A, Schreier G. Methadone in the treatment of neuropathic pain. Pain Res Manag 2003;8(3):149–54.

[58] Berde CB, et al. Comparison of morphine and methadone for prevention of postoperative pain in 3- to 7-year-old children. J Pediatr 1991;119(1 (Pt 1)):136–41.

[59] Shannon M, Berde CB. Pharmacologic management of pain in children and adolescents. Pediatr Clin North Am 1989;36(4):855–71.

[60] Berde CB. Pediatric postoperative pain management. Pediatr Clin North Am 1989;36(4): 921–40.

[61] Hudcova J, et al. Patient controlled opioid analgesia versus conventional opioid analgesia for postoperative pain. Cochrane Database Syst Rev 2006;4:CD003348.

[62] Collins JJ, et al. Patient-controlled analgesia for mucositis pain in children: a three-period crossover study comparing morphine and hydromorphone. J Pediatr 1996;129(5): 722–8.

[63] Coda BA, et al. Comparative efficacy of patient-controlled administration of morphine, hydromorphone, or sufentanil for the treatment of oral mucositis pain following bone marrow transplantation. Pain 1997;72(3):333–46.

[64] Murray A, Hagen NA. Hydromorphone. J Pain Symptom Manage 2005;29(5 Suppl): S57–66.

[65] Ruggiero A, et al. Safety and efficacy of fentanyl administered by patient controlled analgesia in children with cancer pain. Support Care Cancer 2007;15(5):569–73.

[66] Kelly JJ, et al. Postoperative sleep disturbance in pediatric patients using patient-controlled devices (PCA). Paediatr Anaesth 2006;16(10):1051–6.

[67] Anghelescu DL, et al. The safety of patient-controlled analgesia by proxy in pediatric oncology patients. Anesth Analg 2005;101(6):1623–7.

[68] Kost-Byerly S. New concepts in acute and extended postoperative pain management in children. Anesthesiol Clin North America 2002;20(1):115–35.

[69] Arnold JH, et al. Tolerance and dependence in neonates sedated with fentanyl during extracorporeal membrane oxygenation. Anesthesiology 1990;73(6):1136–40.

[70] Borland M, et al. A randomized controlled trial comparing intranasal fentanyl to intravenous morphine for managing acute pain in children in the emergency department. Ann Emerg Med 2007;49(3):335–40.

[71] Mathieu N, et al. Intranasal sufentanil is effective for postoperative analgesia in adults. Can J Anaesth 2006;53(1):60–6.

[72] Borland ML, et al. Intranasal fentanyl is an equivalent analgesic to oral morphine in paediatric burns patients for dressing changes: a randomised double blind crossover study. Burns 2005;31(7):831–7.

[73] Galinkin JL, et al. Use of intranasal fentanyl in children undergoing myringotomy and tube placement during halothane and sevoflurane anesthesia. Anesthesiology 2000;93(6): 1378–83.

[74] Finkel JC, et al. The effect of intranasal fentanyl on the emergence characteristics after sevoflurane anesthesia in children undergoing surgery for bilateral myringotomy tube placement. Anesth Analg 2001;92(5):1164–8.

[75] Haynes G, Brahen NH, Hill HF. Plasma sufentanil concentration after intranasal administration to paediatric outpatients. Can J Anaesth 1993;40(3):286.

[76] Brenchley J, Ramlakhan S. Intranasal alfentanil for acute pain in children. Emerg Med J 2006;23(6):488.

[77] Finkel JC, et al. Transdermal fentanyl in the management of children with chronic severe pain: results from an international study. Cancer 2005;104(12):2847–57.

[78] Christensen ML, et al. Transdermal fentanyl administration in children and adolescents with sickle cell pain crisis. J Pediatr Hematol Oncol 1996;18(4):372–6.

[79] Moffett BS, et al. Safety of ketorolac in neonates and infants after cardiac surgery. Paediatr Anaesth 2006;16(4):424–8.

[80] Gupta A, et al. Ketorolac after congenital heart surgery: does it increase the risk of significant bleeding complications? Paediatr Anaesth 2005;15(2):139–42.

[81] Gunter JB, et al. Recovery and complications after tonsillectomy in children: a comparison of ketorolac and morphine. Anesth Analg 1995;81(6):1136–41.

[82] Buck ML, Norwood VF. Ketorolac-induced acute renal failure in a previously healthy adolescent. Pediatrics 1996;98(2 Pt 1):294–6.

[83] Kallanagowdar C, LeBreton A, Aviles DH. Acute renal failure. Clin Pediatr (Phila) 2006;45(8):771–3.

[84] Simckes AM, et al. Ketorolac-induced irreversible renal failure in sickle cell disease: a case report. Pediatr Nephrol 1999;13(1):63–7.

[85] Reuben SS, Ablett D, Kaye R. High dose nonsteroidal anti-inflammatory drugs compromise spinal fusion. Can J Anaesth 2005;52(5):506–12.

[86] Vitale MG, et al. Use of ketorolac tromethamine in children undergoing scoliosis surgery. An analysis of complications. Spine J 2003;3(1):55–62.

[87] Munro HM, et al. Low-dose ketorolac improves analgesia and reduces morphine requirements following posterior spinal fusion in adolescents. Can J Anaesth 2002;49(5): 461–6.

[88] Lin C, Durieux ME. Ketamine and kids: an update. Paediatr Anaesth 2005;15(2):91–7.

[89] Aspinall RL, Mayor A. A prospective randomized controlled study of the efficacy of ketamine for postoperative pain relief in children after adenotonsillectomy. Paediatr Anaesth 2001;11(3):333–6.

[90] Marcus RJ, et al. Comparison of ketamine and morphine for analgesia after tonsillectomy in children. Br J Anaesth 2000;84(6):739–42.

[91] DA Conceicuo J, Bruggemann CD, Carneiro Leao C. Effect of an intravenous single dose of ketamine on postoperative pain in tonsillectomy patients. Paediatr Anaesth 2006;16(9): 962–7.

[92] Elia N, Tramer MR. Ketamine and postoperative pain—a quantitative systematic review of randomised trials. Pain 2005;113(1–2):61–70.

[93] Bell RF, et al. Perioperative ketamine for acute postoperative pain. Cochrane Database Syst Rev 2006;1:CD004603.

[94] Bozkurt P. Use of tramadol in children. Paediatr Anaesth 2005;15(12):1041–7.

[95] Finkel JC, et al. An evaluation of the efficacy and tolerability of oral tramadol hydrochloride tablets for the treatment of postsurgical pain in children. Anesth Analg 2002;94(6): 1469–73.

[96] Ozalevli M, et al. Comparison of morphine and tramadol by patient-controlled analgesia for postoperative analgesia after tonsillectomy in children. Paediatr Anaesth 2005;15(11):979–84.

[97] Erhan E, et al. Tramadol infusion for the pain management in sickle cell disease: a case report. Paediatr Anaesth 2007;17(1):84–6.

[98] Hullett BJ, et al. Tramadol vs morphine during adenotonsillectomy for obstructive sleep apnea in children. Paediatr Anaesth 2006;16(6):648–53.

[99] Butkovic D, Toljan S, Mihovilovic-Novak B. Experience with gabapentin for neuropathic pain in adolescents: report of five cases. Paediatr Anaesth 2006;16(3):325–9.

[100] Lauder GR, White MC. Neuropathic pain following multilevel surgery in children with cerebral palsy: a case series and review. Paediatr Anaesth 2005;15(5):412–20.

[101] Wheeler DS, Vaux KK, Tam DA. Use of gabapentin in the treatment of childhood reflex sympathetic dystrophy. Pediatr Neurol 2000;22(3):220–1.

[102] Rose MA, Kam PC. Gabapentin: pharmacology and its use in pain management. Anaesthesia 2002;57(5):451–62.

[103] Mendham JE. Gabapentin for the treatment of itching produced by burns and wound healing in children: a pilot study. Burns 2004;30(8):851–3.

[104] Ho KY, Gan TJ, Habib AS. Gabapentin and postoperative pain–a systematic review of randomized controlled trials. Pain 2006;126(1–3):91–101.

[105] Mikawa K, et al. Efficacy of oral clonidine premedication in children. Anesthesiology 1993;79(5):926–31.

[106] Reimer EJ, et al. The effectiveness of clonidine as an analgesic in paediatric adenotonsillectomy. Can J Anaesth 1998;45(12):1162–7.

[107] Orko R, et al. Effect of clonidine on haemodynamic responses to endotracheal intubation and on gastric acidity. Acta Anaesthesiol Scand 1987;31(4):325–9.

[108] Samso E, et al. Comparative assessment of the anaesthetic and analgesic effects of intramuscular and epidural clonidine in humans. Can J Anaesth 1996;43(12):1195–202.

[109] Mukhtar AM, Obayah EM, Hassona AM. Preliminary experience with dexmedetomidine in pediatric anesthesia. Anesth Analg 2006;103(1):250.

[110] Mukhtar AM, Obayah EM, Hassona AM. The use of dexmedetomidine in pediatric cardiac surgery. Anesth Analg 2006;103(1):52–6, Table of contents.

[111] Everett LL, et al. Use of dexmedetomidine in awake craniotomy in adolescents: report of two cases. Paediatr Anaesth 2006;16(3):338–42.

[112] Guler G, et al. Single-dose dexmedetomidine reduces agitation and provides smooth extubation after pediatric adenotonsillectomy. Paediatr Anaesth 2005;15(9):762–6.

[113] Mason KP, et al. Dexmedetomidine for pediatric sedation for computed tomography imaging studies. Anesth Analg 2006;103(1):57–62, Table of contents.

[114] Koroglu A, et al. A comparison of the sedative, hemodynamic, and respiratory effects of dexmedetomidine and propofol in children undergoing magnetic resonance imaging. Anesth Analg 2006;103(1):63–7, Table of contents.

[115] Hammer GB, et al. Prolonged infusion of dexmedetomidine for sedation following tracheal resection. Paediatr Anaesth 2005;15(7):616–20.

[116] Walker J, et al. Sedation using dexmedetomidine in pediatric burn patients. J Burn Care Res 2006;27(2):206–10.

[117] Chrysostomou C, Zeballos T. Use of dexmedetomidine in a pediatric heart transplant patient. Pediatr Cardiol 2005;26(5):651–4.

[118] Finkel JC, Elrefai A. The use of dexmedetomidine to facilitate opioid and benzodiazepine detoxification in an infant. Anesth Analg 2004;98(6):1658–69.

[119] Zub D, Berkenbosch JW, Tobias JD. Preliminary experience with oral dexmedetomidine for procedural and anesthetic premedication. Paediatr Anaesth 2005;15(11):932–8.

[120] Tanelian DL, Brose WG. Neuropathic pain can be relieved by drugs that are use-dependent sodium channel blockers: lidocaine, carbamazepine, and mexiletine. Anesthesiology 1991;74(5):949–51.

[121] Tsai PS, et al. Lidocaine concentrations in plasma and cerebrospinal fluid after systemic bolus administration in humans. Anesth Analg 1998;87(3):601–4.

[122] Nathan A, et al. Primary erythromelalgia in a child responding to intravenous lidocaine and oral mexiletine treatment. Pediatrics 2005;115(4):e504–7.

[123] Wallace MS, et al. Intravenous lidocaine: effects on controlling pain after anti-GD2 antibody therapy in children with neuroblastoma—a report of a series. Anesth Analg 1997;85(4):794–6.

[124] Massey GV, et al. Continuous lidocaine infusion for the relief of refractory malignant pain in a terminally ill pediatric cancer patient. J Pediatr Hematol Oncol 2002;24(7):566–8.

[125] Koppert W, et al. Perioperative intravenous lidocaine has preventive effects on postoperative pain and morphine consumption after major abdominal surgery. Anesth Analg 2004;98(4):1050–5, Table of contents.

[126] Kaba A, et al. Intravenous lidocaine infusion facilitates acute rehabilitation after laparoscopic colectomy. Anesthesiology 2007;106(1):11–8 [discussion: 5–6].

[127] Petersen KL, Rowbotham MC. Will ion-channel blockers be useful for management of nonneuropathic pain? J Pain 2000;1(3 Suppl):26–34.

[128] Rodgers A, et al. Reduction of postoperative mortality and morbidity with epidural or spinal anaesthesia: results from overview of randomised trials. BMJ 2000;321(7275):1493.

[129] Giaufre E, Dalens B, Gombert A. Epidemiology and morbidity of regional anesthesia in children: a one-year prospective survey of the French-Language Society of Pediatric Anesthesiologists. Anesth Analg 1996;83(5):904–12.

[130] Schuepfer G, et al. Generating a learning curve for pediatric caudal epidural blocks: an empirical evaluation of technical skills in novice and experienced anesthetists. Reg Anesth Pain Med 2000;25(4):385–8.

[131] Newman PJ, Bushnell TG, Radford P. The effect of needle size and type in paediatric caudal analgesia. Paediatr Anaesth 1996;6(6):459–61.

[132] Baris S, et al. Is tissue coring a real problem after caudal injection in children. Paediatr Anaesth 2004;14(9):755–8.

[133] Suresh S, Wheeler M. Practical pediatric regional anesthesia. Anesthesiol Clin North America 2002;20(1):83–113.

[134] Wolf AR, et al. Bupivacaine for caudal analgesia in infants and children: the optimal effective concentration. Anesthesiology 1988;69(1):102–6.

[135] Valley RD, Bailey AG. Caudal morphine for postoperative analgesia in infants and children: a report of 138 cases. Anesth Analg 1991;72(1):120–4.

[136] Curatolo M, et al. Epidural fentanyl, adrenaline and clonidine as adjuvants to local anaesthetics for surgical analgesia: meta-analyses of analgesia and side-effects. Acta Anaesthesiol Scand 1998;42(8):910–20.

[137] Campbell FA, et al. Analgesic efficacy and safety of a caudal bupivacaine-fentanyl mixture in children. Can J Anaesth 1992;39(7):661–4.

[138] Jones RD, Gunawardene WM, Yeung CK. A comparison of lignocaine 2% with adrenaline 1:200,000 and lignocaine 2% with adrenaline 1:200,000 plus fentanyl as agents for caudal anaesthesia in children undergoing circumcision. Anaesth Intensive Care 1990;18(2):194–9.

[139] Paalzow L. Analgesia produced by clonidine in mice and rats. J Pharm Pharmacol 1974;26(5):361–3.

[140] De Negri P, et al. New local anesthetics for pediatric anesthesia. Curr Opin Anaesthesiol 2005;18(3):289–92.

[141] Klimscha W, et al. The efficacy and safety of a clonidine/bupivacaine combination in caudal blockade for pediatric hernia repair. Anesth Analg 1998;86(1):54–61.

[142] Weber F, Wulf H. Caudal bupivacaine and s(+)-ketamine for postoperative analgesia in children. Paediatr Anaesth 2003;13(3):244–8.

[143] Lee HM, Sanders GM. Caudal ropivacaine and ketamine for postoperative analgesia in children. Anaesthesia 2000;55(8):806–10.

[144] Johnston P, et al. The effect of ketamine on 0.25% and 0.125% bupivacaine for caudal epidural blockade in children. Paediatr Anaesth 1999;9(1):31–4.

[145] Cook B, et al. Comparison of the effects of adrenaline, clonidine and ketamine on the duration of caudal analgesia produced by bupivacaine in children. Br J Anaesth 1995;75(6):698–701.

[146] White PF, et al. Comparative pharmacology of the ketamine isomers. Studies in volunteers. Br J Anaesth 1985;57(2):197–203.

[147] Marhofer P, et al. S(+)-ketamine for caudal block in paediatric anaesthesia. Br J Anaesth 2000;84(3):341–5.

[148] Baris S, et al. Comparison of fentanyl-bupivacaine or midazolam-bupivacaine mixtures with plain bupivacaine for caudal anaesthesia in children. Paediatr Anaesth 2003;13(2):126–31.

[149] Abdulatif M, El-Sanabary M. Caudal neostigmine, bupivacaine, and their combination for postoperative pain management after hypospadias surgery in children. Anesth Analg 2002;95(5):1215–8.

[150] Tobias JD, et al. Thoracic epidural anaesthesia in infants and children. Can J Anaesth 1993;40(9):879–82.

[151] Bosenberg AT, et al. Thoracic epidural anesthesia via caudal route in infants. Anesthesiology 1988;69(2):265–9.

[152] Seefelder C. The caudal catheter in neonates: where are the restrictions? Curr Opin Anaesthesiol 2002;15(3):343–8.

[153] Kost-Byerly S, et al. Bacterial colonization and infection rate of continuous epidural catheters in children. Anesth Analg 1998;86(4):712–6.

[154] McNeely JK, et al. Culture of bacteria from lumbar and caudal epidural catheters used for postoperative analgesia in children. Reg Anesth 1997;22(5):428–31.

[155] Bubeck J, et al. Subcutaneous tunneling of caudal catheters reduces the rate of bacterial colonization to that of lumbar epidural catheters. Anesth Analg 2004;99(3):689–93, Table of contents.

[156] Abouleish E, Orig T, Amortegui AJ. Bacteriologic comparison between epidural and caudal techniques. Anesthesiology 1980;53(6):511–4.

[157] O'Grady NP, et al. Guidelines for the prevention of intravascular catheter-related infections. Centers for Disease Control and Prevention. MMWR Recomm Rep 2002;51(RR-10):1–29.

[158] Blanco D, et al. [Thoracic epidural anesthesia by the caudal route in pediatric anesthesia: age is a limiting factor]. Rev Esp Anestesiol Reanim 1994;41(4):214–6 [in Spanish].

[159] Rasch DK, et al. Lumbar and thoracic epidural analgesia via the caudal approach for postoperative pain relief in infants and children. Can J Anaesth 1990;37(3):359–62.

[160] van Niekerk J, et al. Epidurography in premature infants. Anaesthesia 1990;45(9):722–5.

[161] Valairucha S, Seefelder C, Houck CS. Thoracic epidural catheters placed by the caudal route in infants: the importance of radiographic confirmation. Paediatr Anaesth 2002;12(5):424–8.

[162] Cork RC, Kryc JJ, Vaughan RW. Ultrasonic localization of the lumbar epidural space. Anesthesiology 1980;52(6):513–6.

[163] Chen CP, et al. Ultrasound guidance in caudal epidural needle placement. Anesthesiology 2004;101(1):181–4.

[164] Rapp HJ, Folger A, Grau T. Ultrasound-guided epidural catheter insertion in children. Anesth Analg 2005;101(2):333–9, Table of contents.

[165] Willschke H, et al. Epidural catheter placement in neonates: sonoanatomy and feasibility of ultrasonographic guidance in term and preterm neonates. Reg Anesth Pain Med 2007;32(1):34–40.

[166] Willschke H, et al. Epidural catheter placement in children: comparing a novel approach using ultrasound guidance and a standard loss-of-resistance technique. Br J Anaesth 2006;97(2):200–7.

[167] Tsui BC. Thoracic epidural catheter placement in infants via the caudal approach under electrocardiographic guidance: simplification of the original technique. Anesth Analg 2004;98(1):273.

[168] Tsui BC. Thoracic epidural catheter placement via the caudal approach under electrocardiographic guidance. Can J Anaesth 2002;49(2):216–7.

[169] Tsui BC, et al. Thoracic and lumbar epidural analgesia via the caudal approach using electrical stimulation guidance in pediatric patients: a review of 289 patients. Anesthesiology 2004;100(3):683–9.

[170] Ivani G, et al. Comparison of ropivacaine with bupivacaine for paediatric caudal block. Br J Anaesth 1998;81(2):247–8.

[171] Foster RH, Markham A. Levobupivacaine: a review of its pharmacology and use as a local anaesthetic. Drugs 2000;59(3):551–79.

[172] Ivani G, et al. Caudal anesthesia for minor pediatric surgery: a prospective randomized comparison of ropivacaine 0.2% vs levobupivacaine 0.2%. Paediatr Anaesth 2005;15(6):491–4.

[173] Breschan C, et al. A prospective study comparing the analgesic efficacy of levobupivacaine, ropivacaine and bupivacaine in pediatric patients undergoing caudal blockade. Paediatr Anaesth 2005;15(4):301–6.

[174] Astuto M, Disma N, Arena C. Levobupivacaine 0.25% compared with ropivacaine 0.25% by the caudal route in children. Eur J Anaesthesiol 2003;20(10):826–30.

[175] Dony P, et al. The comparative toxicity of ropivacaine and bupivacaine at equipotent doses in rats. Anesth Analg 2000;91(6):1489–92.

[176] Bosenberg AT, et al. Pharmacokinetics and efficacy of ropivacaine for continuous epidural infusion in neonates and infants. Paediatr Anaesth 2005;15(9):739–49.

[177] Meunier JF, et al. Pharmacokinetics of bupivacaine after continuous epidural infusion in infants with and without biliary atresia. Anesthesiology 2001;95(1):87–95.

[178] Mazoit JX, Dalens BJ. Pharmacokinetics of local anaesthetics in infants and children. Clin Pharmacokinet 2004;43(1):17–32.

[179] Berde C. Local anesthetics in infants and children: an update. Paediatr Anaesth 2004;14(5):387–93.

[180] Cote CJ, et al. Postoperative apnea in former preterm infants after inguinal herniorrhaphy. A combined analysis. Anesthesiology 1995;82(4):809–22.

[181] Sims C, Johnson CM. Postoperative apnoea in infants. Anaesth Intensive Care 1994;22(1):40–5.

[182] Welborn LG, et al. Postoperative apnea in former preterm infants: prospective comparison of spinal and general anesthesia. Anesthesiology 1990;72(5):838–42.

[183] Krane EJ, Haberkern CM, Jacobson LE. Postoperative apnea, bradycardia, and oxygen desaturation in formerly premature infants: prospective comparison of spinal and general anesthesia. Anesth Analg 1995;80(1):7–13.

[184] Williams RK, et al. The safety and efficacy of spinal anesthesia for surgery in infants: the Vermont Infant Spinal Registry. Anesth Analg 2006;102(1):67–71.

[185] William JM, et al. Post-operative recovery after inguinal herniotomy in ex-premature infants: comparison between sevoflurane and spinal anaesthesia. Br J Anaesth 2001;86(3):366–71.

[186] Craven PD, et al. Regional (spinal, epidural, caudal) versus general anaesthesia in preterm infants undergoing inguinal herniorrhaphy in early infancy. Cochrane Database Syst Rev 2003;3:CD003669.

[187] Somri M, et al. The effectiveness and safety of spinal anaesthesia in the pyloromyotomy procedure. Paediatr Anaesth 2003;13(1):32–7.

[188] Shenkman Z, et al. [Spinal anesthesia in premature infants—indications, technical aspects and results]. Harefuah 2002;141(9):770–4, 860, 859 [in Hebrew].

[189] Abajian JC, et al. Spinal anesthesia for surgery in the high-risk infant. Anesth Analg 1984;63(3):359–62.

[190] Webster AC, et al. Spinal anaesthesia for inguinal hernia repair in high-risk neonates. Can J Anaesth 1991;38(3):281–6.

[191] Marhofer P, Greher M, Kapral S. Ultrasound guidance in regional anaesthesia. Br J Anaesth 2005;94(1):7–17.

[192] Marhofer P, Frickey N. Ultrasonographic guidance in pediatric regional anesthesia part 1: theoretical background. Paediatr Anaesth 2006;16(10):1008–18.

[193] Kovac AL. Management of postoperative nausea and vomiting in children. Paediatr Drugs 2007;9(1):47–69.

[194] Maxwell LG, et al. The effects of a small-dose naloxone infusion on opioid-induced side effects and analgesia in children and adolescents treated with intravenous patient-controlled analgesia: a double-blind, prospective, randomized, controlled study. Anesth Analg 2005;100(4):953–8.

[195] Morray JP, et al. A comparison of pediatric and adult anesthesia closed malpractice claims. Anesthesiology 1993;78(3):461–7.

[196] Rosenblatt MA, et al. Successful use of a 20% lipid emulsion to resuscitate a patient after a presumed bupivacaine-related cardiac arrest. Anesthesiology 2006;105(1):217–8.

[197] Weinberg G, et al. Lipid emulsion infusion rescues dogs from bupivacaine-induced cardiac toxicity. Reg Anesth Pain Med 2003;28(3):198–202.

Advances in Anesthesia 25 (2007) 189–204

ADVANCES IN ANESTHESIA

ELSEVIER
MOSBY

The Use of Ultrasound in Regional Anesthesia

James Benonis, MD, Stuart A. Grant, MBChB, FRCA*

Division of Orthopedics, Plastics, and Regional Anesthesia, Department of Anesthesiology, Duke University Medical Center, Box 3094, Durham, NC 27710, USA

T he use of ultrasound to perform regional anesthesia has become one of the largest changes in the subspecialty in recent years. The publications on ultrasound have changed from case reports and assessments about the feasibility of visualizing a nerve with ultrasound to prospective trials comparing traditional nerve stimulation and landmark techniques with ultrasound. The growth in ultrasound use has been exponential and is mirroring the spread of ultrasound in other medical fields, such as obstetrics, cardiology, emergency medicine, and vascular access. The first publications of the use of ultrasound in regional anesthesia occurred in the late 1990s and corresponded with advances in ultrasound technology. The improvement in ultrasound definition required to discriminate a nerve from the surrounding tissues along with a reduction in cost and size of the units have made ultrasound a viable part of regional anesthesia practice. This article covers the technique and equipment required to perform ultrasound-guided regional anesthesia and summarizes the literature covering the potential advantages of the technique.

GENERAL PRINCIPLES

The ultrasound probe emits varying frequencies of sound waves into the tissues. The frequency of the sound waves is directly proportional to image resolution and inversely proportional to tissue penetration; lower-frequency probes provide greater tissue penetration with less resolution and higher-frequency probes provide greater resolution with less penetration. The image produced on the screen is a function of the time elapsed between the emission and reception of each ultrasound wave and the intensity of the returned signal. Denser materials, such as bone, cause a greater proportion of the sound waves to be reflected back to the probe, resulting in a bright (hyperechoic) image. Most regional anesthesia is performed with broadband transducers in the 5- to 12-MHz range that provide a good combination of penetration and resolution.

*Corresponding author. *E-mail address*: grant021@mc.duke.edu (S.A. Grant).

0737-6146/07/$ – see front matter
doi:10.1016/j.aan.2007.07.010

SPECIFIC EQUIPMENT FOR ANESTHESIA

Probes

Probe choice is crucial to generate the best image of the nerves you are looking at. In the upper limb the brachial plexus is superficial and can be optimally visualized by a high-frequency linear probe of 10 MHz or greater. One exception is the infraclavicular nerve block where the plexus lies deeper and a convex probe with a small radius of curvature may be preferred [1]. The convex probe affords better imaging of the needle because of the sector angle of the beam and also has a smaller footprint that sits comfortably in the infraclavicular fossa. For imaging deeper structures, such as the spine or the sciatic nerve in obese patients, a lower-frequency probe that produces better penetration is preferred.

Machine: portable versus cart-based

The ultrasound machine should fit in your work environment. If the machine position is fixed a cart-based machine works well. If you move the ultrasound machine from preoperative holding area to the operating room then a mobile machine is a better choice. The image quality of cart-based machines can now be found in some portable units so that image quality is not sacrificed for portability.

Probe covers, gel, and infection control

In an effort to keep the field sterile and prevent cross-infection between patients a sterile probe cover can be placed over the probe. Some authors have suggested just covering the probe with a clear adhesive sterile dressing applied to the probe [2] without the need for the full formal probe cover. In our opinion this is satisfactory for a single shot block but not for insertion of a catheter and we encourage the use of a formal probe cover. Infection has been transmitted from patient to patient by way of infected equipment and also large reusable tubs of ultrasound gel. Gel must be applied to the skin to ensure a good transmission of the sound waves through the skin. Air is a poor conductor and gel ensures an optimal image is obtained. If a probe cover is used it comes with a packet of gel in the sterile packaging. Gel must be placed both inside and outside of the probe cover. After performing the block the excess gel should be cleaned off the probe and the probe cleaned with an antimicrobial solution per the manufacturer's recommendations. Probe covers, gel, and cleaning solutions can be purchased from ultrasound supply companies.

TECHNIQUE OF ULTRASOUND-GUIDED NERVE BLOCK: GENERAL PRINCIPLES

Before performing a block we perform a pre-block time out and mark the appropriate site. The patient is positioned appropriately. The ultrasound machine is then positioned in a place where it is easy for the operator to change view from probe and needle to the screen by simply glancing up or down. If the ultrasound machine is placed behind the operator it is difficult to control the probe and needle while looking over the shoulder.

A pre-block nonsterile scan may be performed. This scan allows for optimization of the image on the screen using depth, frequency, and gain control and prevents adjustments being required when the operator is sterile. The skin is cleaned with chlorhexidine and the probe cover applied. Sterile gel from the probe cover is applied to the skin and a skin wheal is made where the needle insertion point is made. As the block needle is inserted a loss of image quality is expected because the indentation of the needle reduces the contact the probe has with the skin. If the needle cannot be visualized in the initial pass there are two options. Either withdraw the needle and redirect it to ensure it is visible or move the probe over the needle to make it appear on the screen. One should avoid moving the needle and the probe simultaneously when searching for the needle. Needle visualization may be facilitated by increasing the deep focus on ultrasound machines with adjustable focal zones. This maneuver results in a wider ultrasound beam more superficially, making reflection of an ultrasound wave off the needle more likely.

Local anesthetic injection is easy to detect on screen and is a reassurance that your injection is not intravascular. One should ensure that the local anesthetic is surrounding all of the nerves and terminate the injection when the spread of local anesthetic is uniform.

Oftentimes the ultrasound image may appear to show the needle in or touching a nerve while attached to a nerve stimulator but no motor response is detected [3]. We see this frequently in our patients. When new to ultrasound-guided regional anesthesia it is often difficult to give up believing the nerve stimulator feedback. Initially, if no motor response is obtained, then it is difficult to accept that the visualized target is a nerve. With an increase in experience, however, a confidence grows in the operator's scanning ability. If the operator is confident that the image on the screen is a nerve then the injection of local anesthetic should be based on the image alone. The lack of nerve stimulation and successful block with an injection based on image alone was first described in the literature by Sites and coworkers [3].

When performing nerve stimulator–guided regional anesthesia it is important to keep the needle completely immobile once the injection has commenced. With ultrasound-guided nerve block it is possible to observe the spread of local anesthetic and redirect the needle to a new position to ensure the nerves are completely surrounded with local anesthetic.

UPPER EXTREMITY NERVE BLOCK

The superficial location of the brachial plexus throughout its course combined with the close proximity of potential hazards, such as the lung and major vessels, make ultrasound guidance particularly useful for neural blockade of the upper extremity. For most of the brachial plexus blocks a linear, high-frequency probe is most suitable because it provides better image resolution [4]. The infraclavicular approach, in which the cords of the brachial plexus lie deep to the pectoralis muscles, may not be best suited for a linear probe. Because of the greater depth of the plexus at this level along with the concavity of the infraclavicular fossa, a curvilinear, low-frequency probe is often most useful for the infraclavicular approach to the brachial plexus [1]. At all levels of the brachial plexus it is best to obtain a short-axis, cross-section image of the nerves. We position the patient in a semi-reclined position with the back of the stretcher at a 45° angle. The person performing the block stands next to the patient on the side to be blocked with the ultrasound machine positioned on the opposite side of the patient. The patient's head is turned away from the side to be blocked, toward the ultrasound screen.

Interscalene
To block the brachial plexus at the level of an interscalene approach one must obtain an ultrasound view of the roots of the brachial plexus. An image of the roots can be acquired by scanning the neck at the level of the cricoid cartilage in an axial oblique plane [5,6]. At the level of the cricoid cartilage the internal jugular vein and carotid artery are located medially. As one moves the probe laterally from the internal jugular vein and carotid artery the triangular sternocleidomastoid muscle is located superficially, with the apex of the triangle pointing laterally. The roots of the brachial plexus are located deep to the sternocleidomastoid muscle and in the interscalene groove between the anterior scalene muscle medially and the middle scalene muscle laterally. The roots of the brachial plexus appear as hypoechoic circles encircled by hyperechoic rings. The bodies of the anterior and middle scalene muscles appear as two large "owl eyes" with the roots lying between them. Depending on the level of the plexus being scanned and the angle of the probe, one or more nerve roots can be seen lying vertically on top of each other (Fig. 1). Two maneuvers help confirm that the structures visualized are nerves. First, pressure applied with the probe ensures that the structures are not compressible, and second, scanning the nerves along their course confirms that the structures in view are continuous in nature. If one cannot identify the brachial plexus at the

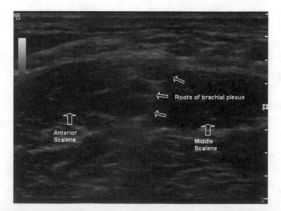

Fig. 1. Ultrasound image of appearance of nerves in the interscalene region.

interscalenc level it is often helpful to first identify the brachial plexus at the supraclavicular level (described later) and trace the image of the nerves proximally to the interscalene level. The bellies of the interscalene muscles are larger and therefore easier to locate on ultrasound in the supraclavicular area than higher up in the classic interscalene region. We use the better definition of the scalene muscles at the supraclavicular level to frame the brachial plexus and then follow the nerves up the neck.

Once a cross-section image of the roots has been identified the block needle is introduced at the end of the probe, in line with the plane of the ultrasound beam. The location of nearby vessels and the handedness of the person placing the block determine whether it is safer and easier to advance the needle from the medial or lateral end of the probe. One should keep in mind that the carotid artery, internal jugular vein, phrenic nerve, and recurrent laryngeal nerve are located medial to the roots of the plexus and the inferior auricular nerve is located laterally. The needle is advanced toward the roots of the brachial plexus under real-time guidance, keeping the tip and shaft of the needle in view at all times. As discussed previously, a nerve stimulator may or may not be used to confirm correct needle placement. When the needle tip is in contact with the plexus the local anesthetic is injected in incremental doses. As the local anesthetic spreads circumferentially around the roots it forms a hypoechoic "donut" around the nerves. If the local anesthetic is not seen to encompass the nerves the needle should be repositioned and advanced through fascial planes as necessary. All needle repositioning and local anesthetic injection should be done under real-time ultrasound guidance to ensure adequate spread of local anesthetic and block success.

Supraclavicular

To obtain an image of a cross section of the trunks of the brachial plexus at the level of a supraclavicular approach [7–10] the probe is placed on the lateral aspect of the neck in the supraclavicular fossa in the coronal oblique plane (Fig. 2). The subclavian artery appears as a circular, hypoechoic, pulsatile structure. Color flow Doppler can be used to confirm the pulsatile flow of an artery. The subclavian vein is located inferior medially to the artery and appears as a circular, hypoechoic structure that varies in size with respiration. Valves, which appear as hyperechoic structures within the vein, can often be seen. Beneath the artery is the first rib, which appears as a horizontal hyperechoic line. The pleura of the dome of the lung, which is located just below the first rib, appears as a hyperechoic parabola that moves with respiration. The trunks of the brachial plexus are found adjacent to the subclavian artery posteriorly, laterally, and cephalad (Fig. 3). The trunks appear as smaller hypoechoic circles that resemble bunches of grapes. The nerves of the brachial plexus are in their closest proximity to each other at this level, which results in the fast block onset and high success rate of the supraclavicular approach [7–9,11–15].

Before needle insertion all structures to be avoided should be identified, specifically the subclavian artery, subclavian vein, and lung. The probe should be

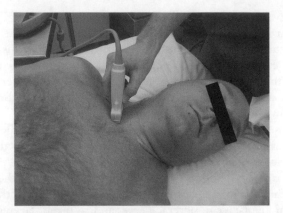

Fig. 2. Probe position for supraclavicular nerve block.

manipulated to provide the best view of the plexus and safest path of approach. Again, the needle is inserted at the end of the probe, in line with the plane of the ultrasound beam, and advanced under real-time guidance. The location of nearby vessels and the handedness of the person placing the block determine whether it is safer and easier to advance the needle from the medial or lateral end of the probe. The needle is directed toward the trunks of the brachial plexus while keeping the tip and shaft of the needle in view at all times. When the needle tip is in contact with the plexus the local anesthetic is injected in incremental doses. Before injection a nerve stimulator may be used to confirm placement. Spread of local anesthetic should be observed adjacent to the artery on the posterior, lateral, and cephalad aspects. If spread of solution does not encompass the nerves immediately adjacent to the artery the needle should be repositioned and advanced through fascial planes as necessary to ensure adequate spread of local anesthetic.

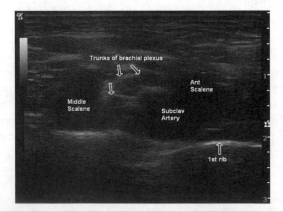

Fig. 3. Ultrasound image of the nerves in the supraclavicular region.

Infraclavicular

Ultrasound images of the cords of the brachial plexus are best obtained by scanning in the parasagittal plane between the coracoid process and mid-clavicle with a low-frequency, curvilinear probe. At this level the cords are located deep to the pectoralis muscles and surround the subclavian artery. The subclavian vein lies just caudad to the artery (Fig. 4). This knowledge was applied in one of the first uses of ultrasound in regional anesthesia, which involved determining the depth of the subclavian artery before block placement [16]. Shortly thereafter, in 2000, Ootaki and colleagues [17] described the first real-time ultrasound-guided infraclavicular block.

The cords of the brachial plexus are positioned around the artery with the lateral cord being superficial and superior or lateral to the artery, the medial cord superficial and inferior or medial to the artery, and the posterior cord deep to the artery (see Fig. 4). By externally rotating the shoulder and abducting the arm 110° the plexus is brought closer to the skin surface and further from the thorax, potentially making the infraclavicular block easier and safer [18]. As with the previous approaches, the needle is advanced and the local anesthetic is injected under ultrasound guidance. Stimulation of the posterior cord has been shown to produce highest block success rate for the infraclavicular block performed with nerve stimulator technique [19,20]. Similarly, our group and others have experienced most success when making the first injection or placing a continuous catheter adjacent to the posterior cord [21]. The needle may be repositioned, if necessary, to ensure local anesthetic spread to the medial and lateral cords.

Axillary

The first series of ultrasound-guided axillary brachial plexus blocks was described by Ting and colleagues [22] in 1989. Guzeldemir and colleagues [23] then described the usefulness of ultrasound in assisting the placement of

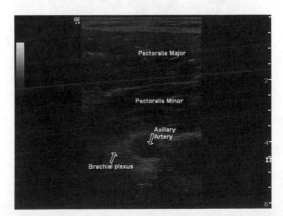

Fig. 4. Ultrasound image of infraclavicular vessels and nerves.

a catheter for continuous axillary brachial plexus blockade. The terminal branches of the brachial plexus can be visualized surrounding the axillary artery by scanning at the axillary fold with the patient's arm abducted 90°, externally rotated, and flexed at the elbow (Fig. 5). The probe should be placed as proximal as possible in the axilla, where the nerves lie in close proximity to the artery. Several vascular structures may be seen, including the axillary artery and vein and their branches. The coracobrachialis, biceps, and triceps muscles may also be seen. The musculocutaneous nerve branches away from the artery high in the axilla and courses away from the artery and deep into the body of the coracobrachialis muscle. Ultrasound can be used to facilitate locating and blocking the nerve [24]. The musculocutaneous nerve appears hyperechoic with honeycombing and as one scans proximally to distally in the axilla the nerve may change in shape from round to oval to triangular [25]. The median, radial, and ulnar nerves may appear as hyper- or hypoechoic circles adjacent to the axillary artery and may vary in their position. The radial nerve is commonly located lateral or anterior lateral to the artery. The median nerve is often located in the anterior medial or posterior medial position and the ulnar nerve in the posterior medial position (Fig. 6) [26]. Blockade of each of the branches of the brachial plexus can be accomplished by directing the needle and injecting the local anesthetic under ultrasound guidance while taking care to avoid puncturing any of the surrounding vessels. Using ultrasound guidance to surround the axillary artery with a donut of local anesthetic can be done more quickly and with an improved overall success rate of blocks when compared with a transarterial axillary block technique [27].

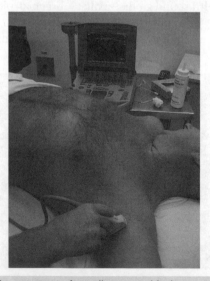

Fig. 5. Patient and probe positioning for axillary nerve block.

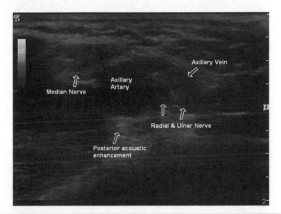

Fig. 6. Ultrasound appearance of nerves in axillary portion of brachial plexus.

LOWER EXTREMITY

Ultrasound-guided regional anesthesia has more limitations and is often more challenging in the lower extremity because of the deeper location of the nerves of the lumbar and sacral plexuses, particularly in obese patients and for blocks at more proximal positions. When choosing between a high-frequency or a low-frequency probe one should consider the depth of the nerve to be blocked.

Lumbar plexus

The limits of current portable ultrasound technology often make visualization of nerves of the lumbar plexus difficult or impossible, except in the thinnest of patients or in pediatric patients [28]. As a result, real-time ultrasound-guided block are not practical. By scanning with a low-frequency probe, however, one can often visualize important surrounding structures, including the vertebral bodies, spinous processes, transverse processes, and kidney. These structures can provide a guide for proper needle insertion site and expected depth to the transverse process, facet joints, and lumbar plexus [29–31].

Femoral

The femoral nerve has a much more superficial location, allowing for real-time ultrasound guided nerve blockade [32–36]. With the patient positioned supine, a linear, high-frequency probe is placed at the level of the inguinal crease. The femoral vein and artery are easily visualized, with the artery lateral to the vein. Pressure applied with the probe and color Doppler can be used to help confirm the artery and vein. The femoral nerve lies approximately 1 cm lateral to the artery. The nerve lies in a triangular-shaped sheath formed by the artery medially; the fascia of the posterior surface of the iliacus muscle, or fascia iliaca, located superior laterally; and the anterior fascia of the rectus femoris muscle located inferior laterally (Fig. 7). The femoral nerve branches as it courses distally down the leg from the level of the inguinal ligament. The motor branch of

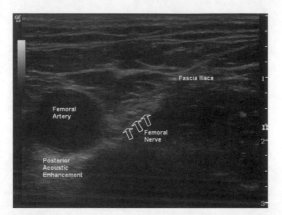

Fig. 7. Femoral nerve appearance on ultrasound.

the femoral nerve, which, when stimulated, produces the classic quadriceps contraction and patellar snap, is usually located at the lateral apex of this fascial triangle. The block needle can be inserted in line with the ultrasound beam, as with the upper extremity blocks, or alternatively the needle may be inserted perpendicular to the probe. Although in-line needle orientation allows for visualization of the needle tip at all times, a perpendicular orientation may allow for technically easier block placement, especially when performing a continuous catheter technique. The needle should be repositioned under ultrasound guidance as necessary to ensure local anesthetic spread within the triangular sheath surrounding the nerve.

Sciatic

The sciatic nerve is deep below the skin in proximal locations, but in more distal locations, such as the subgluteal level [37,38], and in the popliteal [3,39–42] level, it is easily visualized. A low-frequency, curvilinear probe is best suited for the subgluteal approach and a high-frequency, linear probe is best suited for more distal approaches. The sciatic nerve can be scanned through its course from the subgluteal level until it divides into the peroneal and tibial branches at the popliteal level. The nerve can be blocked anywhere along this course.

Subgluteal

To identify an ultrasound image of the sciatic nerve at the subgluteal level, one should scan in the axial plane between the greater trochanter and ischial tuberosity. The patient should be placed in a lateral or Sim's position. The greater trochanter can be identified as a hyperechoic semicircle laterally, and the ischial tuberosity as a hyperechoic semicircle medially. The sciatic nerve lies between these two bony structures, and between the anterior border of the gluteus maximus superficially and the posterior border of the quadratus femoris deep. It may be impossible to visualize the sciatic nerve at this level in obese patients.

Popliteal

To scan and block the sciatic nerve at the popliteal level the patient may be positioned supine, prone, or lateral. As the sciatic nerve descends down the leg it divides into the tibial and peroneal nerves. This division point is highly variable. To locate these nerves at the popliteal level one can trace the sciatic nerve down from the subgluteal level. Alternatively, one can scan in the axial plane at the level of the popliteal fossa with a linear, high-frequency probe. The popliteal artery can be identified as a pulsatile, anechoic circle. The vein often lies posterior lateral to the artery. Color flow Doppler can be used for confirmation. Posterior lateral to the artery and vein is the tibial nerve, which often appears as a hyperechoic circle with hypoechoic honeycombing. The common peroneal nerve is located lateral to the tibial nerve. By tracing these nerves proximally up the leg, the branch point of the sciatic nerve into the tibial and peroneal nerves can be located (Fig. 8). Depending on patient positioning, the block needle can be introduced for the lateral or medial aspect of the thigh, in line with the ultrasound probe. It is best to block the nerve at some point proximal to the branch point.

Saphenous

Ultrasound may be useful for blocking the sciatic nerve because of the close proximity of the sciatic nerve and sciatic vein in the medial thigh and leg, assuming that the saphenous vein is present and has not been removed for coronary artery bypass grafting or in a cosmetic procedure. By scanning with a linear high-frequency probe on the medial aspect of the thigh just proximal to the popliteal crease, one can identify the saphenous vein lying within the body of the sartorius muscle (Fig. 9). Very light pressure should be applied with the probe, because too much pressure can easily occlude the vein and make it impossible to visualize. Once the vein is found, the fascial planes of the belt-like sartorius muscle can be found surrounding the vein. The

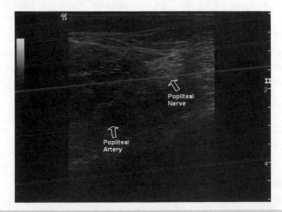

Fig. 8. Ultrasound image of the sciatic nerve in the popliteal region.

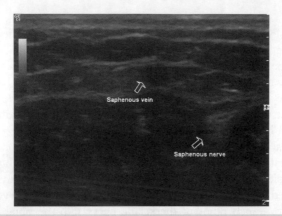

Fig. 9. Image of saphenous vein lying within the sartorius muscle and the saphenous nerve deep to the vein.

saphenous nerve lies posterior to the vein and deep to the sartorius muscle. Often the nerve cannot be easily visualized but by combining ultrasound and tactile sensation, one can see and feel two "pops" as the needle passes through the superficial and deep fascial planes of the sartorius. Ultrasound can then be used to confirm that local anesthetic spread is occurring deep to the sartorius muscle, resulting in the classically described trans-sartorius saphenous nerve block.

Neuraxial and paravertebral

The depth of the vertebral column, especially in obese patients, causes ultrasound-assisted neuraxial and paravertebral blocks to be more technically challenging than peripheral nerve blocks of the upper and lower extremity. As a result, most of the literature involving ultrasound-guided neuraxial blocks pertains to pediatric cases. Ultrasound can also be useful when placing neuraxial and paravertebral block in adults, particularly in identifying vertebral interspaces and depth to the bony landmarks [29,30,43–50]. A low-frequency probe provides deeper tissue penetration allowing visualization of the vertebral structures. By scanning midline in the sagittal plane one can identify the hyperechoic tips of the spinous processes superficially and the hyperechoic lamina and dura at a deeper level (Fig. 10). By scanning lateral from midline, one can visualize and determine the depth of the transverse processes. Although real-time ultrasound guidance may prove difficult in larger patients, knowledge of the location and depth of the appropriate landmarks can make neuraxial and paravertebral blocks easier and possibly safer.

ABDOMINAL WALL

Iliohypogastric/ilioinguinal nerve block

The iliohypogastric/ilioinguinal nerve block is a popular anesthetic technique for procedures in the inguinal area. Unfortunately, this block can have failure

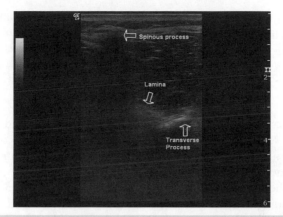

Fig. 10. Transverse image of spinous process and lamina in lumbar region.

rates of 20% to 30% when performed blindly. Ultrasound imaging can be used to ensure that local anesthetic spread is occurring in the desired tissue plane [51,52]. A high-frequency ultrasound probe is placed immediately superior medially to the anterior superior iliac spine in an axial oblique plane. The muscles of the anterior abdominal wall can be identified at this level. The external oblique lies most superficially. The internal oblique lies just deep to the external oblique. The transverse abdominal muscle is the deepest of the three and lies just superficial to the peritoneum. The ilioinguinal and iliohypogastric nerves lie in the fascial plane between the internal oblique and transverse abdominal muscles. By using ultrasound guidance along with tactile sensation, one can feel the pops while watching the block needle transverse the two fascial planes of the external oblique. Injection of local anesthetic between the internal oblique and transverse abdominal muscles is confirmed with ultrasound guidance, which results in higher block success rates.

Transversus abdominus block

This block is useful for lower abdominal procedures. The block is performed bilaterally with the ultrasound probe placed in the anterior axillary line in a coronal plane. The three layers of abdominal muscle can be clearly seen and the local anesthetic is placed in the fascial plane between the internal oblique and transversus abdominus muscles. Local anesthetic (15 mL) placed on each side provides excellent postoperative analgesia following gynecologic or urologic surgeries.

OUTCOME STUDIES

One thrust of studies has been a comparison of ultrasound and nerve stimulation. Is ultrasound quicker and safer, and does it offer a higher success rate than nerve stimulation? Various studies have looked at the onset of the sensory block [1,9,33,34,53] and shown a quicker onset with ultrasound. Other studies have looked at an avoidance of side effects, such as avoiding muscle contraction by using a nerve stimulator [15,53] and avoiding inadvertent intravascular injection [1,54]. Others have reduced the dose of local anesthetic [55,56] and improved the quality of the block [9,33,49].

SUMMARY

The advantages of using ultrasound to visualize a nerve, avoid injection into blood vessels, and monitor the spread of local anesthetic are obvious. Until the advent of ultrasound we had trusted electrons to guide our intervention. Electrons cannot guide local anesthetic. Now local anesthetic spread can be seen around the nerve and we can even pick up intraneural injection [57,58]. Before ultrasound if the patient or needle inadvertently moved after injection of local anesthetic had commenced the operator would not know if the nerve block would work. With ultrasound the needle can be repositioned and the nerve block can proceed with confidence. There are cost issues with the purchase of equipment but if we are to provide the best quality of care for our patients we believe this cost is justified.

References

[1] Sandhu NS, Capan LM. Ultrasound-guided infraclavicular brachial plexus block. Br J Anaesth 2002;89(2):254–9.

[2] Tsui BC, Twomey C, Finucane BT. Visualization of the brachial plexus in the supraclavicular region using a curved ultrasound probe with a sterile transparent dressing. Reg Anesth Pain Med 2006;31(2):182–4.

[3] Sites BD, Gallagher J, Sparks M. Ultrasound-guided popliteal block demonstrates an atypical motor response to nerve stimulation in two patients with diabetes mellitus. Reg Anesth Pain Med 2003;28(5):479–82.

[4] Perlas A, Chan VW, Simons M. Brachial plexus examination and localization using ultrasound and electrical stimulation: a volunteer study. Anesthesiology 2003;99(2):429–35.

[5] Chan VW. Applying ultrasound imaging to interscalene brachial plexus block. Reg Anesth Pain Med 2003;28(4):340–3.

[6] Yang WT, Chui PT, Metreweli C. Anatomy of the normal brachial plexus revealed by sonography and the role of sonographic guidance in anesthesia of the brachial plexus. AJR Am J Roentgenol 1998;171(6):1631–6.

[7] Kapral S, Krafft P, Eibenberger K, et al. Ultrasound-guided supraclavicular approach for regional anesthesia of the brachial plexus. Anesth Analg 1994;78(3):507–13.

[8] Beach ML, Sites BD, Gallagher JD. Use of a nerve stimulator does not improve the efficacy of ultrasound-guided supraclavicular nerve blocks. J Clin Anesth 2006;18(8):580–4.

[9] Williams SR, Chouinard P, Arcand G, et al. Ultrasound guidance speeds execution and improves the quality of supraclavicular block. Anesth Analg 2003;97(5):1518–23.

[10] Royse CE, Sha S, Soeding PF, et al. Anatomical study of the brachial plexus using surface ultrasound. Anaesth Intensive Care 2006;34(2):203–10.

[11] Apan A, Baydar S, Yilmaz S, et al. Surface landmarks of brachial plexus: ultrasound and magnetic resonance imaging for supraclavicular approach with anatomical correlation. Eur J Ultrasound 2001;13(3):191–6.

[12] Cash CJ, Sardesai AM, Berman LH, et al. Spatial mapping of the brachial plexus using three-dimensional ultrasound. Br J Radiol 2005;78(936):1086–94.

[13] Chan VW, Perlas A, Rawson R, et al. Ultrasound-guided supraclavicular brachial plexus block. Anesth Analg 2003;97(5):1514–7.

[14] Collins AB, Gray AT, Kessler J. Ultrasound-guided supraclavicular brachial plexus block: a modified plumb-bob technique. Reg Anesth Pain Med 2006;31(6):591–2.

[15] Plunkett AR, Brown DS, Rogers JM, et al. Supraclavicular continuous peripheral nerve block in a wounded soldier: when ultrasound is the only option. Br J Anaesth 2006;97(5):715–7.

[16] Wu TJ, Lin SY, Liu CC, et al. Ultrasound imaging aids infraclavicular brachial plexus block. Ma Zui Xue Za Zhi 1993;31(2):83–6.

[17] Ootaki C, Hayashi H, Amano M. Ultrasound-guided infraclavicular brachial plexus block: an alternative technique to anatomical landmark-guided approaches. Reg Anesth Pain Med 2000;25(6):600–4.

[18] Bigeleisen P, Wilson M. A comparison of two techniques for ultrasound guided infraclavicular block. Br J Anaesth 2006;96(4):502–7.

[19] Minville V, Fourcade O, Bourdet B, et al. The optimal motor response for infraclavicular brachial plexus block. Anesth Analg 2007;104(2):448–51.

[20] Bloc S, Garnier T, Komly B, et al. Single-stimulation, low-volume infraclavicular plexus block: influence of the evoked distal motor response on success rate. Reg Anesth Pain Med 2006;31(5):433–7.

[21] Porter JM, McCartney CJ, Chan VW. Needle placement and injection posterior to the axillary artery may predict successful infraclavicular brachial plexus block: a report of three cases. Can J Anaesth 2005;52(1):69–73.

[22] Ting PL, Sivagnanaratnam V. Ultrasonographic study of the spread of local anaesthetic during axillary brachial plexus block. Br J Anaesth 1989;63(3):326–9.

[23] Guzeldemir ME, Ustunsoz B. Ultrasonographic guidance in placing a catheter for continuous axillary brachial plexus block. Anesth Analg 1995;81(4):882–3.

[24] Spence BC, Sites BD, Beach ML. Ultrasound-guided musculocutaneous nerve block: a description of a novel technique. Reg Anesth Pain Med 2005;30(2):198–201.

[25] Schafhalter-Zoppoth I, Gray AT. The musculocutaneous nerve: ultrasound appearance for peripheral nerve block. Reg Anesth Pain Med 2005;30(4):385–90.

[26] Retzl G, Kapral S, Greher M, et al. Ultrasonographic findings of the axillary part of the brachial plexus. Anesth Analg 2001;92(5):1271–5.

[27] Sites BD, Beach ML, Spence BC, et al. Ultrasound guidance improves the success rate of a perivascular axillary plexus block. Acta Anaesthesiol Scand 2006;50(6):678–84.

[28] Kirchmair L, Enna B, Mitterschiffthaler G, et al. Lumbar plexus in children. A sonographic study and its relevance to pediatric regional anesthesia. Anesthesiology 2004;101(2): 445–50.

[29] Grau T, Leipold RW, Horter J, et al. Colour Doppler imaging of the interspinous and epidural space. Eur J Anaesthesiol 2001;18(11):706–12.

[30] Greher M, Kirchmair L, Enna B, et al. Ultrasound-guided lumbar facet nerve block: accuracy of a new technique confirmed by computed tomography. Anesthesiology 2004;101(5): 1195–200.

[31] Greher M, Scharbert G, Kamolz LP, et al. Ultrasound-guided lumbar facet nerve block: a sonoanatomic study of a new methodologic approach. Anesthesiology 2004;100(5): 1242–8.

[32] Gruber H, Peer S, Kovacs P, et al. The ultrasonographic appearance of the femoral nerve and cases of iatrogenic impairment. J Ultrasound Med 2003;22(2):163–72.

[33] Marhofer P, Schrogendorfer K, Koinig H, et al. Ultrasonographic guidance improves sensory block and onset time of three-in-one blocks. Anesth Analg 1997;85(4):854–7.

[34] Marhofer P, Schrogendorfer K, Wallner T, et al. Ultrasonographic guidance reduces the amount of local anesthetic for 3-in-1 blocks. Reg Anesth Pain Med 1998;23(6):584–8.

[35] Soong J, Schafhalter-Zoppoth I, Gray AT. The importance of transducer angle to ultrasound visibility of the femoral nerve. Reg Anesth Pain Med 2005;30(5):505.

[36] Sutin KM, Schneider C, Sandhu NS, et al. Deep venous thrombosis revealed during ultrasound-guided femoral nerve block. Br J Anaesth 2005;94(2):247–8.

[37] Chan VW, Nova H, Abbas S, et al. Ultrasound examination and localization of the sciatic nerve: a volunteer study. Anesthesiology 2006;104(2):309–14 [discussion: 5A].

[38] van Geffen GJ, Gielen M. Ultrasound-guided subgluteal sciatic nerve blocks with stimulating catheters in children: a descriptive study. Anesth Analg 2006;103(2):328–33 [table of contents].

[39] McCartney CJ, Brauner I, Chan VW. Ultrasound guidance for a lateral approach to the sciatic nerve in the popliteal fossa. Anaesthesia 2004;59(10):1023–5.

[40] Minville V, Zetlaoui PJ, Fessenmeyer C, et al. Ultrasound guidance for difficult lateral popliteal catheter insertion in a patient with peripheral vascular disease. Reg Anesth Pain Med 2004;29(4):368–70.

[41] Rivas Ferreira E, Sala-Blanch X, Bargallo X, et al. [Ultrasound-guided posterior approach to block the sciatic nerve at the popliteal fossa]. Rev Esp Anestesiol Reanim 2004;51(10): 604–7 [in Spanish].

[42] Sinha A, Chan VW. Ultrasound imaging for popliteal sciatic nerve block. Reg Anesth Pain Med 2004;29(2):130–4.

[43] Watson MJ, Evans S, Thorp JM. Could ultrasonography be used by an anaesthetist to identify a specified lumbar interspace before spinal anaesthesia? Br J Anaesth 2003;90(4):509–11.

[44] Yamauchi M, Honma E, Mimura M, et al. Identification of the lumbar intervertebral level using ultrasound imaging in a post-laminectomy patient. J Anesth 2006;20(3):231–3.

[45] Galiano K, Obwegeser AA, Bodner G, et al. Ultrasound guidance for facet joint injections in the lumbar spine: a computed tomography-controlled feasibility study. Anesth Analg 2005;101(2):579–83 [table of contents].

[46] Ozer Y, Ozer T, Altunkaya H, et al. The posterior lumbar dural depth: an ultrasonographic study in children. Agri 2005;17(3):53–7.

[47] Grau T. [Ultrasound directed punctures in neuro-axial regional anesthesia]. Anasthesiol Intensivmed Notfallmed Schmerzther 2006;41(4):262–5 [in German].

[48] Grau T, Bartusseck E, Conradi R, et al. Ultrasound imaging improves learning curves in obstetric epidural anesthesia: a preliminary study. Can J Anaesth 2003;50(10):1047–50.

[49] Grau T, Leipold RW, Conradi R, et al. Efficacy of ultrasound imaging in obstetric epidural anesthesia. J Clin Anesth 2002;14(3):169–75.

[50] Willschke H, Marhofer P, Bosenberg A, et al. Epidural catheter placement in children: comparing a novel approach using ultrasound guidance and a standard loss-of-resistance technique. Br J Anaesth 2006;97(2):200–7.

[51] Willschke H, Bosenberg A, Marhofer P, et al. Ultrasonographic-guided ilioinguinal/iliohypogastric nerve block in pediatric anesthesia: what is the optimal volume? Anesth Analg 2006;102(6):1680–4.

[52] Willschke H, Marhofer P, Bosenberg A, et al. Ultrasonography for ilioinguinal/iliohypogastric nerve blocks in children. Br J Anaesth 2005;95(2):226–30.

[53] Marhofer P, Sitzwohl C, Greher M, et al. Ultrasound guidance for infraclavicular brachial plexus anaesthesia in children. Anaesthesia 2004;59(7):642–6.

[54] Sandhu NS, Manne JS, Medabalmi PK, et al. Sonographically guided infraclavicular brachial plexus block in adults: a retrospective analysis of 1146 cases. J Ultrasound Med 2006;25(12):1555–61.

[55] Sainz Lopez J, Prat Vallribera A, Segui Pericas M, et al. [Ultrasound-guided supraclavicular brachial plexus block with small volumes of local anesthetic: technical description and analysis of results]. Rev Esp Anestesiol Reanim 2006;53(7):400–7 [in Spanish].

[56] Sandhu NS, Bahniwal CS, Capan LM. Feasibility of an infraclavicular block with a reduced volume of lidocaine with sonographic guidance. J Ultrasound Med 2006;25(1):51–6.

[57] Schafhalter-Zoppoth I, Zeitz ID, Gray AT. Inadvertent femoral nerve impalement and intraneural injection visualized by ultrasound. Anesth Analg 2004;99(2):627–8.

[58] Bigeleisen PE. Nerve puncture and apparent intraneural injection during ultrasound-guided axillary block does not invariably result in neurologic injury. Anesthesiology 2006;105(4): 779–83.

Advances in Anesthesia 25 (2007) 205–232

ELSEVIER
MOSBY

ADVANCES IN ANESTHESIA

Airway Management Devices and Approaches

Anh-Thuy Nguyen, MD*, Keyuri Popat, MD

Department of Anesthesiology and Pain Medicine, The University of Texas M. D. Anderson Cancer Center, 1515 Holcombe Boulevard, Unit 409, Houston, TX 77030, USA

M anagement of the difficult airway has become much safer in the last century, largely because of the proliferation and variety of mechanical devices for ventilation, intubation, and tracheal tube exchange.

This article divides the available devices into those that are placed above the glottic opening to help with ventilation (supraglottic devices) and those used to help place a tube in the trachea (intubation aids) and for emergency surgical airway access. A section on tube exchangers to facilitate changing tracheal tubes is included.

PATIENT ASSESSMENT

There are several assessment tools to show the level of difficulty of intubating a patient. These assessment tools are only guides, however; they are not foolproof. Despite advance preparations, each time tracheal intubation is planned alternate intubation techniques should be ready in case the initial technique does not go as planned. Our experience at a major cancer institution shows that the incidence of a difficult intubation is higher in patients who have had their necks irradiated even when all other criteria seem normal.

SUPRAGLOTTIC AIRWAY DEVICES

Laryngeal mask airway

Since its introduction in 1988, the laryngeal mask airway (LMA; LMA North America, San Diego, CA) has been used in more than 200 million patients worldwide with no reported fatalities [1]. It is the most important airway device since the endotracheal tube (ETT) was developed. It was introduced into use in the United States in 1991 for routine cases involving spontaneous ventilation. In 1995, it was incorporated into the American Society of Anesthesiologists (ASA) Difficult Airway algorithm as a ventilatory device and as a conduit for tracheal intubation [1]. It is indicated for use as an alternative to the face mask but not as a replacement for the ETT. Its use is indicated in routine

*Corresponding author. E-mail address: atnguyen@mdanderson.org (A-T. Nguyen).

0737-6146/07/$ – see front matter
doi:10.1016/j.aan.2007.07.009

Published by Elsevier Inc.

and emergency anesthetic procedures, in patients who have known or unexpected difficult airways, and during emergency resuscitation when intubation is impossible. The LMA is contraindicated in patients undergoing elective surgery who have not fasted and may have retained gastric contents (because it does not protect the patient from aspiration) and in patients who have a fixed decreased pulmonary compliance. It can also be used as a bridge to extubation and with positive-pressure ventilation (up to 20 cm H_2O for all LMAs and up to 30 cm H_2O for the LMA-Proseal) and pressure support [2,3]. It comes in pediatric and adult sizes. All LMA devices are latex-free.

Multiple versions of the LMA are available today, including the LMA Classic, LMA Unique, LMA Fastrach, LMA Proseal, LMA Flexible, and LMA Ctrach. The LMA Classic (Fig. 1) is the standard and original LMA.

The LMA Unique (Fig. 2) is the disposable version of the LMA Classic.

The LMA Fastrach (Fig. 3), also known as the intubating LMA, comes with a curved rigid handle that replicates the natural human anatomy and can accommodate an 8.0-mm cuffed ETT. It can facilitate continuous ventilation during intubation. An LMA ETT, a straight, wire-reinforced, silicone, cuffed ETT, has been developed specifically for use with the LMA Fastrach.

The LMA Proseal (Fig. 4) has a built-in drainage tube designed to channel fluid away and permit gastric access for patients who have reflux or during cases of prolonged duration in which endotracheal intubation is not required.

The LMA Flexible (Fig. 5) has a wire-reinforced, flexible airway. It comes in reusable and disposable forms.

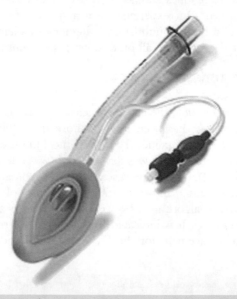

Fig. 1. LMA Classic is latex free and reusable. (*Courtesy of* LMA North America, Inc., http://www.lmana.com; with permission.)

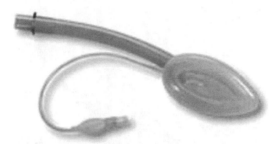

Fig. 2. LMA Unique is a single-use disposable airway. (*Courtesy of* LMA North America, Inc., http://www.lmana.com; with permission.)

The LMA Ctrach (Fig. 6), which enables ventilation during intubation attempts, has built-in fiberoptics that provide a direct view of the larynx and a real-time view of the ETT passing through the vocal cords. As with the LMA FastTrach, the LMA ETT is used when tracheal intubation is performed through the LMA.

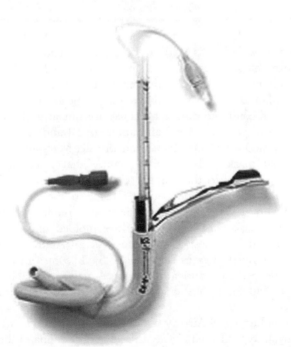

Fig. 3. LMA Fastrach is used for anticipated or unanticipated difficult airway situation and cardiopulmonary resuscitation. (*Courtesy of* LMA North America, Inc., http://www.lmana.com; with permission.)

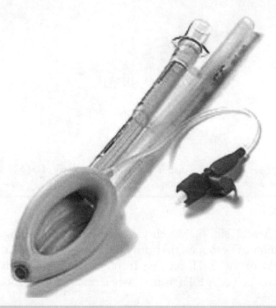

Fig. 4. LMA Porseal enhances supraglottic airway protection. (*Courtesy of* LMA North America, Inc., http://www.lmana.com; with permission.)

The Portex-Soft Seal (Smiths Medical, Portex Ltd, Kent, UK) (Fig. 7) is a disposable laryngeal mask that is designed similarly to the LMA Unique, with the following exceptions: it has no elevating epiglottis bar, no "step" between the tube and the cuff, and a softer cuff that is less permeable to nitrous oxide [4]. Indications for and contraindications to its use are similar to those of the LMA Unique. It comes in pediatric size 3 and adult sizes 4 and 5.

The Ambu AuraOnce (Ambu Inc., Glen Burnie, Maryland, USA) is a disposable laryngeal mask with a built-in curve that replicates the natural human anatomy, similar to the handle of the LMA Fastrach. It allows for placement of the tube with the patient's head in the neutral position. It has a soft cuff, no elevating epiglottis bar, and a reinforced tip to prevent folding; the cuff, mask, and airway tube are molded into a single unit. If intubation is needed, it is best to intubate over an Aintree intubating catheter, which is described later in this article [5]. It comes in seven different sizes that include pediatric and adult sizes. A newer reusable version, the Ambu Aura40 (Fig. 8), is also available and can be steam-autoclaved up to 40 times.

The Intubating Laryngeal Airway (Cookgas LLC, St. Louis, Missouri, USA) (Fig. 9) is an oval, hypercurved airway tube that approximates the anatomy of the oropharyngeal passage. It is designed to decrease airway tube kinking and folding of the cuff tip. The oval shape accommodates standard ETTs (sizes 5.0–8.5 mm). Adult and pediatric sizes are available. A stylet is used to remove the device following intubation.

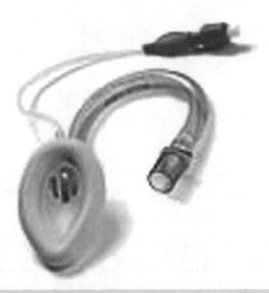

Fig. 5. LMA Flexible is a wire-reinforced, flexible airway. (*Courtesy of* LMA North America, Inc., http://www.lmana.com; with permission.)

The Vital Seal Laryngeal Mask airway (Vital Signs, Totowa, New Jersey) (Fig. 10) is a single-use device used to secure the airway during general anesthesia. The device currently comes in sizes 3, 4, and 5. The product has a reinforced tip that helps prevent rollover on insertion.

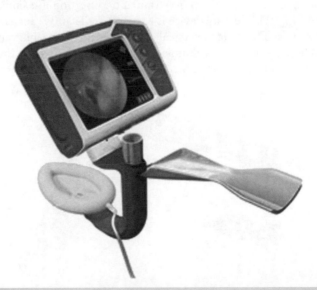

Fig. 6. LMA Ctrach enables ventilation during intubation attempts and has built-in fiberoptics. (*Courtesy of* LMA North America, Inc., http://www.lmana.com; with permission.)

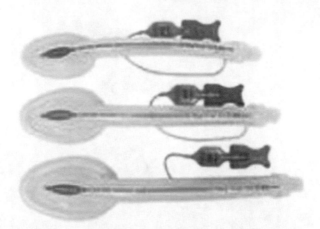

Fig. 7. Portex-Soft Seal is a disposable laryngeal mask. (*Courtesy of* Emergency Medical Product, Inc.; with permission.)

The Laryngeal Tube (VBM Medizintechnik, Sulzam Neckar, Germany) or King Laryngeal Tube (Kings Systems Corp., Noblesville, Indiana) (Fig. 11) is a latex-free, single-lumen, silicone tube with two high-volume, low-pressure cuffs (pharyngeal and esophageal) and a single balloon for pressure control. The proximal cuff lies in the hypopharynx and the distal cuff the upper esophagus. The device has three side eyelets in between the cuffs to provide for ventilation. It can be used for either spontaneous or positive-pressure ventilation. Ventilation, oxygenation, and risk for trauma on insertion are similar to those for the LMA [6,7]. This airway device is easy to handle and is available in adult and pediatric sizes. The King Laryngeal Tube D is the disposable version of the King LT. The LT-suction is a double-lumen laryngeal air tube that incorporates a second esophageal lumen for suction.

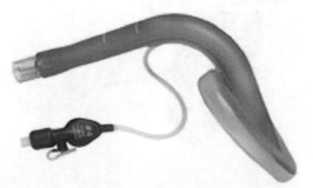

Fig. 8. Ambu Aura40 is reusable (up to 40 times) laryngeal mask with a built-in curve. (*Courtesy of* Ambu, Inc., www.ambuusa.com; with permission.)

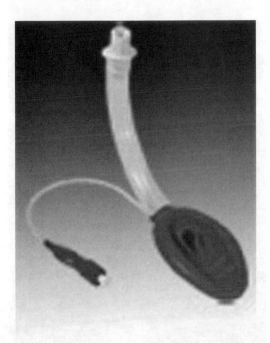

Fig. 9. Intubating Laryngeal Airway is an oval, hypercurved airway tube. (*Courtesy of* Mercury Medical; with permission.)

The Cobra Perilaryngeal Airway

The Cobra Perilaryngeal Airway (PLA; Engineered Medical Systems, Indianapolis, Indiana, USA) is a disposable, single-use tube with a tapered, striated tip that is designed to be positioned in the hypopharynx, where it abuts the laryngeal inlet. The PLA has a high-volume, low-pressure oropharyngeal cuff (Fig. 12). It is placed blindly and provides a higher sealing pressure than the LMA [8]. Available in pediatric and adult sizes, it can be used as a conduit for intubation (accommodates up to an 8.0-mm ETT). The new Cobra PLUS (Engineered Medical Systems) includes a temperature monitor (all sizes) and a distal CO_2 gas sampling monitor (pediatric sizes) (Fig. 13).

The Streamlined Liner of the Pharynx Airway

The Streamlined Liner of the Pharynx Airway (SLIPA) (SLIPA Medical Ltd., London, UK) is a cuffless supralaryngeal airway device with a hollow structure that permits the storage of regurgitated liquids, thereby minimizing aspiration risk (Fig. 14). It has a hollow, blow-molded, soft plastic airway shaped to form a seal in the pharynx. Only adult sizes are available.

The Chou Airway

The Chou Airway (AchiCorp, San Jose, California, USA) was designed by the Wu scope team to overcome an upper airway obstruction resulting from a large

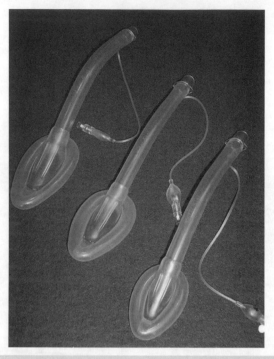

Fig. 10. Vital Seal Laryngeal Mask Airway is a single-use device used to secure the airway. (*Courtesy of* Vital Signs, Inc.; with permission.)

hypopharyngeal tongue, which is often associated with difficult face mask ventilation, obstructive sleep apnea, and difficult intubation (Fig. 15). It is an adjustable oropharyngeal airway with two components: a rigid outer tube that serves as a conduit for and protects the second component, the flexible inner tube that creates a patent air passage from the mouth opening to the glottis. In conjunction with the face mask, it is placed orally to facilitate and maintain spontaneous or assisted breathing. The inner tube is longer than other common oral airways, which makes it capable of reaching beyond the base of the tongue in patients who have a short mandibular ramus or large tongue. By moving the flexible inner tube up or down while ventilating the patient through a face mask, practitioners can find the optimal airway length and maximize air passage. It is available in adult and larger adult sizes.

The esophageal tracheal Combitube

The Combitube (Puritan Bennet, St. Louis, Missouri, and other manufacturers) is a single-use, double-lumen tube that has a unique design that provides an airway for either esophageal or tracheal placement (Fig. 16). It has a large proximal latex oropharyngeal balloon and a distal esophageal low-pressure cuff with multiple holes in between. It is placed blindly without the use of a laryngoscope. It is useful in patients in whom neck movement is contraindicated

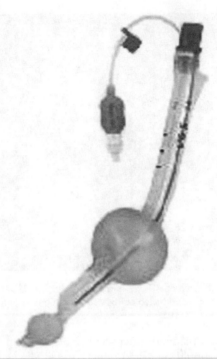

Fig. 11. The laryngeal Tube/King Laryngeal Tube is a latex-free, single-lumen, silicone tube. (*Courtesy of* SP Services; with permission.)

and in those whose vocal cords cannot be visualized because of a limited airway or massive bleeding.

INTUBATION AIDS

Some of the devices described in this section may also be useful for placing an ETT in an awake and spontaneously breathing patient.

Patient preparation

If a difficult airway is anticipated, it is important to communicate your plan to the patient and win their trust because only then will they cooperate. If an awake intubation is planned, then you must provide more details to the patient regarding what you are going to do. Awake intubations are approached with a fiberoptic scope and only rarely with awake tracheotomy. For awake fiberoptic intubations, we apply a topical anesthetic (4% lidocaine) to the upper airway using an atomizer. An anti-sialagogue (eg, glycopyrrolate) may also be given. During the procedure mild sedation, consisting of dexmedetomidine, midazolam (Versed), ketamine, or propofol, is given as needed. A bite block or Ovassapian airway should be placed if oral intubation is planned so the patient does not bite the fiberscope.

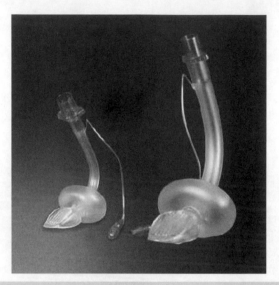

Fig. 12. The Cobra Perilaryngeal Airway is a disposable, single-use tube with a tapered, striated tip. (*Courtesy of* Engineered Medical System; with permission.)

If nasal intubation is planned, phenylephrine spray can be applied to both nostrils. The patient should be asked which nostril allows better air flow and the better one is sprayed with 2% to 4% lidocaine.

Another method of preparation is a transtracheal injection in which a 20-gauge angiocatheter is inserted through the cricothyroid membrane, the needle is removed, and 5 mL of 2% to 4% lidocaine is injected.

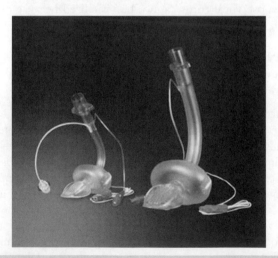

Fig. 13. The Cobra PLUS includes a temperature monitor and a distal CO_2 gas sampling monitor. (*Courtesy of* Engineered Medical System; with permission.)

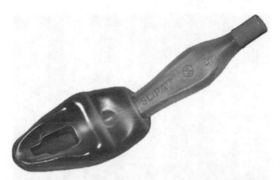

Fig. 14. SLIPA is a cuffless supralaryngeal airway device. (*Courtesy of* ARC Medical Inc.; with permission.)

Types of intubation aids

Box 1 lists various intubation aids.

Fiberoptic bronchoscopy

The art of fiberoptic bronchoscopy (FOB) requires skilled training and practice and has a steep learning curve. It can be used in an awake or an anesthetized

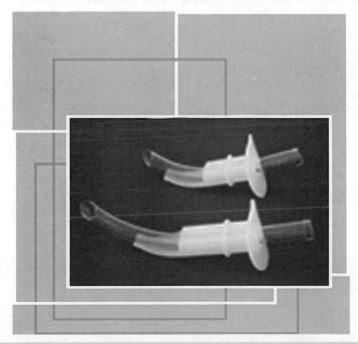

Fig. 15. The Chou Airway is an adjustable oropharyngeal airway with two components. (*Courtesy of* Achi Corporation; with permission.)

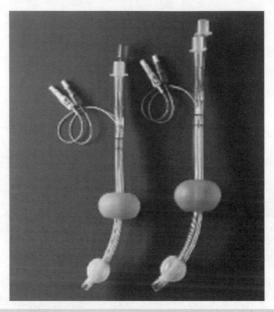

Fig. 16. Esophageal Tracheal Combitube is a single-use, double-lumen tube. (*Courtesy of* Nellcor; with permission.)

patient. If FOB is to be used in an anesthetized patient, an open airway and adequate mask ventilation must be assured after induction. Fiberoptic bronchoscopy is then performed as described below.

Technique
In an awake patient, the patient's airway is prepared as described earlier. Before starting, all parts of the equipment (eg, light source, suction port) should be tested for function. The anesthesiologist stands at the head of the patient with the bed as low as possible. The scope should be lubricated so that the ETT can slide over it easily. The connector of the ETT is removed and the desired size of tube fed on the fiberscope. If the desired tube is small so that the fit is snug, a smaller (neonatal) scope can be used. For endotracheal intubation with an average-sized adult tube, a pediatric scope is most suitable. Before

Box 1: Intubation aids

Fiberscope
Shikani scope
Bullard scope
Mac videoscope
Intubating stylets

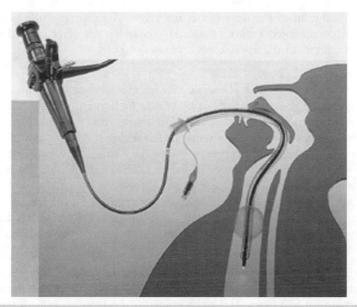

Fig. 17. The technique of fiberoptic bronchoscopy. The carina is visualized through the fiberoptic scope before the tracheal tube is advanced through the cords and carinal visualization is reconfirmed after tube advancement before removal of the fiberoptic scope.

starting, also orient yourself to the movement of the lever that moves the tip of the scope up or down.

Enter the patient's mouth in the midline and proceed farther under vision by way of the scope; similarly enter the desired nostril and proceed farther inside under vision using the lever on the scope to move the tip of the scope up or down. Advance the tip below the epiglottis until the vocal cords are visualized. If you lose orientation, withdraw the scope until you see familiar landmarks, reorient yourself, and advance again. Once you see the vocal cords, advance the fiberscope until the carina is seen. Then, loosen the ETT and advance it through the cords. The tube tends to get caught on the arytenoids. To facilitate passage, it is helpful to turn the tube before advancement so that the Murphy's eye is anterior and then withdraw only the fiberscope slowly under direct

Table 1		
Fiberoptic intubations		
Patient condition	Awake technique of choice	Anesthetized rescue technique
Orifice	Oral	Nasal (easier than oral)
Pediatric	Available for neonatal, pediatric, and adult	
Advantages	Relatively safe for difficult airways	
Disadvantages	Difficult to use with bleeding in the airway	

vision until the tip of the tube comes into view. Appropriate tube placement should be documented before completely removing the fiberscope (Fig. 17). Table 1 summarizes the approaches and uses of FOB.

Recent findings

An adaptation of the awake fiberoptic intubation technique called awake fiber-capnic intubation was recently described in the literature [9]. In this technique, a catheter is placed at the suction channel that measures end-tidal CO_2, and the user uses this measurement as a guide to advancing the ETT, using only the fiberscope for visual identification of the tracheal ring. The investigators had success with this approach in 98% of patients. The study population consisted of patients who had head and neck cancer [9].

In a recent randomized controlled trial conducted in a pediatric population comparing hemodynamic changes between fiberoptic oral versus nasal intubation, the authors found that the hemodynamic changes were less and the changes were of shorter duration in patients who underwent nasal intubation [10].

Optical stylets

Intubating optical stylets (Fig. 18) are being used increasingly to help manage the difficult airway. Optical stylets combine fiberoptic imaging with the traditional stylet design. There are several versions of optical stylets on the market. It is relatively easy to learn to use the optical stylet, and it can be a particularly useful intubating device in patients who have a reduced mouth opening. In addition, the patient's neck does not need to be extended during intubation. A disadvantage of the device is that it can only be used by way of the oral route, so it is not very useful in the presence of copious blood in the airway.

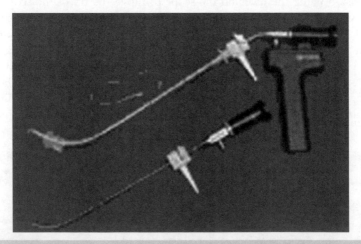

Fig. 18. Optical Stylets are used increasingly to help manage the difficult airway. (*Courtesy of* University of Florida Dept. of Anesthesiology; with permission.)

Technique
The ETT is loaded on the stylet. With the head of the anesthetized patient in a neutral position the stylet and tube are inserted midline and advanced with little movement of the neck. The vocal cords are visualized and the ETT is advanced through the cords. This is not the device of choice for an awake intubation. In the hands of someone skilled in its use, however, it can be used for an awake intubation. The oral optical stylet is the most useful type. There is a report in the literature of the insertion of this device to assist with tracheostomy placement. A fiberscope is a better device for a nasal intubation. Some of these optical stylets come in pediatric sizes.

Recent findings
In a comparison of optical stylets and a gum elastic bougie, the authors found the optical stylet to be superior to the bougie as an intubation device [11].

Newer devices
Several newer devices have been introduced commercially for intubation.

VideoMAC scope
The VideoMAC scope (Karl Storz, Tuttlingen, Germany) is a version of the Macintosh blade, but it is attached to a fiberoptic light source instead of a regular handle. This feature enables an observer to see what the person intubating is seeing, a feature that makes the device useful in teaching programs for residents.

Flexible-tip laryngoscope blades
Flexible-tip Macintosh scopes are made by several manufacturers and fit on a regular laryngoscope handle, but the tip can be lifted up to 70 degrees by squeezing a lever at the proximal end. This maneuver helps to lift the epiglottis, which gives a clear view to the vocal cords.

Airtraq scope
The Airtraq scope (Prodol Meditec SA, LLC, Vizcaya, Spain) (Fig. 19) is a modified single-use optical laryngoscope. It permits practitioners to view the glottis without much manipulation of the neck. This scope has a Macintosh-type blade with two channels, one for the ETT and another that ends in a lens. The scope is battery operated with a life of 90 minutes. This scope comes in two sizes, small and regular.

Trachlight
The Trachlight (Laerdal Medical, Wappingers Falls, New York) is an intubation device that can be used in awake or asleep patients and for oral or nasal intubation.

The smallest ETT that can accommodate a Trachlight is 5.5 mm in diameter. A lubricant should first be applied to the ETT, which is then threaded over the Trachlight. The room needs to be darkened during placement so that it is possible to visualize the translucence and thus the progression of the scope through the airway. The assembly consisting of the stylet and ETT should

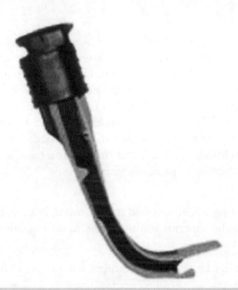

Fig. 19. The AirTraq Scope is a modified single-use optical laryngoscope. (*Courtesy of* University of Florida Dept. of Anesthesiology; with permission.)

be introduced starting midline and, staying midline, advanced until a pretracheal glow is seen in the midline. Occasionally as the ETT is advanced the pretracheal glow can be seen traveling down with the tube. Once the tube is in the trachea the lighted stylet should be withdrawn. The user should then confirm that the light bulb is still in place and confirm tube placement by auscultation and end-tidal CO_2 tracing.

There are several advantages and disadvantages to using a Trachlight. One advantage is that it can be used in awake and anesthetized patients with a success rate of 99% in trained hands. It can also be used in managing a difficult airway when conventional methods have failed. Because it requires minimal manipulation of the head, the Trachlight is particularly useful in patients who have blood in the airway or an anterior larynx.

The Trachlight is also associated with several disadvantages. Because the device requires transillumination, it may not be suited to use in an outdoor environment. It may also be difficult to appreciate the glow of the light in patients who have a thick neck or darkly pigmented skin. Because there is no direct visualization of the airway, the device should be avoided in patients suspected of having airway tumors or a foreign body in the airway.

Because the Trachlight can only be accommodated in an ETT with a diameter of 5.5 mm or greater, it cannot be used in the pediatric population.

Rigid laryngoscopes

Bullard laryngoscope

The Bullard laryngoscope (Fig. 20) is one of the rigid laryngoscopes that can aid in the intubation of patients who have a small mouth opening or in

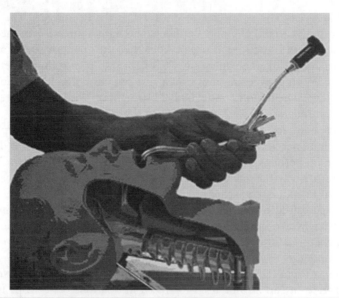

Fig. 20. A Bullard laryngoscope. (*Courtesy of* University of Florida Dept. of Anesthesiology; with permission.)

whom the oral and pharyngeal axis cannot be aligned. The Upsher scope (Fig. 21), another version of a rigid laryngoscope, has similar uses. Disadvantages of these scopes are that they must be used orally and thus cannot be used in patients without oral access.

Technique. The adult or pediatric size is chosen depending on the patient's height (adult and pediatric sizes for patients > and ≤5 ft [1.5 m] in height, respectively). To begin the intubation, the appropriate size of ETT is lubricated and attached to the scope by way of the dedicated nonmalleable stylet or

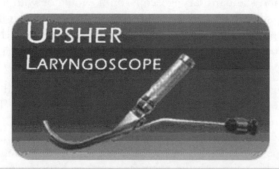

Fig. 21. An Upsher Scope. (*Courtesy of* University of Florida Dept. of Anesthesiology; with permission.)

a malleable stylet. The connector of the ETT is then removed. The scope is also lubricated at the blade, and the fiberoptic light source is attached to the scope. The patient is induced as usual. After this, the operator stands at the patient's head and, while the patient's neck is kept stable, introduces the scope in the midline. With a sweeping movement, the operator should be able to visualize the glottis. The handle should be held straight up with some degree of suspension required.

The most common reason the cords cannot be visualized is that the scope is not in the midline. Sometimes the tube cannot be advanced even if the cords are identified, perhaps because of close proximity to the cords. Once the ETT is advanced, the scope is withdrawn using an opposite movement to that used to introduce the scope.

This scope can also be used in awake patients, but it is not the method of choice for an awake intubation, which requires a great deal of expertise and good patient preparation. It is an ideal scope, however, for asleep patients who can undergo regular induction. With practice, this technique can also be used for a rapid-sequence induction. Although this scope is well suited for oral intubation, it can also be used for nasal intubations. The scope is still introduced orally and the ETT has to be guided through the vocal cords. This scope is also appropriate for pediatric use because there is a pediatric size available.

Recent findings. In a recent review of a teaching institution's 7-year experience with the management of 447 patients who had an unexpected difficult airway, all the patients were successfully ventilated with an LMA and about 50% were intubated blindly by way of an LMA. The Bullard laryngoscope was the technique of choice for managing a difficult airway at this institution. Fiberoptic intubations failed 10% of the time. These authors thus emphasized the importance of learning different techniques of managing difficult airways [12].

In a study in which the ease of Bullard laryngoscopy performed by inexperienced residents was examined, the residents were asked to perform Bullard laryngoscopy and standard laryngoscopy on a simulator with a rigid cervical spine. The investigators found that the ease of intubation with the Bullard laryngoscope improved significantly with repeated attempts, which showed that Bullard laryngoscopy is an easily mastered art [13].

Wu laryngoscope
The Wu laryngoscope was designed by an anesthesiologist and combines the technology of a rigid laryngoscope with a fiberoptic light source. This scope has a built-in channel for the ETT and an oxygen channel.

To insert the Wu laryngoscope, the operator stands at the head of the patient. The scope is introduced in the midline, and at this point the operator should start looking through the eyepiece. As the glottic opening comes into view, the tracheal tube should be aligned with the glottis by moving the blade sideways. The tube is advanced and the scope withdrawn.

An advantage of the Wu laryngoscope is that it is easy for one person to use. An additional advantage is that the fiberoptic source is protected and thus the view of the airway is not obstructed by blood or mucus. A disadvantage of the scope is that it requires at least a 25-mm mouth opening.

The Wu laryngoscope has been used successfully for awake intubation in experienced hands and a well-prepared patient (Figs. 22 and 23). It can also be inserted in an asleep patient after regular induction. Because the scope does not come in a pediatric size, it cannot be used in children.

OTHER AIRWAY TECHNIQUES
Retrograde intubation
Retrograde intubation is particularly useful in patients in whom orotracheal intubation is technically impossible or contraindicated (Fig. 24) [18]. It can be performed despite the presence of blood or secretions in the upper airway. It is also an alternative to cricothyroidotomy in patients who have short, obese, or anatomically distorted necks [14]. After appropriate nasal, oral, and tracheal anesthesia, an 18-gauge intravenous catheter with syringe attached is inserted through the cricothyroid membrane into the trachea. Air is aspirated and the stylet removed. A 110- to 120-cm guidewire of 0.32- to 0.38-in diameter is passed through the catheter and angled cephalad. The wire is advanced until it is seen in the mouth or nose. The wire is clamped at the cricothyroid entrance point and a tracheal tube threaded over the wire. Various options are available, including placing an exchange stylet or fiberoptic bronchoscope over the wire and then passing the tracheal tube using the exchange stylet or FOB.

Percutaneous transtracheal jet ventilation
Percutaneous transtracheal jet ventilation with a large-bore angiocath that is inserted through the cricothyroid membrane can provide immediate oxygenation

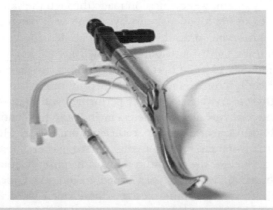

Fig. 22. Wu Laryngoscope (*Courtesy of* Achi Corporation; with permission.)

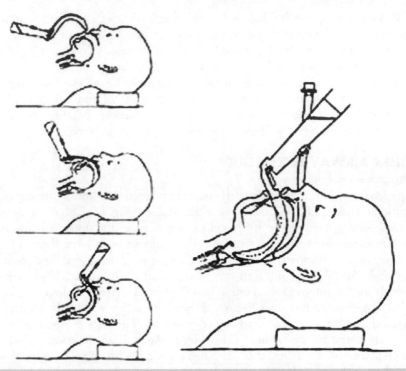

Fig. 23. Wu Laryngoscope (*Courtesy of* Achi Corporation; with permission.)

from a high-pressure (50 lb per square inch) oxygen wall outlet and ventilation by means of manual triggering. There are several commercial manual jet ventilation devices currently available.

Cricothyrotomy

Cricothyrotomy is an emergency incision made through the skin and cricothyroid membrane to secure a patient's airway. Along with percutaneous tracheostomy, it is a life-saving procedure in the final step in the ASA Difficult Airway algorithm for failed intubation and failed ventilation attempts. There are several techniques of cricothyrotomy, including needle cricothyrotomy, percutaneous cricothyrotomy, and surgical cricothyrotomy.

Needle cricothyrotomy (Fig. 25) can be performed with 4- to14-cm catheters in adults. Commercially available catheters include the Jet Ventilator Catheter and a 6-French transtracheal airway catheter from Cook Medical Critical Care that is more resistant to kinking than standard plastic catheters. Commercially available kits include the cricothyrotomy catheter set (Cook Critical Care, Bloomington, Indiana), which is user friendly, and the Quicktrach (VBM Medizintechnik). Surgical cricothyrotomy is performed by making incisions through the cricothyroid membrane using a scalpel, followed by the insertion of an ETT.

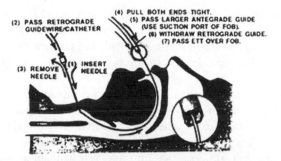

Fig. 24. Retrograde intubation is useful in patients in whom orotracheal intubation is technically impossible or contraindicated. A catheter over the needle device is placed through the cricothyroid membrane (1) and the needle stylet removed. A guidewire is placed through the catheter (2). The catheter is removed (3). Both ends of the wire are pulled tight (4). A fiberoptic bronchoscope is threaded over the wire and passed into the trachea (5). The guidewire (6) is removed and the tracheal tube is advanced over the fiberoptic bronchoscope (7). (*Courtesy of* Greg Gordon, MD.)

Tracheostomy

Tracheostomy is a surgical procedure performed to open a direct airway through an incision in the trachea below the level of the cricoid cartilage. It can be done percutaneously or surgically. The Seldinger technique is used in percutaneous cricothyrotomy, but there are several adaptations. These include

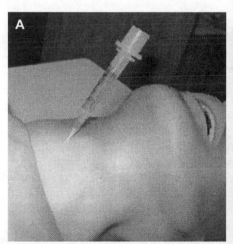
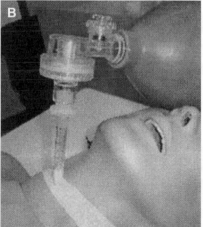

Fig. 25. (A) Needle cricothyrotomy is performed with a 14-gauge catheter attached to a syringe inserted through the cricothyroid membrane. A transtracheal jet ventilation system can be attached to the catheter or a guidewire can be inserted over which a large dilator-cannula assembly is threaded (B) A cannula has been inserted (special cricothyrotomy sets include 3.5-, 4-, and 6-mm cannulas). (*Courtesy of* Cook Critical Care, Bloomington, IN; with permission.)

the use of a wire-guided sharp forceps (Griggs technique) [15], performance of the procedure under bronchoscopic control, the use of a single tapered dilator (Blue Rhino), passage of the dilator from inside the trachea to the outside (Fantoni's technique) [16], and the use of a screw-like device to open the trachea wall (PercTwist) [17].

Surgical tracheotomy is performed in a sterile environment, usually with the patient under general anesthesia, but can be done with the patient awake in an emergent situation. Surgical tracheotomy is favored over the percutaneous techniques for patients who have coagulation abnormalities, a need for high levels of oxygenation support, an unstable cervical spine, or unfavorable neck anatomy. There is no absolute contraindication to a tracheotomy because it is a life-saving procedure.

AIRWAY EXCHANGE CATHETERS

Numerous airway exchange catheters have been developed to aid in tracheal intubation and extubation.

The Aintree Intubation Catheter (Fig. 26) (Cook Medical Critical Care) is a 56-cm catheter used for the fiberoptic guided placement and exchange of ETTs (inner diameter larger than 7.0 mm), nasotracheal tubes, and LMAs. The catheter has a 4.7-mm inner diameter to accept a fiberoptic bronchoscope, and the use of a removable Rapi-Fit adapter permits ventilation (including jet ventilation) during the exchange procedure if that proves necessary. The

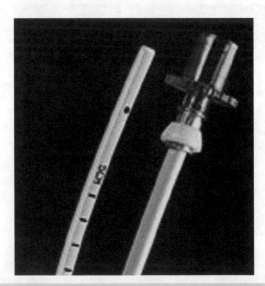

Fig. 26. Aintree Intubation Catheter is a single-use, 56-cm catheter used for the fiberoptic-guided placement and exchange of ETTs, nasotracheal tubes, and LMAs. (*Courtesy of* Cook Medical Critical Care, Bloomington, IN; with permission.)

Aintree catheter has a through-lumen design with distal side ports for airflow and a blunt tip to minimize trauma. These devices are for single use only.

The Arndt Airway Exchange Catheter Set (Fig. 27) (Cook Medical Critical Care) is used for the exchange of LMAs and ETTs using fiberoptic bronchoscopy. It comes with a removable Rapi-Fit adapter that permits ventilation, if necessary, during the exchange procedure. It also has multiple side ports, a bronchoscopic port, a guide wire, and a catheter. It is used with an ETT with an inner diameter of 5 mm or larger. It has a tapered end and comes in various lengths (50–78 cm). It is a single-use device only.

The Cook Airway Exchange Catheter (Fig. 28) (Cook Medical Critical Care) is used for uncomplicated, atraumatic ETT exchange. It comes with a Rapi-Fit adapter, has a through-lumen design with side ports and a blunt tip, and comes in multiple lengths that can accommodate various sizes of ETTs (3- to 7-mm inner diameter) (Fig. 29). The Cook Airway Exchange Catheter EF is an extra-firm catheter designed to be used for uncomplicated, atraumatic ETT or double-lumen endobronchial tube exchange. It comes in two sizes, both 100 cm long, that can accommodate ETTs with an inner diameter of 4 or 5 mm or larger. The Cook Airway Exchange Catheter EF Soft Tip (Fig. 30) is similar to the EF except that it has a 7-cm, flexible distal tip.

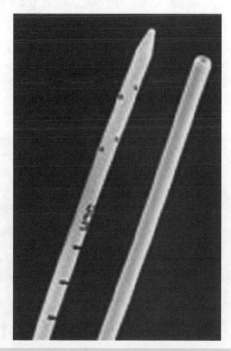

Fig. 27. The Arndt Airway Exchange Catheter Set is used for the exchange of LMAs and ETTs. (*Courtesy of* Cook Medical Critical Care; with permission.)

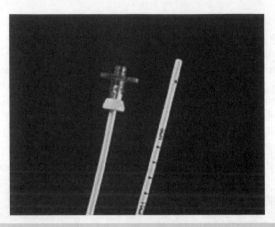

Fig. 28. The Cook Airway Exchange Catheter is used for uncomplicated, atraumatic ETT exchange. (*Courtesy of* Cook Medical Critical Care; with permission.)

The Frova Intubating Introducer (Fig. 31) (Cook Medical Critical Care) is used to facilitate endotracheal intubation. It has an angled tip similar to the gum elastic bougie. It comes with a hollow lumen, a Rapi-Fit adapter, and an optional stiffening cannula. There are two sizes of the introducer: pediatric (35 cm, for replacement of ETTs with a 3-mm inner diameter or larger) and adult (65 cm, for 6-mm ETTs or larger).

The Portex Venn Tracheal Tube Introducer (Fig. 32) (Smiths Medical International Limited, Hythe, Kent, UK), also known as the gum elastic bougie or Eschmann introducer, is designed to assist with tube placement during difficult intubations, such as in patients who have an anterior larynx or a small mouth

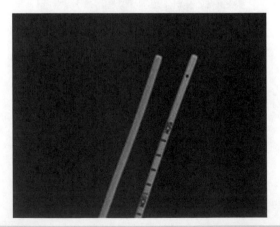

Fig. 29. Rapi-Fit adapter is used with various sizes of ETTs (3- to 7-mm inner diameter). (*Courtesy of* Cook Medical Critical Care; with permission.)

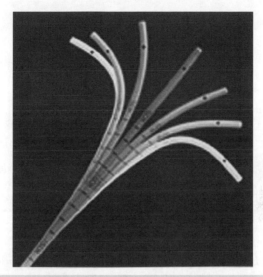

Fig. 30. The Airway Exchange Catheter EF Soft Tip is similar to the EF except that it has a 7-cm, flexible distal tip. (*Courtesy of* Cook Medical Critical Care; with permission.)

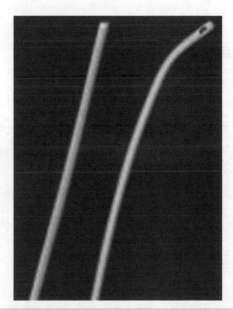

Fig. 31. The Frova Intubating Introducer facilitates endotracheal intubation. (*Courtesy of* Cook Medical Critical Care; with permission.)

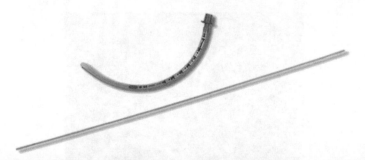

Fig. 32. The Portex Venn Tracheal Tube Introducer assists with tube placement in patients who have an anterior larynx or a small mouth opening. (*Courtesy of* Smiths Medical International Limited, Hythe, Kent, UK; with permission.)

opening [18,19]. It has an angled tip. The straight tip or the guide is designed to assist in tube exchange. These introducers are made from a woven polyester base and not gum. There is also a reusable bougie that is made of polyvinylchloride. The introducers come in various lengths, and all lengths can accommodate ETTs ranging from 2.5 to 11.0 mm.

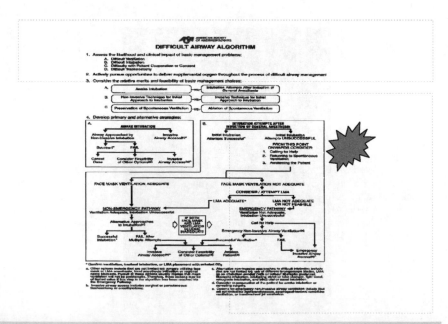

Fig. 33. ASA Airway Algorithm was first published in 1993 and updated in 2003. (*From* The American Society of Anesthesiologists; with permission.)

SUMMARY

Adverse outcomes associated with the management of a difficult airway include death, hypoxic injury, myocardial infarction, cardiopulmonary arrest, unnecessary tracheostomy, airway trauma, and dental injury. The ASA published its first version of the ASA Difficult Airway algorithm in 1993, which the ASA Task Force on the Management of the Difficult Airway updated in 2003 (see algorithm below). The goal of the ASA Algorithm (Fig. 33) is to facilitate the management of the difficult airway and reduce the likelihood of an adverse outcome [20].

With so many devices and techniques for dealing with the difficult airway, many airway problems can now be overcome. This requires good clinical judgment, experience, and familiarity with the use of the airway devices and techniques. In the face of an emergency, the practitioner tends to revert to the use of the technique with which he or she is most familiar. Practitioners should familiarize themselves with several techniques for managing the difficult airway other than direct laryngoscopy, however. With repeated practice, the practitioner will increase his or her chances of success. Ultimately, it is more important to know how to use a few devices well than to barely know how to use them all. And do not forget, call for help.

Reference

[1] Benumof JL. Laryngeal mask airway and the ASA difficult airway algorithm. Anesthesiology 1996;84(3):686 99.

[2] Brian A, Denman W, Goudsouzian N. LMA-Classic and LMA-Flexible instruction manual: LMA North America, Inc.

[3] Brimacombe J, AIJ B. The laryngeal mask airway. A review and practical guide. Philadelphia: WB Saunders; 1997.

[4] van Zundert AA, Fonck K, Al-Shaikh B, et al. Comparison of cuff-pressure changes in LMA-Classic and the new Soft Seal laryngeal masks during nitrous oxide anaesthesia in spontaneous breathing patients. Eur J Anaesthesiol 2004;21(7):547–52.

[5] Hagberg K. Current concepts in the management of the difficult airway. Available at: www.asahq.org/rcls. Accessed October 14, 2007.

[6] Ocker H, Wenzel V, Schmucker P, et al. A comparison of the laryngeal tube with the laryngeal mask airway during routine surgical procedures. Anesth Analg 2002;95(4):1094–7.

[7] Ferson DZ, Tamm E, Chi LT, et al. Comparative anatomical study of supraglottic airways. Anesthesiology 2004;101:A602.

[8] Akca O, Wadhwa A, Sengupta P, et al. The new perilaryngeal airway (CobraPLA) is as efficient as the laryngeal mask airway (LMA) but provides better airway sealing pressures. Anesth Analg 2004;99(1):272–8.

[9] Huitink JM, Balm AJ, Keijzer C, et al. Awake fibrecapnic intubation in head and neck cancer patients with difficult airways: new findings and refinements to the technique. Anaesthesia 2007;62(3):214–9.

[10] Xue FS, Li CW, Liu KP, et al. Circulatory responses to fiberoptic intubation in anesthetized children: a comparison of oral and nasal routes. Anesth Analg 2007;104(2):283–8.

[11] Evans A, Morris S, Petterson J, et al. A comparison of the Seeing Optical Stylet and the gum elastic bougie in simulated difficult tracheal intubation: a manikin study. Anaesthesia 2006;61(5):478–81.

[12] Connelly NR, Ghandour K, Robbins L, et al. Management of unexpected difficult airway at a teaching institution over a 7-year period. J Clin Anesth 2006;18(3):198–204.

[13] Wackett A, Anderson K, Thode H. Bullard laryngoscopy by naive operators in the cervical spine immobilized patient. J Emerg Med 2005;29(3):253–7.

[14] McNamara RM. Retrograde intubation of the trachea. Ann Emerg Med 1987;16(6): 680–2.

[15] Griggs WM, Korthley LIG, Gilligan JE, et al. A simple percutaneous tracheostomy technique. Surg Gynecol Obstet 1990;170:543–5.

[16] Fantoni A, Ripamonti D. A non-derivative, non surgical tracheostomy: the translaryngeal method. Intensive Care Med 1997;23:386–92.

[17] Durbin CG Jr. Techniques for performing tracheostomy. Respir Care 2005;50(4):488–96.

[18] Venn P. The gum elastic bougie. Anaesthesia 1993;48:274–5.

[19] Henderson JJ. Development of the "gum-elastic bougie." Anaesthesia 2003;58(1):103–4.

[20] Practice guidelines for management of the difficult airway: an updated report by the American Society of Anesthesiologists Task Force on Management of the Difficult Airway. Anesthesiology 2003;98(5):1269–77.

Advances in Anesthesia 25 (2007) 233–239

ADVANCES IN ANESTHESIA

INDEX

0737-6146/07/$ – see front matter
doi:10.1016/S0737-6146(07)00020-2